Advances in Neurosurgery 13

Extra-Intracranial Vascular Anastomoses

Microsurgery at the Edge of the Tentorium

Edited by
H. Dietz M. Brock M. Klinger

With 179 Figures and 71 Tables

Springer-Verlag
Berlin Heidelberg New York Tokyo

Proceedings of the 35th Annual Meeting of the
Deutsche Gesellschaft für Neurochirurgie
Hannover, June 13–16, 1984

Prof. Dr. med. Hermann Dietz
Neurochirurgische Klinik der
Medizinischen Hochschule Hannover
Konstanty-Gutschow-Str. 8, D-3000 Hannover 61

Prof. Dr. Mario Brock
Neurochirurgische Klinik und Poliklinik
Universitätsklinikum Steglitz, Freie Universität Berlin
Hindenburgdamm 30, D-1000 Berlin 45

Priv.-Doz. Dr. Margareta Klinger
Neurochirurgische Klinik der Universität Erlangen-Nürnberg
Schwabachanlage 6 (Kopfklinikum), D-8520 Erlangen

ISBN-13:978-3-540-15615-4 e-ISBN-13:978-3-642-70603-5
DOI: 10.1007/978-3-642-70603-5

Library of Congress Cataloging in Publication Data. Main entry under title: Deutsche Gesellschaft für Neurochirurgie. Tagung (35th: 1984: Hannover, Germany)
Extra-intracranial vascular anastomoses. (Advances in neurosurgery; 13)
"Proceedings of 35th Annual Meeting of the Deutsche Gesellschaft für Neurochirurgie, Hannover, Juni 13–16, 1984" – T.p. verso. Includes bibliographies and index. 1. Cerebral arteries – Surgery. 2. Cerebral revascularization. 3. Microsurgery. I. Dietz, H. (Hermann), 1925– .II.Brock, M. (Mario), 1938– .III. Klinger, M. (Margareta), 1943– .VI. Title. V. Series. [DNLM: 1. Cerebral Revascularization – congresses. 2. Microsurgery – congresses. W1 AD684N v. 13/ WG 595.C37 D486 1984e] RD 594.2.D484 1984 617'.481 85-17244
ISBN-13:978-3-540-15615-4 (U.S.)

2122/3130-543210

Preface

This 13th volume of *Advances in Neurosurgery* presents those papers held at the 35th Annual Meeting of the German Society of Neurosurgery in Hannover, June 13-16, 1984. Of 150 papers submitted, the program committee of the Society chose 69 for presentation. I would like to thank Professors Bock, Brock, Jensen, Wenker, and Wüllenweber for their assistance in the selection.

It was the intention of the President of the Congress at this meeting to lay special scientific emphasis on *discussion*. For this reason the number of papers had to be limited even more than usual in order to give all participants the opportunity for questions and the presentation of their own experience.

The main topic of the first day was *Extra-Intracranial Anastomoses*. Here the operative experience and the long-term results of these operations in the German-speaking countries were reviewed. This discussion was preceded a day earlier by a satellite symposium on the possibilities of the prophylaxis and treatment of ischemic neurological deficits following subarachnoid hemorrhage by means of calcium antagonists.

Microsurgery at the Edge of the Tentorium was the second main topic. In cooperation with the Society's microneurosurgery working group, only a small number of lectures were planned, but the topic was covered thoroughly in a round-table discussion.

The last topic, *Forum of Young Neurosurgeons*, consisted of three scientific sessions with short papers, where the results of clinical observations and experimental research from different centers were presented. The scientific meeting ended with an extensive round-table discussion on the currently very interesting topic of chemonucleolysis of lumbar discs.

The annual meeting of the Society was held in Hannover for the first time since the foundation in 1965 of the Medizinische Hochschule Hannover, where the Department of Neurosurgery has been working for 13 years. In recognition of his services in planning this department in the early 1960s, Professor Pia was invited to hold a special lecture, and I would like to thank him here once more for all his efforts towards the realization of the department.

At the same time, and in close proximity, the German Association of Neurosurgical Nursing also held its annual meeting. I would like to thank its administrative council for the cooperation with our Society.

Finally, I would like to thank all colleagues who contributed to the success of the 35th Annual Meeting with their presentations and their discussions. Last but not least, I want to thank Dr. Margareta Klinger for her untiring help in editing this volume, and Springer-Verlag for their cooperation and technical assistance.

Hannover — Hermann Dietz

Contents

Microsurgery at the Edge of the Tentorium

New Research

List of Contributors*

* The addresses are given at the beginning of each contribution

Extra-Intracranial Vascular Anastomoses

Pathophysiological Aspects of Cerebral Blood Flow in Respect of Extracranial-Intracranial Anastomosis

A. Hartmann

Abteilung für Neurologie, Universitäts-Nervenklinik und Poliklinik, Sigmund-Freud-Straße 25, D-5300 Bonn 1

Introduction

It is a constant wish of neurologists to treat successfully patients suffering from acute ischemia of the brain. An increase of regional cerebral blood flow (rCBF) in the ischemic area by hyperventilation may reduce the size of infarction under experimental conditions (1). At present, however, it is not known whether this effect leads to clinical improvement. Neurosurgeons have provided us with a technique which may increase blood supply to certain regions with reduced flow, i.e., the connection of an extracranial artery to an intracranial branch – so-called extracranial-intracranial anastomosis (EICA). To understand the logic of bypassing narrowed arteries it seems necessary to bear in mind certain physiological and pathophysiological principles in respect of the blood flow and metabolism of the brain in acute ischemia. Here I will summarize certain observations which might be important in understanding the physiological basis of EICA.

CBF may vary considerably during acute ischemia of the brain. The intensity of flow reduction depends on the following factors:

1. *The cause of ischemia:* Slowly developing arterial thrombosis may be bypassed by collateral circulation, where the total intravascular resistance is increased but may be low enough to allow sufficient perfusion of the dependent tissue. Sudden arterio-arterial emboli, however, lead to a sudden drop in perfusion pressure and collaterals cannot open.

2. *The location of the territory:* Watershed infarction along the borderzone of two major intracerebral arteries might suffer first if, for instance, during a hemodynamic crisis the local perfusion pressure worsens. However, in some cases microemboli are responsible for this type of ischemia. Occlusion of the internal carotid artery with subsequent watershed infarction is predominantly due to microemboli from the stump. In other cases hematogenous disorders may cause watershed infarction by obstructing small vessels. EICA might be of help in preventing watershed infarction if damage to autoregulation is assumed to be the cause. Microemboli and rheological disturbances must be treated by other techniques.

3. *The degree of vascular narrowing:* Under usual circumstances narrowing of the arterial branches may be neutralized by poststenotic vasodilatation. However, if the stenosis approaches a high degree, rCBF is affected. Figure 1 indicates that after endarterectomy of the internal carotid artery, rCBF increases only if the stenosis is of 90%. This proves that prior to surgery this type of stenosis did influence tissue perfusion. However, in patients with previous strokes, endarterec-

Advances in Neurosurgery, Vol. 13
Edited by H. Dietz, M. Brock, and M. Klinger

tomy improves the blood flow even in low-degree stenosis, since autoregulation is disturbed.

4. The condition of blood flow regulation: If autoregulation (constancy of rCBF despite changing perfusion pressure) is intact, decreased blood pressure (or perfusion pressure) can be compensated for by vasodilatation. By contrast, if autoregulation is damaged due to longstanding systemic hypertension or foregoing episodes of ischemia, the tissue will not tolerate a mild reduction of perfusion pressure (Fig. 2).

5. The cardiac condition: In acute cerebral ischemia tissue perfusion depends passively on cardiac output, since autoregulation is impaired.

6. The development of brain edema: Brain edema increases total intracranial volume and thus intracranial pressure. This again lowers perfusion pressure and rCBF.

7. The rheological condition: Increased hematocrit, elevated fibrinogen level, reduction of local perfusion pressure, alteration of erythrocyte deformability, red cell and platelet aggregation and alteration of plasma viscosity by abnormal proteins (alpha-2-macroglobulins) may affect blood flow. In areas with reduced CBF, tissue perfusion is further impaired by alterations in the rheological condition which themselves depend on sufficient perfusion: circulus vitiosus (Fig. 3).

Besides alteration of rCBF due to these parameters, flow varies considerably over time, since reactive hyperemia (2), the no-reflow phenomenon (3), and time-dependent development of brain edema may affect basis flow and flow regulation.

In the very acute phase of ischemia, CBF in the affected hemisphere tends to be reduced compared with that in the other hemisphere (Fig. 4). Blood flow reduction concerns predominantly the area of direct ischemia. However, ischemia spreads to neighboring areas and may lead to general involvement of the hemisphere. The directly involved tissue (the ischemic core) is surrounded by areas which might suffer from reduction of functional metabolism but not from damage to the basic metabolism, which is necessary for survival of the tissue (penumbra) (4, 5). Development of infarction requires not only a certain intensity of flow reduction but also a certain time (6, 7). Animal experiments have indicated that below a level of about 12 ml $\cdot$ 100 g^{-1} $\cdot$ min, the ischemic tolerance decreases significantly (8-14). In respect of the clinical situation it is obvious that ischemic attacks must be treated as emergencies, where any additional fall in rCBF (due to heart failure, reduction of perfusion pressure by increase of intracranial pressure, etc.) may lead to a further CBF reduction in the ischemic tissue. One of the aims of EICA is to restore flow to this tissue. As our own studies in patients with transient ischemic attacks have shown, rCBF restoration does not always correspond to clinical symptomatology and may even be delayed until the 3rd day (symptoms of TIA always vanish within 24 h) (Fig. 5). In these and in other patients with transient symptoms of cerebral ischemia, EICA might increase rCBF above the critical threshold to prevent further attacks.

The acute clinical improvement of patients with an EICA (15) probably reflects the existence of a penumbra-like area which takes advantage of the offer of blood. EICA may allow the transition of an area with signs of penumbra to one with full function. Further, it may protect the brain from further damage in the case of impaired autoregulation if perfusion pressure drops transiently. The observation that during the chronic state of stroke the lower flow threshold may be as high as 17-18 ml $\cdot$ 100 g^{-1} $\cdot$ min^{-1} indicates that an area with signs of penumbra in the acute phase of ischemia might be transformed to a tissue with characteristics of permanent damage. An EICA might be able to prevent this deleterious course. However, since other means of increasing flow to ischemic tissue exist (like improvement of rheological parameters), at present it has not been definitely established which method of rCBF enhancement in patients with chronic ischemic stroke should be used. The advantage of EICA is that it may target exactly to the area where ischemia is present.

In addition to spreading ischemia in unilateral brain infarction, CBF might be reduced in the contralateral side: transneural depression or diaschisis. The authors who have thus far reported on this phenomenon have measured CBF only once and therefore have not been able to separate a contralateral acute flow decrease from one due to the basic chronic vascular process (16). Our own studies in patients with acute infarction of the brain who were subjected to measurement of rCBF over both hemispheres of the brain have shown that diaschisis is a phenomenon of limited duration (17). Only in cases in which the development of brain edema – as indicated by computer tomography – complicated the course, was contralateral flow reduction observed for a longer period. Since diaschisis does not complicate the chronic course of unilateral ischemic infarction, it is not reasonable to instal a unilateral EICA with the aim of improving the blood flow of the contralateral side. Transneural depression of blood flow is not confined only to stroke patients but has also been observed in patients suffering from unilateral brain tumors (18).

In the acute state of stroke, ischemia is mostly confined to the area where the focal neurological symptoms originate. Interestingly, diaschisis is not only a mirror focus with contralateral flow reduction in the area exactly opposite to the homolateral ischemia but a widespread phenomenon involving the total contralateral hemisphere. We have never observed a case where diaschisis was more pronounced than ischemia in the homolateral side.

Considering therapeutic concepts for acute and chronic cerebral ischemia, one should not only strive for improvement of *basic* blood flow. The sensitive mechanism of autoregulation is impaired by the development of brain ischemia and may even be damaged in the chronic state of infarction (Fig. 1). A slight reduction of blood pressure then leads to a decrease in regional blood flow and indicates that reactive vasodilatation for compensation of the fall in perfusion pressure has failed. In areas with critical basic rCBF the tissue perfusion may be kept constant only by excessive vasodilatation and subsequent normalization of the cerebrovascular resistance. If blood pressure further decreases, an additional compensating vasodilatation might not be possible, resulting in a perfusion pressure dependent decrease of blood flow. An EICA might deliver more blood to that area and thus allow some slight vasoconstriction. Thereafter reduction of perfusion pressure can be compensated for by some mild vasodilatation. The consequence is stabilization of blood flow despite fluctuating blood pressure (or perfusion pressure) (Fig. 6).

The mechanism of autoregulation is probably myogenic in nature, following the alteration of transmural pressure in the resistance vessel (19). The role of adenosine on autoregulatory capacity has not yet been clearly established (20). The autonomic nervous system plays an additional role (21) despite the fact that this system acts on the larger rather than the smaller resistance vessels. Dilatation of the vessels due to excessive lowering of perfusion pressure (below 60 mmHg) may even be increased by vasodilatating agents or hypercapnia (22). On the other hand, autoregulation shifts to the right in chronic hypertension (23, 24), probably due to wall structural alteration. The consequence is that in patients with chronic hypertension a mild reduction of systemic blood pressure within the physiological limits may reduce rCBF. The damage to autoregulation caused by tissue ischemia is not limited to the area of direct ischemia. Transorbital clipping of the middle cerebral artery in monkeys leads to spread of autoregulation damage (and even reactivity to altered blood gases) to areas where initial ischemia was not measured (Fig. 7). This can even happen in areas with normal basic flow (posterior cerebral artery). Any improvement of flow, e.g., by an EICA, may improve the reactivity of the tissue and the vascular system. Since autoregulation seems to be one of the most important factors for survival of the brain tissue (Fig. 8), it is desirable to improve this parameter in acute and chronic ischemia.

An EICA will be of no help for tissue which has suffered structural damage. However, tissue with a penumbra-like character might benefit. Computer tomography (including studies of contrast medium enhancement) to identify possible damage to the blood-brain barrier measurement with control of the autoregulatory capacity forms a basis for the selection of patients for surgery. On the other hand, the existence of an rCBF increase in the area of the anastomosis does not necessarily indicate that tissue metabolism has actually been normalized; rather it might just reflect a luxury perfusion with increased flow but without metabolic improvement. Studies of metabolism are highly important, but with the systems available at present (such as positron emission tomography) the evaluation is far too expensive and impractical for daily clinical use. The following patients should not be selected for EICA anastomosis:

1. Patients with complete infarction and severe symptoms: increase of flow would result in luxury perfusion.
2. Patients with one single ischemic attack and no recognizable tissue or vascular lesion. If rCBF, autoregulation studies and CT are normal, there is no reason why bypass surgery should be performed.

Furthermore it should be kept in mind that additional supply of blood to a vascular area behind a moderate stenosis lowers the perfusion pressure gradient across the stenosis and therefore might favor the complete occlusion of the vessel (Fig. 9). Patients with stenosis of high degree in the proximal part of the middle cerebral artery should be selected carefully for bypass surgery (25).

Other methods of preventing further tissue damage by reduced rCBF concern the blocking of certain metabolic mechanisms in the brain. Since the back transport of Na^+K^+ after membrane leakage consumes a large part of energy, blocking of membrane leakage prevents excessive energy consumption. Hypothermia and lidocaine (26) are stated to possess a membrane-stabilizing effect (whereas barbiturate blocks only synaptic transmission). Lidocaine delays the extracellular K^+ accumulation after brain ischemia (27) and partially blocks the Ca^+ channel (28). However, the action of lidocaine has not been checked in patients with cerebral infarction, nor are there sufficient data from animal experiments.

Rheological changes might alter CBF by influencing viscosity and other parameters. This might be of importance, since rCBF falls in areas with increased viscosity when autoregulation and other regulatory processes are impaired. This results in rCBF being affected primarily in ischemic tissue. From the therapeutic point of view, improvement of rheological parameters alters rCBF more in areas with foregoing ischemia. Since rheological therapy can be carried out using both parenterally and orally administered agents, this method should be considered in patients with EICA, above all when the bypass does not result in an increase of focal flow or improvement of autoregulation.

References

1. Soloway, M., Nadel, W., Albin, M.S. et al.: The effect of hyperventilation on subsequent cerebral infarction. Anesthesiology 29, 975-980 (1968)
2. Crockard, H.A., Symon, L., Branston, N.M., Juhasz, J.: Changes in regional cortical tissue tension and cerebral blood flow during temporary middle cerebral artery occlusion in baboons. J. Neurolog. Sc. 27, 29-44 (1976)
3. Ames III, A., Wright, R.L., Kowada, M., Thurston, J.M., Majno, G.: Cerebral ischemia. II. The no-reflow phenomenon. Am. J. Pathol. 52, 437-453 (1968)
4. Astrup, J., Siesjö, B.K., Symon, L.: Threshold in cerebral ischemia – the ischemic penumbra. Stroke 12, 723-725 (1981)
5. Branston, N.M., Symon, L., Crockard, H.A. et al.: Relationship between the cortical evoked potential and local cortical blood flow following acute middle cerebral artery occlusion in the baboon. Exp. Neurol. 45, 195-208 (1974)
6. Heiss, W.S., Hayakawa, T., Waltz, A.G.: Cortical neuronal function during ischemia. Effects of occlusion of one middle cerebral artery on single-unit activity in cats. Arch. Neurol. 33, 813-820 (1976)
7. Branston, N.M., Strong, A.J., Symon, L.: Extracellular potassium activity, evoked potential and tissue blood flow. Relationships during progressive ischemia in baboon cerebral cortex. J. Neurol. Sci. 32, 305-321 (1977)
8. Symon, L., Brierly, J.B.: Morphological changes in cerebral blood vessels in chronic ischemic infarction: Flow correlation obtained by the hydrogen clearance method. In: Cérvos-Navarro, J., Betz, E., Matakas, F. et al. (eds.) The cerebral vessel wall. New York, Raven Press, pp. 165-174 (1976)
9. Symon, L., Crockard, H.A., Dorsch, N.W.C. et al.: Local cerebral blood flow and vascular reactivity in a chronic stable stroke model in baboons. Stroke 6, 482-492 (1975)
10. Tamura, A., Asano, T., Sano, K.: Correlation between rCBF and histological changes following temporary middle cerebral artery occlusion. Stroke 11, 487-493 (1980)
11. Nicholson, D., ten Bruggencate, G., Steinberg, R. et al.: Calcium modulation in brain extracellular microenvironment demonstrated with ion-selective micropipette. Proc. Natl. Acad. Sci. USA 74, 1287-1290 (1977)
12. Symon, L., Pasztor, E., Branston, N.M.: The distribution and density of reduced cerebral blood flow following acute middle cerebral artery occlusion: An experimental study by the technique of hydrogen clearance in baboons. Stroke 5, 355-364 (1974)
13. Morawitz, R.B., De Girolami, U., Ojemann, R.G. et al.: Cerebral blood flow determined by hydrogen clearance during middle cerebral artery occlusion in unanesthetized monkeys. Stroke 9, 143-149 (1978)

14. Morawitz, R.B., Marcoux, F.W., Crowell, R.M. et al.: Identical thresholds for cerebral ischemia in white and gray matter. Acta Neurol. Scand. 60 (Suppl. 72), 282-283 (1979)

15. Gratzl, O., Schmiedeck, P., Spetzler, R. et al.: Clinical experience with extra-intracranial arterial anastomosis in 65 cases. J. Neurosurg. 44, 313-324 (1976)

16. Sokoloff, L.: Aspects of cerebral circulatory physiology of relevance to cerebrovascular disease. Neurology 11, 34 (1961)

17. Hartmann, A.: Diaschisis and its course in patients with ischemic infarction. In: Betz, E. et al. (eds.) Pathophysiology and pharmacotherapy of cerebrovascular diseases. Witzstrock, pp. 241-245 (1980)

18. Cronquist, S., Agee, F.: Regional cerebral blood flow in intracranial tumors. Acta Radiol. (Diagn.) 7, 393 (1968)

19. Symon, L., Held, K., Dorsch, N.W.C.: A study of regional autoregulation in the cerebral circulation to increased perfusion pressure in normocapnia and hypercapnia. Stroke 4, 139-147 (1973)

20. Winn, H.K., Welsh, J.E., Rubio, R., Berne, R.M.: Brain adenosine production in rat during sustained alteration of systemic blood pressure. Am. J. Physiol. 239, H636-H641 (1980)

21. Klocke, F.J., Mates, R.E., Copley, D.P., Orlick, A.E.: Physiology of the coronary circulation in health and coronary artery disease. In: Klocke, F.J., Yu, P.N., Goodwin, J.T. (eds.) Symposium on Coronary Circulation. Lea & Febiger, Philadelphia, Chapter 1, pp. 1-17 (1976)

22. Häggendal, E., Johanson, B.: Effects of arterial carbon dioxide tension and oxygen saturation on cerebral blood flow autoregulation in dogs. Acta Physiol. Scand. 66 (Suppl. 258), 27-53 (1965)

23. Strandgaard, S.: Autoregulation of cerebral blood flow in hypertensive patients. The modifying influence of prolonged antihypertensive treatment on the tolerance to acute, drug-induced hypotension. Circulation 53, 720-727 (1976)

24. Jones, J.V., Fitch, W., MacKenzie, E.T., Strandgaard, S., Harper, A.M.: Lower limit of cerebral blood flow autoregulation in the baboon. Circ. Res. 39, 555-557 (1976)

25. Gumerlock, M.K., Ono, H., Neuwelt, E.A.: Can a patent extracranial-intracranial bypass provoke the conversion of an intracranial arterial stenosis to a symptomatic occlusion? Neurosurgery 12, 391-400 (1983)

26. Astrup, J., Møller Sørensen, P., Rahbek Sørensen, H.: Oxygen and glucose consumption related to Na^+-K^+ transport in the canine brain. Stroke 12, 726-730 (1981)

27. Astrup, J., Skovsted, P., Gjerris, F. et al.: Increase in extracellular potassium in the brain during circulatory arrest: Effects of hypothermia, lidocaine and thiopental. Anesthesiology 55, 256-262 (1981)

28. Astrup, J., Møller Sørensen, P., Rahbek Sørensen, H.: Inhibition of cerebral oxygen and glucose consumption in the dog by hypothermia, pentobarbital and lidocaine. Anesthesiology 55, 263-268 (1981)

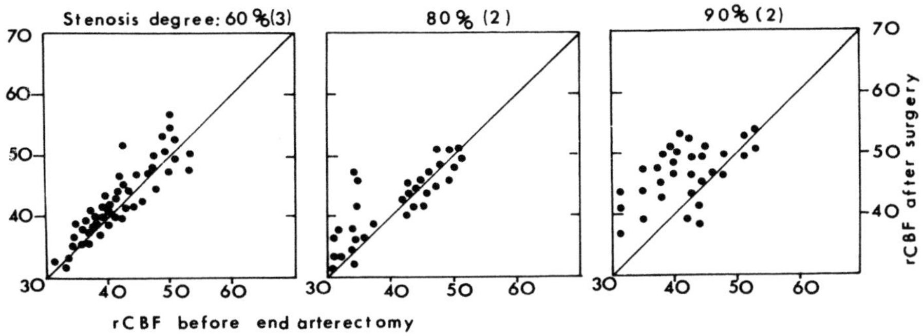

Fig. 1. Effect of endarterectomy on regional cerebral blood flow. Blood flow indicated as initial slope index (normal value about 52 s^{-1}). *Black points* indicate flow before *(abscissa)* and after *(ordinate)* surgery. In patients with stenosis of about 60%-80%, endarterectomy led to an increase of regional flow only in some detectors. In two patients with 90% stenosis, endarterectomy led to an increase of flow in most of the areas with reduced flow. This indicates that only a stenosis degree of 90% may influence blood flow hemodynamics

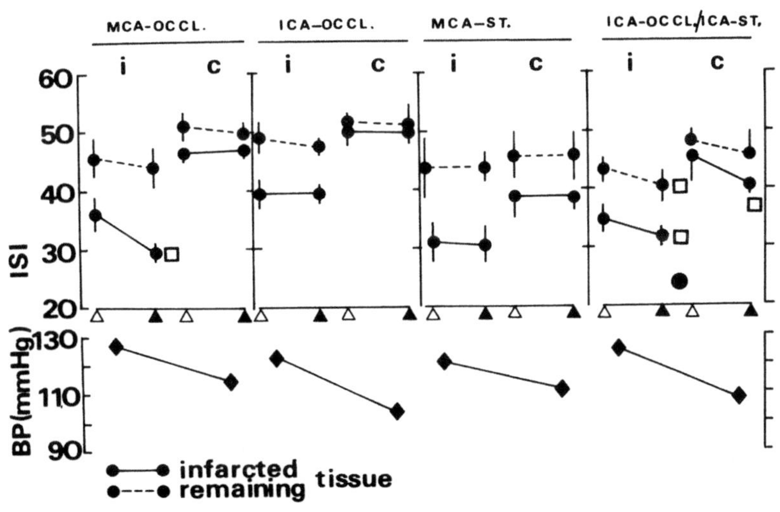

Fig. 2. Effect of induced blood pressure reduction on regional cerebral blood flow in four patients with chronic cerebral infarction. Blood flow is indicated as initial slope index (ISI, normal value about 52 s^{-1}). ISI is indicated as flow values in the involved ("ischemic") *(i)* and in the contralateral *(c)* hemisphere. The tissue of each hemisphere was classified as infarcted *(solid line)* and remaining *(dashed line)*. ISI was measured before *(open triangles)* and after *(black triangles)* lowering of systemic blood pressure to within the normal limits of autoregulation. In two patients blood pressure decrease led to a reduction of blood flow within the infarcted tissue (indicated by *open squares*), and in one patient to a reduction of flow in the remaining tissue. This indicates impaired autoregulation even in the chronic state of ischemic infarction

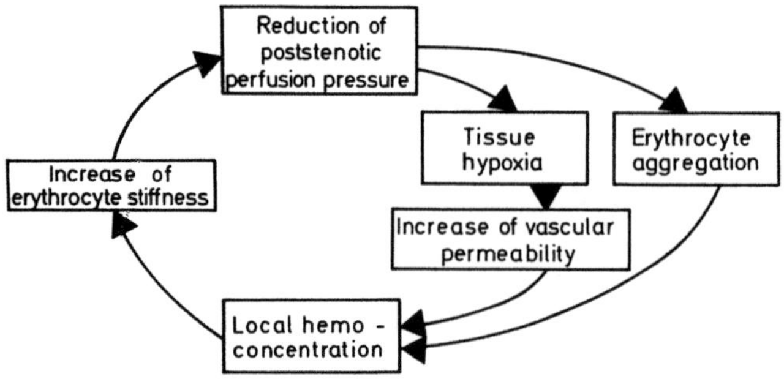

Fig. 3. Alteration of rheological parameters by vascular stenosis

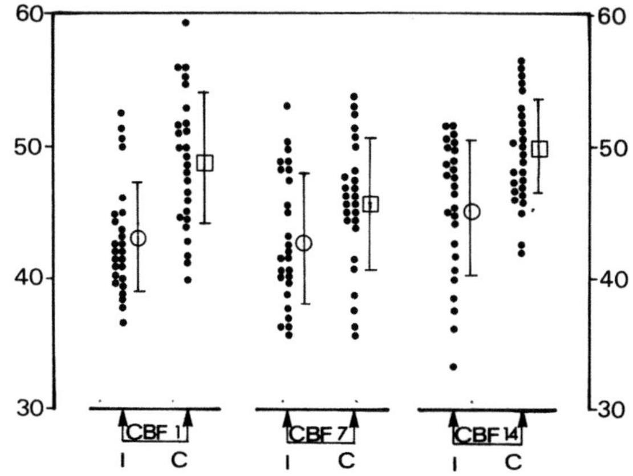

Fig. 4. Mean regional cerebral blood flow in ischemic stroke. Blood flow is expressed as initial slope index (ISI, normal value about 52 s^{-1}) on the ordinate. CBF was measured on the day of ischemic stroke (CBF 1), on day 7, and on day 14. *I* indicates all hemispheric flows of the ischemic side, *C* all data of the contralateral hemispheres. During all three CBF measurements, the mean rCBF of the ischemic side was lower than that of the contralateral side

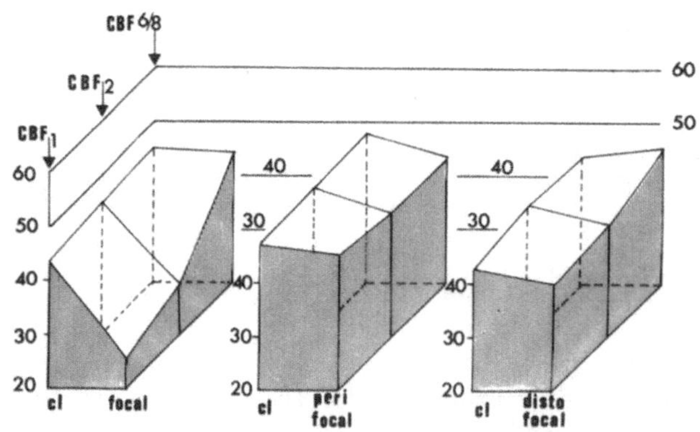

Fig. 5. Regional cerebral blood flow in patients with transient ischemic attacks. The data were drawn from 20 patients with TIA. This figure represents focal, perifocal, and distofocal rCBF of three patients in whom focal flow on CBF^{2} (1 day after TIA) was lower than on $CBF^{6/8}$ (days 6-8). CBF^{1} represents flow on the day of the attack. Perifocal and distofocal flow were not affected by the TIA. The figure indicates that in some patients with TIA, CBF might be reduced on day 2, i.e., on a day when clinical symptoms have disappeared. CBF is expressed as initial slope index (normal values about 52 s^{-1})

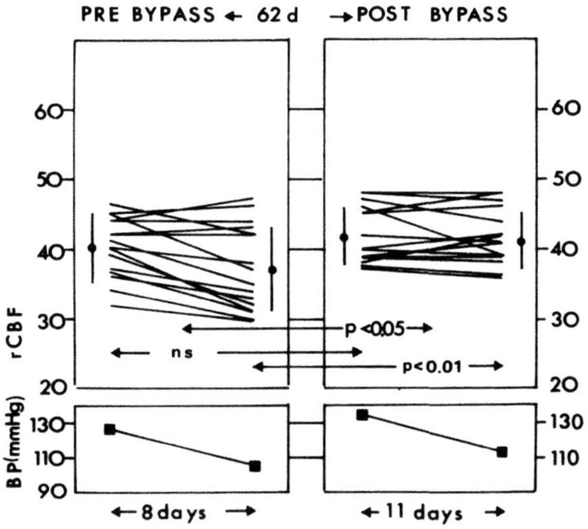

Fig. 6. rCBF before and after EICA and its alteration by blood pressure reduction. The *left column* indicates that rCBF falls after reduction of increased blood pressure. This is a consequence of impaired autoregulation. After bypass surgery (EICA) *(right column)* reduction of blood pressure does not reduce rCBF. This indicates that EICA has restored normal autoregulation. rCBF is expressed as initial slope index (ISI, normal values 52^{-1})

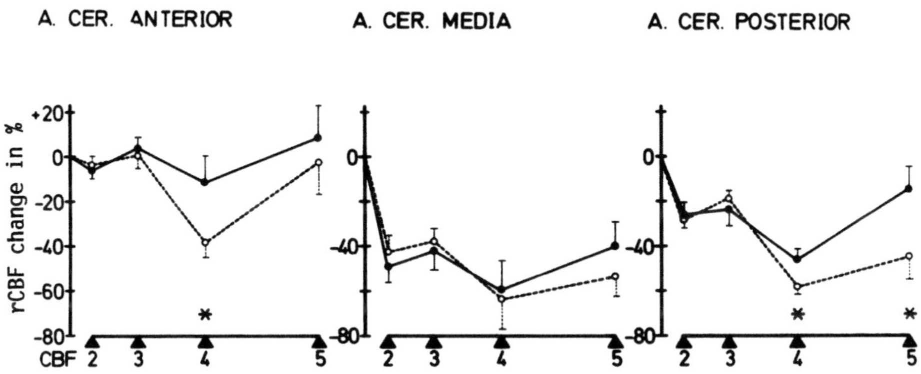

Fig. 7. Regional cerebral blood flow in monkeys after permanent clipping of the middle cerebral artery. rCBF indicated as percentage difference from CBF before clipping. *CBF 2* and *CBF 3*, day of infarction; *CBF 4*, 7 days after clipping; *CBF 5*, 28 days after clipping. In the territory of the posterior and anterior cerebral artery, rCBF falls on day 7 (CBF 4). This indicates that even tissue which is not involved in the process of primary ischemia (by the clip) might suffer from secondary ischemia. However, since rCBF recovers in the territory of the anterior cerebral artery from CBF 4 to CBF 5, the tissue is part of the penumbra. *Solid line*, animals treated with steroids; *broken line*, untreated control animals

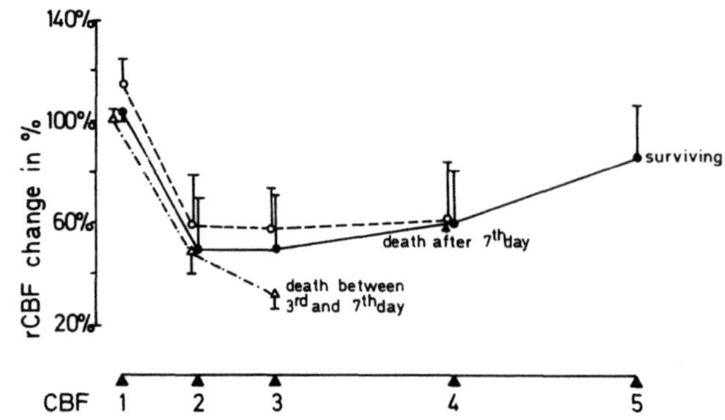

Fig. 8. Autoregulation in monkeys with infarction of the middle cerebral artery. CBF was measured five times (day 1 of the stroke: *CBF 1-3*; day 7: *CBF 4*; day 28: *CBF 5*). Autoregulation was tested by reduction of blood pressure within the physiological limit. The data indicate that all monkeys which died after the 3rd day (between CBF 3 and CBF 4) already had a worse autoregulatory capacity at CBF 3 compared with monkeys which survived the 3rd day. Therefore autoregulation is one of the determinant factors for the fate of the ischemic tissue

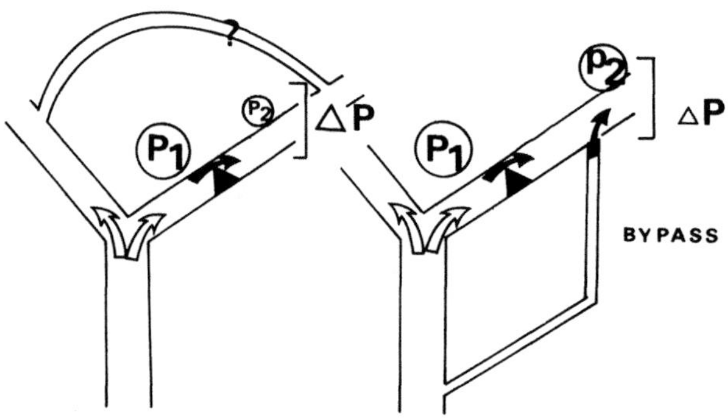

Fig. 9. Effect of bypass on perfusion pressure gradient. The *left-hand drawing* shows the pressure gradient ΔP, which is a consequence of the high pressure before the stenosis *(black triangle)*, and the low pressure, P^2, behind the stenosis. The pressure gradient is lowered if a bypass increases the poststenosis pressure, P^2 *(right-hand drawing)*. This might worsen the flow at the point of the stenosis but improves it (and the pressure gradient) downstream

The STA-MCA Bypass Procedure

O. Gratzl and H. R. Müller

Departements für Neurochirurgie und Neurologie, Neurochirurgische Universitätsklinik, Kantonsspital Basel, CH-4031 Basel

Reconstructive surgery of the cerebral arteries must be considered preventive. The clinical experience of most groups indicates that persistent residual neurological impairment cannot be significantly better alleviated by surgery than by allowing spontaneous recovery. The patient best suited for bypass surgery is one who has had transient ischemic attacks. These demonstrate the difference between physiological paralysis and anatomical infarction.

Bypass Function

Bypass function, the postoperative dilatation of the donor artery, depends on the hemodynamic disturbance. The bypass function is not correlated to the selection of the bypass feeder or its diameter (3). For patency and quality control we use Doppler sonographic tests (4, 5). The diastolic current indicating the connection of the extracranial to the intracranial vessel rises during the first few days postoperatively. Occluding the frontal branch of the superficial temporal artery, we measure flow velocity of the STA minus a natural collateral supply via the ophthalmic artery, i.e., the current in the bypass (branch occlusion test). By measuring the velocity and the vessel diameter over the common carotid artery sonographically (QFM ultrasonic flowmeter), we can calculate the bypass volume flow by performing the bypass compression test.

Differential flow ranged between 5 ml/min and 231 ml/min in our series, with a mean of 83 ml/min. An ophthalmic collateral vessel fed by the STA appears to limit the total increase of flow produced by an STA-MCA bypass. In cases of proven carotid cross-flow the bypass resulted in a redistribution of common carotid flow: this means an increase on the operated side and a decrease in the contralateral vessel. In about 50% of our bypass series we observed a marked true increase of hemispheric flow without incidence of redistribution. Moreover, nearly 25% of the cases studied showed an increase of volume flow on both sides, which indicates a decrease of pressure in the external carotid system and an external carotid cross-flow from the nonoperated side due to the bypass.

Bypass Risk and Clinical Results

To evaluate the risk of our bypass surgery we assessed the clinical results of two series. The first 100 patients were operated on between 1970 and 1975 and in a second series of 100 patients the procedure was performed between 1978 and 1983. The combined operative risk was 7%

Advances in Neurosurgery, Vol. 13
Edited by H. Dietz, M. Brock, and M. Klinger

in the earlier series, but only 3% in the later series. [Combined risk stands for the surgical mortality rate (death within one month following the operation) plus the percentage of morbidity with neurological deterioration during the same period.] CROFT et al. (1) calculated that endarterectomy and extra-intracranial bypass surgery versus conservative medical treatment would appear to be the procedure of choice, provided the combined morbidity and mortality is less than 4%. Thus our data showed that this kind of low-risk surgery is feasible for an experienced team. To evaluate the long-term clinical results of STA-MCA bypass surgery, we reported a follow-up study over 10 years in a small group of 23 patients (2). These were operated on between 1970 and 1972. Even the most recent case has been followed-up for over 10 years. We found that 17 patients were doing well and were free of ischemic attacks. Two, however, showed a temporary deterioration due to a myocardial infarction. There were five deaths, three of them caused by myocardial infarctions. Only one patient suffered complications related to cerebral vascular disease: he died from a cerebral infarction. The stroke incidence is thus 0.5% per year in our study. The mortality from arteriosclerotic disease, however, is high in this group: the long-term clinical effect is probably a lower morbidity compared with that without surgical intervention.

Summary

Extra-intracranial bypass procedures are being used successfully in the prevention of cerebral ischemia. Function of the bypass has been demonstrated by Doppler tests. We have presented series of patients with clinical findings to evaluate the risk of the procedure and the long-term results.

References

1. Croft, R.J., Harrison, M.J.G., Marston, A., Chapple, C.H., Thakkar, R.: Surgery for stroke. J. R. Soc. Med. 74, 330-332 (1981)
2. Gratzl, O., Schmiedek, P.: STA-MCA bypass: results 10 years postoperatively. Neurol. Res. 5, 11-18 (1983
3. Moritake, K., Gratzl, O.: Morphological and clinical analysis of extra-intracranial bypass. Arch. Psychiatr. Nervenkr. 232, 325-357 (1982)
4. Müller, H.R., Gratzl, O.: Quantitative Funktionsprüfung des ATS/ACM-Bypasses mittels eines neuartigen Ultraschall-Flowmeters. Ultraschall 1, 217-222 (1980)
5. Müller, H.R., Radü, E., Pallotti, C., Gratzl, O.: Common carotid CW Doppler flow measurement in neurovascular surgery. In: A. Kurjak, G. Kossoff (eds.) Recent advances in ultrasound diagnosis (4). Elsevier, Amsterdam 1984

Risk and Benefit of STA/MCA Anastomoses

G. Meinig, P. Ulrich, and E. Köster
Abteilung für Neurochirurgie, Klinikum der Johannes Gutenberg-Universität Mainz, Langenbeckstraße 1, D-6500 Mainz

Introduction

The advantage of EC/IC operation has not yet been proved unequivocally enough. We therefore attempted to analyze our cases in order to establish the possible benefit and risk of the operation. We compared the outcome of the operated and nonoperated patients with reference to the literature.

Patients and Methods

Since 1976, we have performed EC/IC anastomosis in 177 patients (Table 1) aged from 16 to 78 years (mean, 50 years). Thirty-nine of our patients had a history of reversible cerebral ischemic symptoms (TIA, PRIND). Thirty-five were suffering from severe stroke (CSs) and 85 from minor stroke (CSm). Most of our patients showed occlusion of the internal carotid artery (ICA); only 36 showed obstruction of the middle cerebral artery (MCA), as shown in Table 2. Pre- and postoperative bilateral cerebral blood flow measurements were carried out in all patients using the ^{133}Xe-inhalation technique (nrCBF).

Table 1. Neurological findings in 177 EC/IC patients

TIA	13
PRIND	26
Completed stroke (m)	85
Completed stroke (s)	39
	163
ICA ligation before EC/IC	11
Basal tumor	3
	177

Results

Of our 177 patients, seven died of heart failure or pulmonary embolism (Table 3). In all of these patients there were evident severe signs of generalized vascular sclerotic disease (three patients had bilateral ICA occlusion and three had myocardial infarction some years previously). They all had a high risk of anesthesia (grades III or IV).

Advances in Neurosurgery, Vol. 13
Edited by H. Dietz, M. Brock, and M. Klinger

Table 2. Angiographic findings in 177 EC/IC patients

1. ICA occlusion	105
2. Bilateral ICA occlusion	(15)
3. Ligation of ICA	14
4. Coiling	2
5. Stenosis of ICA	7
6. Siphon stenosis	10
7. Partial MCA occlusion	21
8. MCA occlusion	11
9. Moya-Moya syndrome	4
10. Basal tumors	3
	177

Table 3. Cause of death after 177 EC/IC operations since 1976

Serial number	Age	Risk of anesthesia	Preoperative findings	Time of death/ cause of death
11	68	IV	Cardiac infarction (2x) ICA prosthesis right ICA occlusion left 8 x stroke	3rd postoperative day, cardiac insufficiency
90	59	IV	Bilateral ICA occlusion Thromboangiitis obliterans	11th postoperative day, pulmonary embolism
108	73	IV	Bilateral ICA occlusion	41st postoperative day, severe pulmonary embolism (8th postop. day, small pulmonary embolism)
1	55	III	ICA occlusion Chron. general art. disease	3 years postoperatively
14	64	III	Right ICA occlusion Cardiac infarction	1 year postoperatively, 2nd cardiac infarction
16	62	III	Bilateral ICA occlusion	4 years postoperatively, pulmonary embolism (suspicion)
73	65	III	Partial MCA occlusion Cardiac infarction	4 months postoperatively, cardiac insufficiency

In our 177 patients there were no surgical complications (Table 4), only one scalp flap necrosis after a large craniotomy, no wound infection, and no rebleeding. Further ischemic events were extremely seldom postoperatively. As Table 5 shows, three patients suffered a minor stroke, one a PRIND, and seven TIAs. On the other hand, of the 158 patients who were questioned by a neutral person, 70 reported improvement of the neurological deficit and felt they had profited from the operation. Eighty-four patients reported stabilization at the preoperative level, while four patients deteriorated (Table 6). In the group of 60 patients with ICA occlusion who could be examined over a period of three years, only three died and only three suffered minor strokes (Table 7).

Table 4. Surgical complications (177 EC/IC patients)

Wound hematoma	0
Infections	0
Scalp flap necrosis	1
CSF fistula	0

Table 5. Cerebral ischemic events after EC/IC (*n* = 177)

TIA	7 patients
PRIND	1 patient
CS (m)	3 patients
	1. Anesthetic incident
	2. Brain edema, 4th postop. day
	3. Reinsult

Table 6. State of health 1 year after EC/IC (questioning by a neutral person)

Better	70 patients
Unchanged	84 patients
Worse	4 patients
	158

Table 7. Outcome 3 years after EC/IC (ICA occlusion)

3 patients dead	5%
3 patients completed stroke (m)	5%

In addition to the clinical observations, we performed nrCBF follow-up measurements. During the first year, we found a slight increase of mean CBF on average (3). Later, CBF seemed to decline gradually while the interhemispheric difference between the affected and nonaffected hemisphere continued to improve.

In contrast to the clinical improvement and the angiographic finding of a patent and hemodynamic effective bypass, we sometimes did not find an increase of resting flow. This observation stimulated us to pay more attention to cerebrovascular reserve capacity, which we tested by CO_2 inhalation. Figure 1 shows the results of our preoperative and postoperative hypercapnia test. We registered an improved CO_2 reactivity factor within one year in nearly all cases.

Discussion

The EC/IC operation is characterized by a very low surgical mortality. Complications primarily depend on the preexistent general internal medical situation or on the risk of anesthesia, and can be lowered to less than 1% by observing a strict indication. Accordingly, the surgical mortality in the anesthesia risk groups I and II is zero among our own patients. The early surgical complications are also very slight, and almost negligible. If the overall risk of stroke and death is about 30% in a period of approximately three years in patients with carotid artery occlusion not operated upon (2), the prognosis after STA/MCA bypass operation seems to be more favorable.

It is our impression that the value of the EC/IC operation consists in an improvement of the survival time and a reduction of the rate of reinsult. The cause of this improved prognosis is an ameliorated cerebral blood flow situation which reflects less an improvement of the resting cerebral blood flow than an improvement of the reserve capacity which enables the patient to adapt to critical situations, like a fall of blood pressure, stress, etc.

Patients with a slight brain substance defect and lowered brain blood flow may profit most from the operation. Nevertheless, we also carry out the operation in patients with manifest insult, e.g., bilateral carotid occlusion. According to our results these patients also receive protection against imminent reinsult or spreading of ischemia. In a very high percentage an improvement of the neurological deficit is to be expected.

Summary

Since 1976, 177 patients aged from 16 to 78 years (mean, 50 years) have been given STA/MCA anastomoses. The patients were analyzed in accordance with the neurological situation, angiographic findings, and pre-existing internal medical situation. The surgical mortality and morbidity were extremely low, especially when the indication was strict. In our own patients, the surgical mortality in the anesthesiological risk groups I and II was zero. The early complications were also exceedingly slight and almost negligible. According to our results, the value of the EC/IC operation consists in an improvement of the survival time and a reduction in the reinsult rate. This is caused by an improvement of the brain blood flow situation, and especially an improvement of the reserve capacity.

The patient with a slight brain substance defect and lowered brain blood flow profits most from the operation. Nevertheless, we carry out the operation even in patients with manifest insult, e.g., bilateral internal carotid occlusion. According to our observations, these patients also receive protection against reinsult or spreading of ischemia. In a very high percentage an improvement of the neurological deficit is to be expected.

References

1. Barnett, H.J.M.: Progress towards stroke prevention: Robert Wartenberg Lecture. Neurology 30, 1212-1225 (1980)
2. Cote, R., Barnett, H.J.M., Taylor, D.W.: Internal carotid occlusion: A prospective study. Stroke 14, 6, 898-902 (1983)
3. Meinig, G., Ulrich, P., Köster, E., Schürmann, K.: Ergebnisse der atraumatischen Hirndurchblutungsmessung. Akt. Neurol. 10, 203-211 (1983)

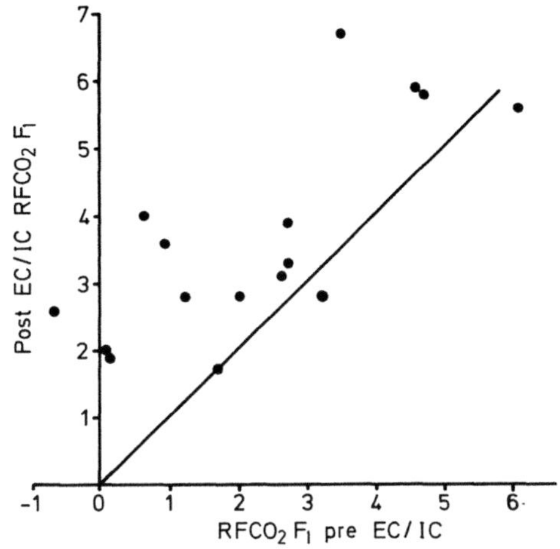

Fig. 1. Pre- and postoperative CBF changes in %/mmHg $PaCO_2$ difference (= $RFCO_2$) (F_1, gray matter flow)

Clinical Experience with Anastomoses Between the Superficial Temporal Artery and the Middle Cerebral Artery: A Survey of 15 Years

H. G. Imhof, H. M. Keller, and M. G. Yasargil
Neurologische Klinik, Universitätsspital, Rämistraße 100, CH-8091 Zürich

Introduction

The rationale behind extra-intracranial arterial bypass (EIAB), developed and successfully applied to an inaccessible regional vascular obstructive lesion by DONAGHY and YASARGIL in 1966/67, is augmentation, of collateral blood flow to the brain (11, 12). This may ameliorate ischemic neurologic deficit and reduce the incidence of stroke or recurrent stroke. With the help of EIAB a prophylactic collateral blood supply can be established in order to allow therapeutic occlusion of a major intracranial vessel.

Method, Analysis of Cases, and Results

Between 1967 and December 1982, we performed 162 EIABs in 158 patients. In 15 patients the EIAB was performed as a conjoint treatment in managing aneurysms of intra- or extracranial cerebral vessels, carotid artery-sinus cavernosus fistulas, or basal tumors with vascular compromise. These cases will not be analyzed here.

One hundred and forty-three patients were operated on because of obstructive cerebrovascular disease (CVD). The age and sex distribution in this series is summarized in Table 1. Thirty-five patients (24%) suffered from transient ischemic attacks (TIA) or prolonged reversible ischemic neurologic deficits (PRIND), and 108 (76%) from completed stroke (CS). Neurologic deficits resulting from CS were mild in 78 (55%), moderate in 27 (19%), and severe in 3 (2%). Of these 143 patients 68% suffered two or even several ischemic events prior to surgery. The sites of the vascular obstructions, documented by angiography, are summarized in Table 2. These obstructions were thought to be of atherosclerotic origin in most of the patients. The operative technique has been described exactly elsewhere (13). Patency of the anastomosis was documented angiographically or by Doppler sonography. Thirty-nine patients were controlled by both methods; the results corresponded in every patient. Ninety-two percent of the anastomoses were patent.

Table 1. Sex and age distribution (n=143)

Age (years)	0-9	10-19	20-29	30-39	40-49	50-59	60-69	70-
Female (29)	1	2	2	6	7	6	5	0
Male (114)	2	6	1	14	22	40	26	3
Total (143)	3	8	3	20	29	46	31	3

Advances in Neurosurgery, Vol. 13
Edited by H. Dietz, M. Brock, and M. Klinger

Table 2. Site of the obstructive lesion, established by angiography (n = 143)

Internal carotid artery (85.3%):	- Occlusion	
	unilateral	47 (32.9%)
	unilateral with contralateral stenosis	32 (22.4%)
	bilateral	15 (10.4%)
	- Stenosis, distal (inaccessible)	27 (18.9%)
Middle cerebral artery (14.7%)	- Occlusion	9 (6.3%)
	- Stenosis	13 (9.1%)

Of the nine occluded anastomoses, four were in patients suffering from skin flap necrosis/infection or from intracranial hematoma.

Of 103 patients presenting preoperatively with an ischemic neurologic deficit, 23 (22%) were improved within some days after surgery, and 39 (38%) within 3-6 months. Early and rapid improvement was seen only in patients with preoperatively mild neurologic ischemic deficits. Severely disabled patients remained unchanged. Of the 135 patients who tolerated surgery without major complication, 16 (11.8%) suffered another ischemic event (follow-up period ranging from 4 months to 13 years): eight patients TIA and eight patients CS with persisting ischemic deficit (Table 3). Of 35 patients presenting preoperatively with TIA, 32 tolerated surgery well. None of these 32 patients developed a CS during follow-up; TIAs stopped in 81%. Of 108 patients presenting preoperatively with CS, 103 tolerated surgery well.Of these 103 patients, four suffered during follow-up from a recurrent stroke homolaterally to the EIAB, and three from a recurrent stroke. In one of the former patients, the EIAB was occluded.

Table 3. Type and number of postoperative ischemic events in 135 patients (94.4% of 143 patients) who tolerated surgery without major complication (mean follow-up period: 4 years)

Type of preoperative ischemic event	Type of postoperative ischemic event	
	TIA	CS with persistent neurologic deficit
TIA: 32 patients	5	1 (contralateral)[a]
CS with persistent neurologic deficit: 103 patients	3 (contralat.)[a]	7-4 homolateral[a] (EIAB not patent) -3 contralateral[a]

a In relation to the operative procedure

Postoperatively four patients showed worsening of the preoperative condition and recovered only partially (Table 4): two developed an acute subdural hematoma, and one bleeding into the preoperatively infarcted temporal lobe; recraniotomy was mandatory in all three. The fourth patient developed an infarct during surgery.

During the postoperative course, eight patients suffered from epileptic seizures. Antiepileptic therapy stopped the seizures promptly. In three patients,a slowly progressive worsening was seen some weeks after the bypass procedure. CT scans showed subdural hematomas. The hematomas were evacuated; all three anastomoses were found to be patent during and after recraniotomy. The complication seen most frequently was marginal skin flap necrosis. Four patients died from complications of surgery: Two patients suffering from known hypertension showed a postoperative hypertonic crisis resistant to therapy and died 28 h after surgery. Autopsy revealed intracerebellar hematomas in both (CT scan was not yet available). One patient expired from an intracerebral hematoma diagnosed immediately after surgery in spite of recraniotomy. The fourth patient died several months after surgery from septicemia subsequent to infection of the skin flap.

Table 4. Complications in STA-MCA bypass surgery (n = 143)

Type of complication	Number	Pertinent deficit	Death
Subdural hematoma			
- acute	3	2	-
- chronic	3	-	-
Intracerebral hematoma	2	1	1
Intracerebellar hematoma	2	-	2
Subarachnoid hemorrhage	1	-	-
Subgaleal hematoma	4	-	-
Ischemic infarct	1	1	-
Transient increase of neurological deficit	5	-	-
Infection (skin, galea, bone)	5	-	1
Epileptic seizures	8	-	-
Marginal skin flap necrosis	13	-	-
Pulmonary embolism	1	-	-
	48	4	4

Overall morbidity: 33.6% Serious morbidity: 2.8%
Mortality: 2.8%

Discussion

The course of ischemic cerebrovascular disease is hardly predictable. Evaluation of patients profiting by augmentaton of collateral blood flow to a symptomatic or potentially symptomatic territory of the brain is difficult (12). In our series the procedure was performed in patients with obstructive CVD only when they had suffered previously from one or several ischemic events - TIA, PRIND, or CS. A prerequisite was that the patient was not severely disabled in daily life activity and that his angiograms revealed a hemodynamically significant and poorly collateralized obstructive vascular lesion, corresponding with his neurologic symptomatology and not treatable by conventional endarterectomy.

To avoid undue cerebral angiography, carotid artery Doppler sonography and dynamic ^{99m}Tc-brain scan were done regularly. Angiography may be withheld from patients in whom both tests reveal normal results (14).

Generally we did not operate on patients presenting with persistent neurologic deficits or computed tomographically assessed large infarcts within 4 weeks from the last ischemic event, because of the risk of converting an ischemic to a hemorrhagic infarct and the technical problems involved in operating on a swollen brain. For the same reason we did not operate on patients suffering from stroke in evolution. Bypass surgery was considered to be contraindicated if obstruction was of embolic origin, if microangiopathy was present, if severely disabling neurologic deficits persisted, and if the general condition of the patient was poor and made the risk of surgery high.

The rates of mortality and serious morbidity were each 2.8%, which is comparable with other series. These not unimportant percentages express the risk of intracranial surgery and of advanced age and multisystem pathology in many patients presenting with systemic cerebral ischemia.

It is possible that prompt recovery from mild neurologic deficit is the result of reactivating "idling" neurons in the penumbra zone. Indeed, there seems to be a correlation between augmentation of blood flow and amelioration of neurologic deficits; inversely, augmentation of blood flow does not necessarily mean amelioration of the clinical condition of the patient. We saw neither a rapid recovery from moderate neurologic deficits nor any amelioration of severe neurologic deficits after bypass surgery. It is possible that in patients presenting with large infarcts, microvasculature is destroyed, resulting in lack of amelioration of microcirculation even after successful revascularization (8). Slowly progressing amelioration of mild or moderate neurologic deficits occurring over several months is likely to correspond to the natural history of ischemic stroke.

It is said that without therapy one-fourth to one-third of patients who have experienced an ischemic event will develop a major stroke or suffer from recurrent stroke, usually within 1 year from the initial event (1, 9, 10). During mean follow-up of 4 years, only 2.8% (4/143) of our patiens operated on experienced a further ischemic event homolaterally to the bypass. In spite of these promising results, the prophylactic effect of EIAB in preventing stroke or recurrent stroke in patients suffering from obstructive CVD is not yet established. Real control groups are lacking. Comparison of highly selected surgical series with unselected series of patients identified solely by the clinical diagnosis is not efficient. A comparison may be possible if patients operated on are compared with patients suffering from an identically localized obstructive vascular lesion. Occlusion of the proximal ICA is thought to have an annual rate of stroke of 2-5% (2, 4) and obstruction of the distal ICA a rate of 4.6-7.6% (2, 7); persistent obstruction of the MCA seems not to have good prognosis because of leptomeningeal collaterals being marginal in their protective capabilities (6, 3).

Conclusion

Initially EIAB was developed to be performed before therapeutic ligature of a major cerebral vessel (12). This is done in the case of insufficient collaterals, the least controversial indication, even though a patent bypass does not guarantee safe occlusion. Complications, probably of embolic origin, during or after therapeutic occlusion of the ICA are well known. Today EIAB is most often used in obstructive cerebrovascular disease of atherosclerotic origin. Given the lack of readily available methods of assessing the viability of brain tissue, its value in amelioration of the postinfarct neurologic condition is controversial. Certainly it is not a method to bring dead tissue back to life. In view of the often very impressive demonstration of anatomic revascularization, EIAB may help to lower the rate of the dramatically disabling event of ischemic stroke. Yet the indications for EIAB in treatment of obstructive CVD have to be restrictive, even though the technical problems of the procedure, at least in STA-MCA anastomosis, have practically been resolved.

References

1. CARTLIDGE, N.E.F., WHISNANT, J.P., ELVEBACK, L.R.: Carotid and vertebral-basilar transient cerebral ischemic attacks. A community study, Rochester, Minnesota. Mayo Clin Proc 52: 117-120, 1977.
2. CRAIG, D.R., MEGURO, K., WATRIDGE, C., ROBERTSON, J.T., BARNETT, H.J.M., FOX, A.J.: Intracranial internal carotid artery stenosis. Stroke 13: 825-828, 1982.
3. DAY, A.L.: Indications for surgical intervention in middle cerebral artery obstruction. J. Neurosurg 60: 296-304, 1984.
4. FURLAN, A.J., WHISNANT, J.P., BAKER, H.L.: Long-term prognosis after carotid artery occlusion. Neurology 30: 986-988, 1980.
5. HEROS, R.C.: Thromboembolic complications after combined internal carotid ligation and extra- to intracranial bypass. Surg Neurol 21: 75-79, 1984.
6. HINTON, R.C., MOHR, J.P., ACKERMANN, R.H., ADAIR, L.B., FISHER,C.M.: Symptomatic middle cerebral artery stenosis. Ann Neurol 5: 152-157, 1979.
7. MARZEWSKI, D.J., FURLAN, A.J., St. LOUIS, Ph., LITTLE, J.R., MODIC, M.T.: Intracranial internal carotid artery stenosis: Long-term prognosis. Stroke 13: 821-824, 1982.
8. NISHIKAWA, M., YASARGIL, M.G., YAGI, N., FISCH, U.: Experimental extracranial-intracranial anastomosis. Surg. Neurol 8: 249-253, 1977.
9. SACCO, R.L., WOLF, Ph.A., KANNEL, W.B., McNAMARA, P.: Survival and recurrence following stroke. The Framingham study. Stroke 13: 290-295, 1982.
10. WIEBERS, D.O., WHISNANT, J.P., O'FALLON, W.M.: Reversible ischemic neurologic deficit (RIND) in a community: Rochester, Minnesota, 1955-1974.

11. YASARGIL, M.G.: Experimental small vessel surgery in the dog, including patching and grafting of cerebral vessels, and for formation of functioning extra-intracranial shunts. In: DONAGHY, R.M.P., YASARGIL, M.G.: Microvascular surgery. pp 87-126, G. Thieme Verlag, Stuttgart, 1967.

12. YASARGIL, M.G.: Diagnosis and indications for operations in cerebrovascular occlusive disease. In: YASARGIL, M.G. (ed): Microsurgery applied to neurosurgery. pp 95-119. G. Thieme Verlag, Stuttgart, 1969.

13. YONEKAWA, Y.,YASARGIL, M.G.: Extra-intracranial arterial anastomosis. Clinical and technical aspects. Results. In: KRAYENBUEHL, H. (ed): Advances and technical standards in neurosurgery, pp 47-78. Springer Verlag, Wien, New York, 1976.

14. ZUMSTEIN, B., KELLER, H.M., LUETOLF, U.: Noninvasive management of stroke patients by Doppler sonography and dynamic radionuclide brain scanning. In: PEERLESS, S.J., MOCCORMICK, C.W.(ed): Microsurgery for cerebral ischemia, pp 89-94. Springer, New York, 1980.

Clinical Findings and Operative Results in 250 Patients Who Underwent EIAB Operations

K. Piscol, H. Meyer, V. Palm, Ch. Friedrichsen, and J. Janus

Kliniken der Freien Hansestadt Bremen, Zentralkrankenhaus St.-Jürgen-Straße, Neurochirurgische Klinik, D-2800 Bremen 1

The technical data, the clinical findings, and the postoperative courses in 250 patients who underwent EIAB procedures are reviewed. Of these 250, 220 underwent standardized procedures (=88%), with a branch of the superficial temporal artery (STA) as the donor vessel and a branch of the middle cerebral artery (MCA) as the recipient. In 25 procedures (= 10%), the occipital artery (OA) was used: 7 times (3%) to create a bypass to the posterior inferior cerebellar artery (PICA) in patients with a vertebral artery syndrome, and 18 times to create a bypass to an angular branch of the MCA when the occipital artery possessed a larger caliber than the STA or when frontal natural anastomosis was to be spared. In five procedures (=2%) grafts were used: in two cases Goretex tubes between either the subclavian artery or the common carotid artery and the MCA, and in three cases venous grafts between the superior thyroid artery (2x) or the proximal STA and the MCA (Fig. 1). Following GRATZL's critical observations on the importance of flow capacity, procedures using long-distance grafts should be reserved for particular patients.

Double bypass on the same side led to a good result if the operations were done at different times and with different donor vessels, e.g., superficial temporal artery and occipital artery (two patients). The procedure had less effect if it was done in one session with two branches of the same donor vessel, for there was no increase in flow rate. The bilateral EIAB procedures show favorable results and therefore are being performed with increasing frequency by our team (as yet, upon 20 patients). Another question is use of the STA as the donor vessel following disobliterating and widening procedures on the external carotid artery; our results in 12 cases are very good, and there has so far been no case of reobliteration. (Other special cases are listed in an earlier publication (4).) Evaluating the patency of the anastomoses at intervals between 6 months and five years with the help of angiography, the HAM-scan method, and (in most cases), Doppler sonography, flow ranged from sufficient to very good in 92% of the patients (Fig. 2). A questionable or weak flow was demonstrated in 5%, mostly in patients with stenosis of the internal carotid artery (ICA) or with well-established natural anastomosis. In 3% an occlusion was found, mostly in cases with diffuse vascular processes.

Regarding the affected vessels, in 1984 lesions of the ICA were seen in 76% (1980: 68%), of the MCA in 15% (1980: 19%), and of the vertebral artery (VA) in 3.5% (1980: 3.3%), and multiple or diffuse lesions in 1.5% (1980: 6.6%). EIAB in connection with giant aneurysm was carried out in 4.0% (1980: 3.3%) of the patients (Table 1). In the anterior part of cervicocranial circulation unilateral lesions dominated, while the posterior part lesions were usually found in both sides. In the carotid artery obliteration was usually found, while in the middle or vertebral artery obliteration and stenosis were equally seen.

Advances in Neurosurgery, Vol. 13
Edited by H. Dietz, M. Brock, and M. Klinger

Table 1. Angiographic findings on cervicocra..ial vessels leading to operative indication. Statistical results of 1984 compared with those of 1980

	1980			1984		
A. carotis int.:						
Obliteration, bilateral	6.6			6.0		
Oblit., unilat.; stenosis, contralat.	3.3	41.0		13.7	60.2	
Obliteration, unilateral	31.1			40.5		
Stenosis, bilateral			68%	3.5	15.8	76%
Stenosis, unilateral	27.0	27.0		12.3		
A. cerebri med.:						
Obliteraiton, bilateral				0.5		
Obliteration, unilateral	11.0	12.1		5.4	7.4	
Oblit., ramus unilateral	1.1		19%	1.5		15%
Stenosis, bilateral	1.1	6.7		1.0	7.6	
Stenosis, unilateral	5.6			6.6		
A. vertebralis:						
Oblit., unilat., stenosis contralat.				1.0		
Obliteration, unilateral				0.5		
Stenosis, bilateral		3.3		1.0	3.5	
Stenosis, unilat.; stenosis, a. bas.				0.5		
Hypoparesia; kinking, contralat.				0.5		
Other:			13%			9%
Multiple vessel lesions		6.6		1.5	5.5	
Giant aneurysms		3.3		4.0		

Of the patients, 70% were male. The average age was 52.5 years. Nevertheless, 91% of the patients were younger than 65 years, about 40% were younger than 50 years, and eight patients were between 19 and 29 years of age (Fig. 3)!

Results

Altogether 77.8% of the patients exhibited improvement of their complaints or deficits. The neurological status remained unchanged in about 17% and deterioration occurred in only 5.3%.

Figure 4 shows the detailed results in the various groups according to the clinical indication for surgery. As expected, patients in 0-stage or those with reversible neurological deficit profited more from operation than did those with completed stroke: the former showed improvement in 93% of cases and deterioration in 1.7%, while the latter showed improvement in 61% of cases and deterioration in 8.5%.

The results in patients with vertebral insufficiency syndrome are really better than is suggested by the percentage figures. Five patients with severe disorder of balance, drop attacks, and other pontocerebellar symptoms are now fully capable of working, and two of them are absolutely free of symptoms.In one patient with unchanged status an old cerebellar infarct was detected during operation. One death was due to sepsis preceded by thrombophlebitis.

Dysphasia and aphasia are symptoms of special importance and were the decisive factor indicating surgery in 19% of the cases. Among these patients the speech disorder disappeared in 16%, improved in 65%, and remained unchanged in 18%.

It is difficult to assess complaints like headaches, dizziness, sleep disturbances, difficulties in concentration etc., although these symptoms are often of great importance for the patients. These complaints are mentioned as very disturbing by 5%-15%. With surprising constancy, these disturbances subside in about 60% after operation and remain unchanged in 10%. On the other hand in 30% they first appear after operation.

We tried to compare our last results (1984) with those of 1980 and with those presented in the literature (Table 2). Our early results correlate well with those in the literature. Follow-up investigations are done at intervals between 1 year and 6 years, so that we are not able to speak generally of "late results", but can give some follow-up assessments.

Looking at the results of 1984, there are three columns in Table 2. In the left-hand column are only the operative results, in the middle column are results at the time of discharge, and in the right-hand column are follow-up results. There was a very low operative mortality and morbidity. The higher mortality at the time of discharge demonstrates the unfavorable influence of general arteriosclerosis: three additional deaths due to myocardial infarction.

The most important results are those in the right-hand column. In the TIA + PRIND group, one patient died as a result of carotid disobliteration surgery on the contralateral side. Two patients later experienced stroke on the contralateral side; one patient suffered from epileptic seizures and another one from myocardial infarction. On the other hand greater activeness was recently shown in two cases. In one the symptoms of headache had subsided and in one further case there was complete cessation of ischemic attacks.

Table 2. Results (%) for 1984 listed according to main clinical groups, compared with results from 1980 and those reported in the literature (Lit)

	Lit	1980	1984[a]		
TIA + PRIND + O					
Asymptomatic	81.4	83.1	83.5	83.5	79.4
Improved	12.6	8.0	10.4	9.5	8.6
Isolat. attacks	3.3	2.6	2.6	2.6	2.6
Heterol. attacks		5.3	2.6	2.6	2.6
Worse			0.9	0.9	5.1
Deceased	2.7	1.0	0	0.9	1.7
COST 1 + COST 2					
Asymptomatic			6.9	6.9	5.2
Improved	50-70	60	55.5	54.1	48.0
Unchanged	25-50	38	31.6	30.5	32.0
Worse	2.8-6.5	2	5.0	5.5	9.8
Deceased			1.0	3.0	5.0

a Left-hand column = only operative results; middle column = results at time of discharge; right-hand column = follow-up results

In the group with completed strokes there were two additional cases of death after discharge: myocardial infarction was again the cause in one case while in the other death was due to serious contralateral stroke. It was only in this group that in one case, despite bypass operation, homolateral recurrence of ischemic attack was noticed. One patient experienced TIAs on the contralateral side, one psychopathological disturbances, and a third grand mal epileptic seizures. Altogether about 54% of the patients in this group were very satisfied at the time of follow-up examination. On the other hand, about 60% with objective improvement of neurological status did not agree with this assessment, because they did not see any benefit in their daily activities.

In the TIA + PRIND group about 80% of patients should be able to work, but only 55% undertook full-time jobs. In the group with completed strokes nearly 20% are working full-time and 6% half-time or less. Despite this decrease in the early very good results, we can be very satisfied with the later results, for they are significantly better than those of conservative treatment. This correlates with the results of a randomized study by HERRSCHAFT in which, after 2 years, 42 operated patients altogether showed much better results than 40 who were not operated.

The number of complications has been very low and does not need to be mentioned in our study.

Bruit at Site of Anastomosis

A special problem to be discussed is bruit at the site of anastomosis. We first dealt with this phenomenon in 1981 (3). According to our preliminary phonographic analysis, the characteristics of the bruit are as follows: it is a loud, systolic "decrescendo" sound, synchronous with the pulse, reaching the diastole and containing high frequency elements (maximum frequency between 14 and 250 Hz). The bruit, when auscultated, sounds like that of AV fistulas in a weaker form.

In 1981 we reported eight cases. The number has now risen to 11 patients (4% of all)(Table 3). In seven patients the bruit was registered without complaint; two patients described it as annoying and two others did not hear anything. In these latter bruit was detected by auscultaion during follow-up examination. One patient can hear the sound but it could not be objectively detected. In most cases the bruit has appeared months after operation and has lasted weeks or months. In at least three cases it can still be observed. In one case the bruit was heard only from the 6th to the 12th postoperative day.

Phonography is able to analyse the bruit but not to give an explanation. We presume that formation of turbulences at the site of anastomosis, where pulsating and laminar flow meet, could be the cause under special circumstances (e.g., one patient could only hear the bruit at the time of local CSF accumulation). Stenosis can be excluded as a cause, for there have been no signs of it under angiographic control.

Finally our prognostic statement in 1980 regarding the development of EIAB surgery will be reviewed: We concluded at that time, that in future 80% of patients will have TIA and PRIND. Now, in 1984, we can see that we made an error in this respect. Only 52% of our patients are in this group (Table 4). One reason is that patients with completed stroke are more willing to undergo operation than those with TIA or PRIND. But another important reason seems to be that in serveral recent publications assessment of the results of EIAB operation on completed stroke has been too optimistic, leading to a higher admission of completed stroke patients. According to our results, however, there is no doubt that the

Table 3. Patients (11 of 250 = 4.4%) with bruit at site of anastomosis
Ø = not found

No. of patients	Bruit obj.	Bruit subj.	Contin-uous	Spo-radic	Onset postop.	Dura-tion	Comments
2	+	++	+		6 months	Still present	Duration 1x2.5 yr. 1x hyper-tension
5	+	+		+	4-6 months	12-24 months	2xØ con-trols
1	+	+	+		6th day	6th-12th day	CSF cushion!
2	+	Ø	?	?	?	Weeks?	Observed in outpa-tient dept.
1	Ø	+	+		5 months	Still present	Not con-firmed

Table 4. Percentage of patients in the clinical groups[a]. Arrows show 1980 prognostic statement

1980				1984		
TIA	38%	68% → 80%		TIA + O	32%	52%
PRIND	30%			PRIND	20%	
COST 1	13%	28% → 20%		COST 1	30.5%	44%
COST 2	15%			COST 2	13.5%	
VERT	4%	4% → ? / Ø		VERT	3%	4%
SIE	1%			SIE	1%	

a Abbreviations: see Fig. 4; SIE = stroke in evolution

operative and neurological results are far better in younger patients, in patients with less cardiovascular processes, and in patients with reversible or slight cerebral dysfunction. We are therefore of the opinion that these factors should be given greater consideration when assessing the indication for operation.

References

1. GRATZL, O.: Technik und Ergebnisse extra-intrakranieller mikrovaskulärer Eingriffe. Arbeitstagung "Der zerebrale Notfall", Port el Kantaoui, Tunesien, 31.5-4.6.1984
2. HERRSCHAFT, H.: Diagnose und Therapie zerebrovasculärer Insuffizienz. Fortb. Tagung. Med. Kliniken Bremen, 28.3.1984.
3. PALM, K.V., CUEVAS-SOLORANZO, A., KLEIN, J., MEYER, H., PISCOL, K., TRAPPE, H.-J.: Some special experiences with extracranial-intracranial arterial bypass operations with particular attention to fistulous bruits. In: Neurological surgery. Stuttgart, New York: Thieme, 1981
4. PISCOL, K.: Die extra-intrakraniellen arteriellen Bypass-Operationen. Therapiewoche 31, 8082 (1981)

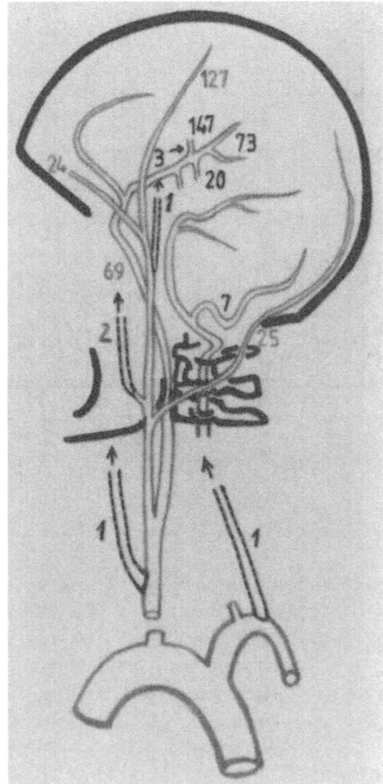

Fig. 1. The different donor vessels (*gray numbers*) with grafts (*gray numbers* and *punctated lines*) and recipient vessels (*black numbers*) in 250 EIAB operations. Superficial temporal artery (STA), 69 cases; parietal branch of STA, 127 cases; frontal branch of STA, 24 cases; occipital artery, 25 cases; subclavian artery (Goretex), 1 case; common carotid artery (Goretex), 1 case; proximal STA (Vena), 1 case; superior thyroid artery (Vena), 2 cases; middle cerebral artery, 147 cases; angular artery, 73 cases; internal temporal artery, 20 cases; central artery, 3 cases; posterior inferior cerebellar artery, 7 cases

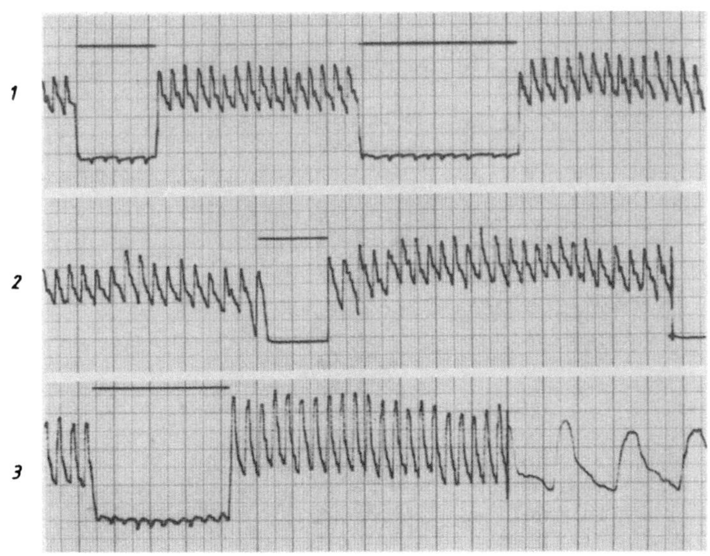

Fig. 2. Doppler sonograms at the site of anastomosis of 3 patients. The lines above indicate the effect of compression of the proximal STA (*1* and *3*) and of CCA (*2*)

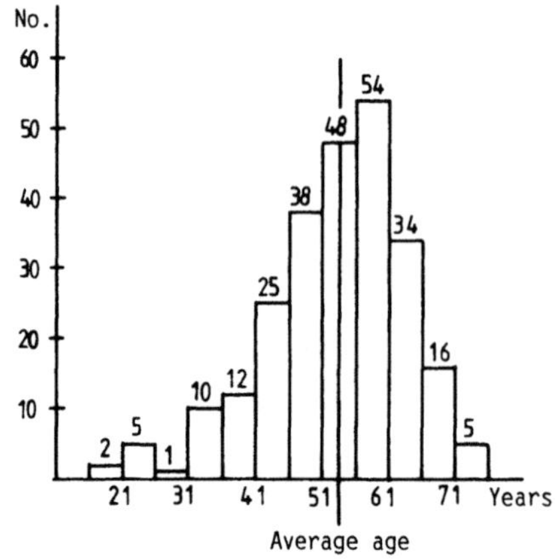

Fig. 3. Age of 250 EIAB patients. The *vertical line* marks the average age

52%

TIA=0 = 73 = 32.0%	
Asymptomat.	62 = 85.0%
Improved	6 = 8.3%
Isol. Att.	2 = 2.7%
Heterol. Att.	2 = 2.7%
Worse	0 = 0
Deceased	1 = 1.3%

PRIND = 43 = 20.0%	
Asymptomat.	35 = 81.4%
Improved	5 = 11.6%
Isol. Att.	1 = 2.3%
Heterol. Att.	1 = 2.3%
Worse	1 = 2.3%
Deceased	0 = 0

Asymptomatic:	83.5%	93.1%
Improved:	9.5%	
Isolat. Att.:	2.6%	5.2%
Heterol. Att.:	2.6%	
Worse:	0.9%	1.7%
Deceased:	0.9%	

45%

COST 1= 68 = 30.5%	
Asymptomat.	7 = 10.2%
Improved	38 = 55.0%
Unchanged	20 = 29.0%
Worse	2 = 2.9%
Deceased	2 = 2.9%

COST 2= 33 = 14.5%	
Asymptomat.	0 = 0
Improved	17 = 51.5%
Unchanged	11 = 33.5%
Worse	4 = 11.7%
Deceased	1 = 3.3%

Asymptomatic:	6.9%	61.0%
Improved:	54.1%	
Unchanged:	30.5%	30.5%
Worse:	5.5%	8.5%
Deceased:	3.0%	

3%

VERT = 7 = 3.0%	
Asymptomat.	2 = 29.0%
Improved	3 = 43.0%
Unchanged	1 = 14.0%
Deceased	1 = 14.0%

Asymptomat. + Improved — 72%

Fig. 4. Results listed according to clinical indications. *TIA*, transient ischemic attacks; *PRIND*, prolonged reversible ischemic neurological deficit; *COST 1*, completed stroke, lighter form; *COST 2*, completed stroke, severer form; *VERT*, vertebral artery syndrome

Late Results of Extra-Intracranial Bypass Surgery – 119 Cases

H. Müller and F. Oppel

Neurochirurgische Klinik, Klinikum Steglitz, Freie Universität Berlin, Hindenburgdamm 30, D-1000 Berlin 45

Many late follow-up studies after extra-intracranial (EC/IC) bypass have been performed recently (2, 4-6, 8, 11-15, 18), all of them based on results from cases ranging in number from 46 (18) to 100 (6). Here we report on 119 EC/IC bypass patients whose outcome was assessed both clinically and by (repeated) angiography.

Patients and Methods

Between 1977 and 1982, EC/IC bypass operations were performed in 119 patients, using the superficial temporal artery (STA) to middle cerebral artery (MCA) end-to-side anastomosis by a combined fibrin clot-suture technique in recent cases. (9). Ninety male and 29 female patients were operated on; their average age was 51 years. Prior to admission, 34 patients had suffered transient ischemic attack(s) (TIA), 46 (prolonged) reversible ischemic deficits (PRIND), and 39 (completed) stroke (Table 1).

Preoperative angiography revealed complete occlusion of the internal carotid artery (ICA) in 95 cases and MCA occlusion in 4. ICA stenosis was found in 13 and MCA stenosis in 7 patients (Table 2).

Figure 1 shows the correlation between the preoperative clinical and the angiographic findings. As could be expected, TIAs corresponded more often to stenosis, as did stroke to occlusion, but in many cases this correlation could not be observed (cf. 1). Arterial occlusion was also diagnosed better than stenosis by other procedures (computed tomography, Doppler sonography, EEG, scintigram). We noticed a better validity

Table 1. Preoperative syndromes

TIA	PRIND	Compl. stroke	Total
34	46	39	119

Table 2. Preoperative angiography

Occlusion of		Stenosis of		Total
ICA	MCA	ICA	MCA	
95	4	13	7	119

Advances in Neurosurgery, Vol. 13
Edited by H. Dietz, M. Brock, and M. Klinger

of Doppler sonography compared with computed tomography.

Results

Immediately after surgery, the neurological deficit increased in 11 cases (9.2%). One patient (0.8%) died after 10 days due to hemorrhagic infarction.

A hundred and eight patients could be followed-up for periods ranging from 6 months to 6 years. In the late results, the number of patients with residual neurological deterioration was only 4 (3.7%). Mortality was 4.6% (Table 3) due to the generalized vascular disease. Six patients had further ischemic cerebrovascular events; two of them died. Figure 2 shows the correlation between preoperative diagnosis and postoperative clinical course. All four patients with clinical deterioration had suffered PRINDs or stroke preoperatively.

Angiographic controls were performed in 78 patients, in 6 of them twice. Forty-eight patients were reexamined 1-2 weeks after surgery, and another 30 patients after 4-8 months. The EC/IC bypass patency rate thus determined was 88%. Comparison of the long-term clinical course with the angiographic findings in detail made it possible to distinguish five groups of patients (Table 4):

1. Patients with clinical improvement or unchanged symptoms, in whom follow-up angiography demonstrates a patent anastomosis with sufficient blood flow (Fig. 3). This was the largest patient group.
2. Patients with equally good clinical long-term results, in whom early control angiography showed a patent but poorly functioning anastomosis, which, however, improved in late angiography (Fig. 4).
3. Patients with an unchanged symptomatology but angiographic demonstration of a nonpatent bypass as well as an adequate collateral blood flow. In these cases, indication for EC/IC bypass surgery might be reconsidered.
4. Patients with recurrent ischemic deficits but angiographically proven patency of the anastomosis. In these cases, reocclusion of the bypass might have occurred. The cause of reocclusion might be thrombosis at the anastomosis site, embolization from a thrombotic carotid bifurcation, or progressive arteriosclerosis of the donor vessel itself.
5. A small group of patients with clinical deterioration and a nonpatent bypass, which may be due to technical deficiencies or reocclusion of the bypass before angiographic evaluation.

Table 3. Postoperative findings

	Immediately after surgery (n = 119)	Late follow-up (n = 108)
Deterioration	11 (9.2%)	4 (3.7%)
Mortality	1 (0.8%)	5 (4.6%)
Bypass patency		88%

Table 4. Patient groups after EC/IC bypass

Clinical course	Angiography
1. Improved or unchanged	Patent anastomosis with good flow
2. Improved or unchanged	Patent anastomosis with poor flow, but improved late angiography
3. Unchanged	Anastomosis not patent, but demonstration of collateral blood flow
4. Deteriorated (recurrent ischemia)	Patent anastomosis
5. Deteriorated (recurrent ischemia)	Anastomosis not patent

Discussion and Conclusions

A survey of our late results showed that EC/IC bypass surgery was of value for the majority of cases, especially when TIA or PRIND was diagnosed preoperatively. The patency and mortality rates are in good agreement with the ligature (2, 3, 7, 11, 15, 17). We had no cases of subdural hematoma (cf. 10).

Reocclusion of the anastomosis and/or recurrent ischemia despite a patent bypass were the most interesting complications in our series. It must be considered that EC/IC bypass procedures can create new routes for an embolism originating from an ICA stump at the bifurcation level, an atherosclerotic plaque, and/or stenosis of the external carotid artery (ECA) at its origin. Therefore, in special cases we decided to operate upon the carotid bifurcation and the EC/IC bypass in a single session in cooperation with the vascular surgeon. This method was introduced in a previously pzblished article (16), and our results will be presented in the future.

References

1. AUSMAN, J.I., LATCHAW, R.E., LEE, M.C. et al.: Results of multiple angiographic studies on cerebal revascularization patients. In: Microsurgery for stroke. SCHMIEDEK, P. (ed.), pp. 222-229. New York, Heidelberg, Berlin: Springer 1977.
2. CHATER, N.L., PEERLESS, S.J., WEINSTEIN, P.R.: Review of experience with 50 consecutive cases of superficial temporal artery to middle cerebral artery anastomosis for treatment of cerebrovascular occlusive disease. In: Microvascular anastomoses for cerebral ischemia. FEIN, J.M., REICHMAN, O.H. (eds.), pp. 290-304. New York, Heidelberg, Berlin: Springer 1978.
3. DONAGHY, R.M.P.: Evaluation of extra-intracranial blood flow diversion. In: Microneurosurgical anastomoses for cerebral ischemia. AUSTIN, G.M. (ed.), pp. 256-274. Springfield, Ill.: Ch.C. Thomas 1976.
4. GRATZL, O., SCHMIEDEK, P., STEINHOFF, H.: Five years follow-up of 65 patients treated with extra-intracranial arterial bypass for cerebral ischemia. In: Advances in Neurosurgery, Vol. 3. PENZHOLZ, H., BROCK, M., HAMER, J., et al. (eds.), pp. 115-119. Berlin, Heidelberg, New York: Springer 1975.

5. GRATZL, O., SCHMIEDEK, P., SPETZLER, R. et al.: Clinical experience with extra-intracranial arterial anastomosis in 65 cases. J. Neurosurg. 44, 313 (1976)

6. GRATZL, O., SCHMIEDEK, P., OLTEANU-NERBE, V.: Long-term clinical results following extra-intracranial arterial bypass surgery. In: Microsurgery for stroke. SCHMIEDEK, P. (ed.), pp. 271-275. Berlin, Heidelberg, New York: Springer 1977.

7. HALSEY, J.H., MORAWETZ Jr., R.B., BLAUENSTEIN, U.W.: The hemodynamic effect of STA-MCA bypass. Stroke 13/2, 163-167 (1982)

8. KIKUCHI, H., KARASAWA, J.: Clinical experiences with STA-MCA anastomosis in 54 cases. In: Microvascular anastomoses for cerebral ischemia. FEIN, J.M., REICHMAN, O.H. (eds.), pp 278-283. New York, Heidelberg, Berlin: Springer 1978.

9. KLETTER, G.: The extra-intracranial bypass operation for prevention and treatment of stroke. Wien, New York: Springer 1979.

10. KOOS, W.T., KLETTER, G., SCHUSTER, H.: Microsurgical extra-intracranial arterial bypass in patients with completed stroke. Excerpta med. Cerebral vascular disease, 2nd ed. (1979).

11. MEINIG, G.: Der extra-intrakranielle Bypass für das Karotisstromgebiet. Akt. Neurol. 10, 196-202 (1983)

12. MÉREI, T.F., BODOSI, M.:Microsurgical anastomosis for cerebral ischemia in ninety patients. In: Microsurgery for stroke. SCHMIEDEK, P. (ed.), pp. 264-270. New York, Heidelberg, Berlin: Springer 1977.

13. OLTEANU-NERBE, V., SCHMIEDEK, P., GRATZL, O. et al.: Late follow-up studies in a selected group of patients with extra-intracranial arterial bypass. In: Microsurgery for stroke. SCHMIEDEK, P. (ed.), pp. 276-280. New York, Heidelberg, Berlin: Springer 1977.

14. OPPEL, F., SCHRAMM, J., BRADAĈ, G.B., BROCK, M.: Extra-intracranial bypass surgery: Correlation between long-term results and angiographic findings (Abstract). In: 7th Europ. Congress of Neurosurg. BRIHAYE, J., VIGOUROUX, R., ACHSLOGH, J. et al. (eds.), p 222. Brussels: E.A.N.S. 1983.

15. SCHMIEDEK, P., GRATZL, O., OLTEANU-NERBE, V. et al.: Nine years of experience with extra-intracranial bypass surgery for cerebral ischemia. In: Advances in neurosurgery, Vol. 7. MARGUTH, F., BROCK, M., KAZNER, E. et al. (eds.), pp. 32-39. Berlin, Heidelberg, New York: Springer 1979.

16. WONDZINSKI, A, OPPEL, F., BROCK, M. et al.: Kombiniertes einseitiges extra- und intracranielles Vorgehen bei der Behandlung der cerebrovasculären Insuffizienz. 6. Münchner Gefäßchirurgisches Gespräch, 2.-3.12.1983.

17. YASARGIL, M.G.,: Microsurgery applied to neurosurgery. Stuttgart: G. Thieme 1969.

18. YASARGIL, M.G., YONEKAWA, Y.: Experiences with STA-cortical anastomosis in 46 cases. In: Microvascular anastomoses for cerebral ischemia. FEIN, J.M., REICHMAN, O.H. (eds.), pp. 272-277. New York, Heidelberg, Berlin: Springer 1978.

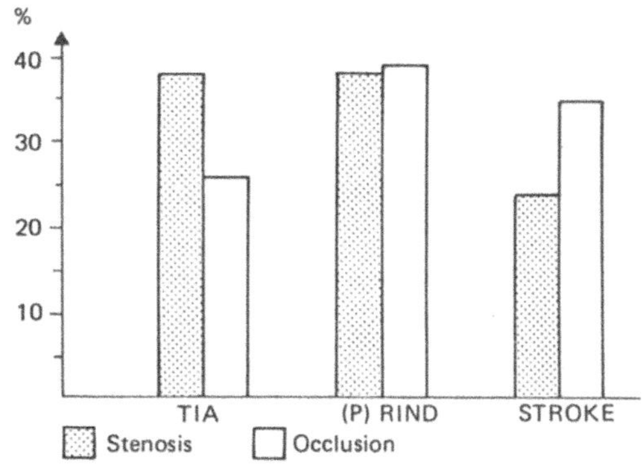

Fig. 1. Correlation between neurological syndrome and morphology

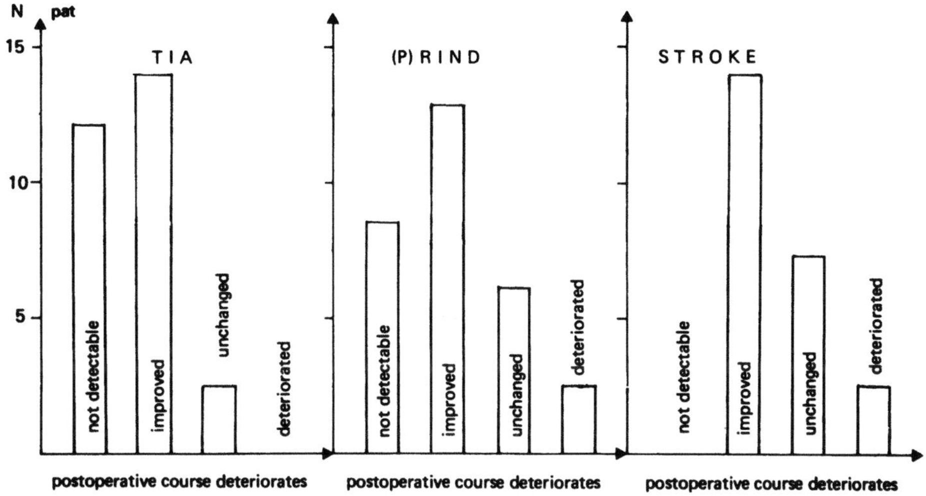

Fig. 2. Postoperative clinical course according to the preoperative diagnosis

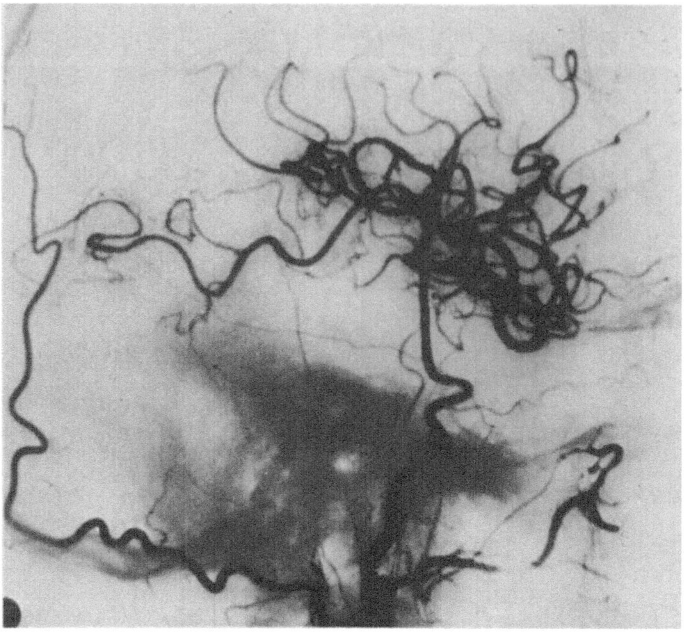

Fig. 3. Patent STA-MCA bypass with good flow

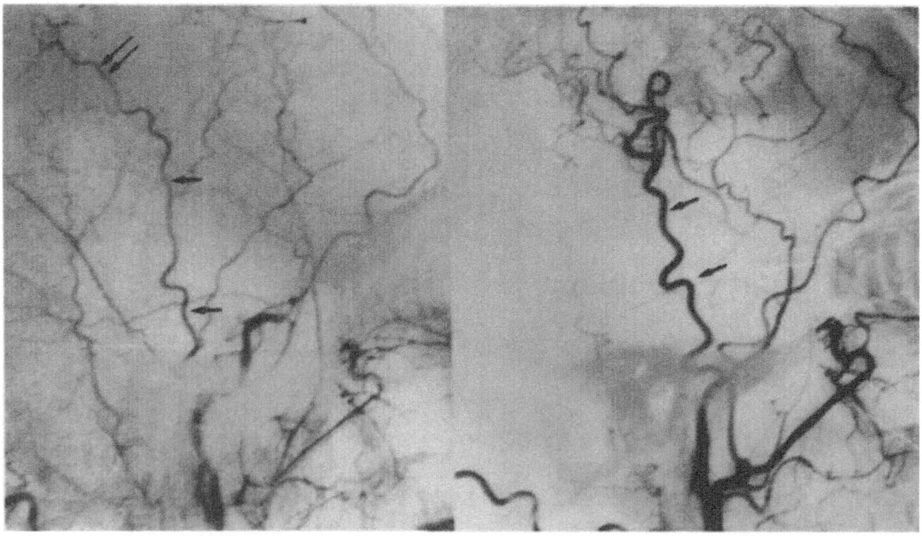

Fig. 4. *Left:* Patent EC/IC bypass with poor function. *Right:* Improved blood flow in the late angiographic control

Protective EIAB in Intracranial High-Risk Operations

D. Terhaag and R. A. Frowein

Neurochirurgische Universitätsklinik Köln, Josef-Stelzmann-Straße 9, D-5000 Köln 41

The beneficial effect of an EIAB for the prevention of an acute cerebrovascular accident during intracranial operations has already been reported on. Whether or not an anastomosis can be created as a precautionary measure and whether this then remains well supplied with blood is the subject of further discussion.

Model anastomoses created in dogs between the superficial temporal artery and the middle cerebral artery remained well supplied with blood for several months when the opening of the anastomosis had been designed with wide lumina, even when normal blood circulation was allowed to continue via the internal carotid artery.

After these observations in animal experiments were recorded, 30 patients (Table 1) with giant aneurysms, angiograms of the temporal lobes, carotid-sinus cavernosus fistulas, and tumors of the median line have, since 1979, been given anastomoses at an average of 3 weeks (2-90 days) prior to surgery. Treatment continued after healing of the anastomosis or after a further improvement of the general condition. All EIABs remained well supplied with blood.

Table 1. Basic disease in patients with protective EIAB

Basic disease	Number
Giant aneurysm	
- Middle cerebral artery	8
- Internal carotid artery (supraclinoidal)	7
- Internal carotid artery (infraclinoidal)	5
Multiple aneurysms	2
A-V angiogram	2
Carotid-sinus cavernosus fistula	2
Midline tumors	4
	30

Advances in Neurosurgery, Vol. 13
Edited by H. Dietz, M. Brock, and M. Klinger

The extra-intracranial anastomoses were to ensure further circulation in a brain artery if one of the following situations were to occur:

1. If, in order to render a vascular deformity ineffective or to remove an angioma/tumor, it were necessary to block the supplying brain artery temporarily, yet for a longer period than the maximum ischemia time.
2. If, after an operation on or near a brain artery, this artery spotaneously closed due to a thrombosis.
3. If definitely eliminating a vascular or similar deformity were possible only by means of blocking the brain artery for a longer period of time.

In five of eight patients (Fig. 1) with giant aneurysms of the middle cerebral artery, it was possible to completely remove this artery from blood circulation without creating focal neurological disorders. These also did not occur in an almost 60-year-old patient in whom the middle cerebral artery closed spontaneously due to a thrombosis 1 day after the extirpation of a media aneurysm. A 52-year-old patient in whom hemiplegia had already occurred during a cerebral hemorrhage recuperated only incompletely.

The occurrence of fatal recurring hemorrhages 12, 20, and 26 days after the creation of an extra-intracranial anastomosis, but still prior to aneurysm surgery, gave reason to select a time interval between the two operations which was as short as possible, i.e. to perform the intracranial operation as soon as the patient's general condition allowed. In one patient, whose anterior cerebral artery was inadequately supplied with blood from the opposite side, there was a sufficient supply of blood via the extra-intracranial anastomosis. When blocking the internal carotid artery at the neck with the Selverstone clamp was attempted, this resulted in focal neurological and electroencephalographic disorders. Although it was possible to reduce the size of the aneurysm by one-half by means of coagulation and circular ligatures and to surround it with muscular tissue, it could not be eliminated altogether. A subarachnoid hemorrhage 4 months later was fatal.

The necessity of definitively closing the intracranial vascular deformity was also recognized in the adverse progression of the illness of a 44-year-old patient, in whom an aneurysm of the internal carotid artery had been supplied with a ligature 10 years earlier. Postoperative angiography had confirmed that the deformity had been eliminated. Upon the patient's readmission, the aneurysm revealed in the angiogram was larger than it had been earlier. Since the beginning section of the anterior cerebral artery was included in the aneurysm wall, the deformity could not be eliminated completely. The recurring hemorrhage 3 days later was fatal.

In five of the seven patients (Fig. 1) with giant aneurysms of the internal carotid artery that were located supraclinoidally, it was possible to definitely eliminate the deformity without causing focal disorders. These also did not occur in a 36-year-old patient in whom the extirpation of the aneurysm required intracranial blockage of the internal carotid artery for a duration of 38 min.

In one patient the hemiplegia which had existed since the beginning of the illness grew more severe.

Among the five patients with giant intraclinoidal aneurysm who had received a additional blood supply via previously installed anastomoses, a hemiparesis occurred in our first patient 10 h after the neck carotid artery had been blocked by means of ligature. In the other patient, who were treated later, the blockage was achieved by means of a Selverstone clamp placed at the neck; the carotid artery was blocked intracranially with a clip and the ophthalmic artery with a ligature. No focal neurological disorders occurred. In all of these patients the anterior cerebral artery could also be supplied with blood from the opposite side.

If intracranial angiomas are not totally extirpated, there is a 2% annual risk of recurring hemorrhage. For this reason it is particularly desirable that a complete extirpation of the angioma be achieved in younger patients. In two patients, aged 14 and 17, who had arteriovenous angiomas of the temporal lobe affecting the media bifurcation point, total extirpation of the vascular deformity without the occurrence of focal neurological disorders was possible both below and above the sylvian fissure 2 and 8 weeks after an extra-intracranial anastomosis had been created.

Since in two patients with post-traumatic carotid-sinus cavernosus fistulas focal neurological disorders were revealed by the EEG, an anastomosis was created below the ligature of the ophthalmic artery in front of the intra- and extracranial blockages of the carotid artery. In both cases the procedure, with the additional blood supply via the extra-intracranial anastomosis, was uninterrupted and the regional measurements of blood supply of the brain resulted in normal findings.

Extra-intracranial anastomoses were created in four patients with compressive lesions of the midline. In the two patients with gliomas, further procedures depended on the biological valence of the glioma.

It was possible, in a 60-year old patient, to completely extirpate a medial meningeal tumor of the sphenoid bone surrounding the internal carotid artery; the patient, in whom an extra-intracranial anastomosis had been created 9 weeks earlier, enjoyed an undisturbed postoperative recovery.

Because of the small numbers of patients in the various groups, the observation of 30 patients with such widely differing clinical pictures allows us only to state that extra-intracranial anastomoses remain supplied with blood even in cases of relatively low pressure differences and that they also have a protective effect in high-risk intracranial operations.

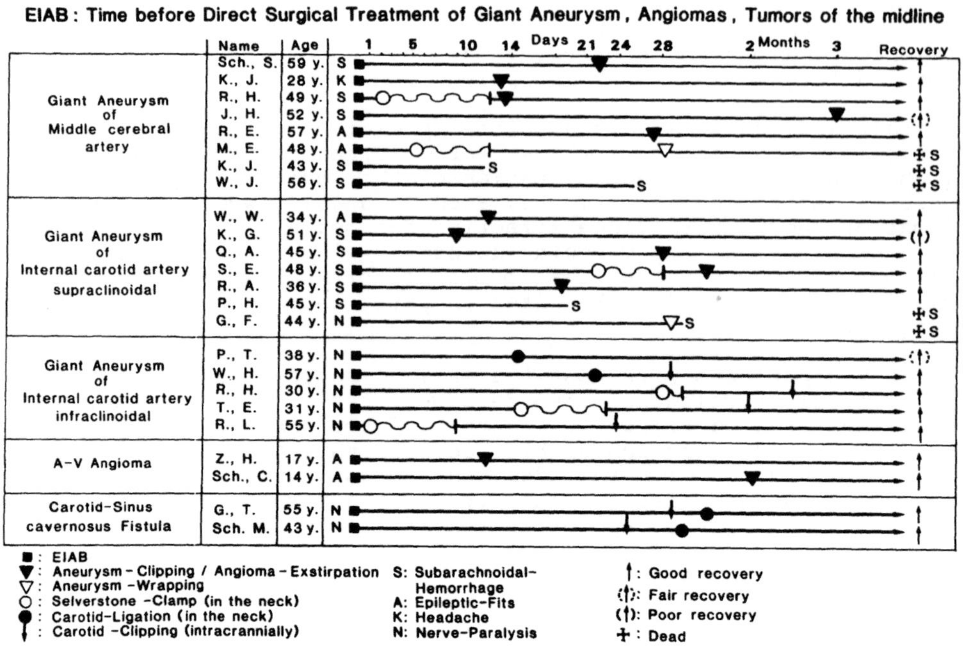

Fig. 1. Outcome and time of EIAB prior to intracranial surgery

Recovery After Stroke – Improvement by Extra-Intracranial Arterial Bypass (EIAB)? A 7-Year Follow-up Study

H. Wassmann[1], K. H. Holbach[2], and Z. Czernicki[1]

[1] Neurochirurgische Universitätsklinik, D-5300 Bonn-Venusberg
[2] Neurochirurgische Abteilung des Katharinen-Hospitals, D-7000 Stuttgart

Introduction

The natural history of recovery after completed stroke, its speed, its duration, and its final extent are still not accurately known. Most authors have observed neurological improvement in the chronic postapoplectic state until the third or sixth month after stroke. If this improvement is caused by recovery of brain function, metabolism in a perifocal, still reversible altered brain area must be investigated by neurological and brain metabolism follow-up studies.

The aim of this study was to answer the question of whether recovery after stroke is improved by extra-intracranial arterial bypass (EIAB) surgery.

Methods and Patients

In our clinic EIAB has been carried out since 1974 in certain patients with internal carotid artery or middle cerebral artery occlusion. To assess the long-term effectiveness of this operation, all such patients have been subjected to neurological investigations at 6-month to 1-year intervals. Thirty-three patients had this operation in the chronic post-stroke stage, and their follow-up over 6 to 8 years with regard to neurological function and the significance of EEG studies is the subject of this study. Of these 33 patients, 26 were men and 7 woman; the median age was 50.3 years. The cause of vascular insufficiency was carotid occlusion in 28 cases and middle cerebral artery occlusion in 5 cases. The indication for bypass operation in this stage was improvement under hyperbaric oxygen therapy in all cases (1, 5). The operation was performed on average 3.2 months after stroke. All the patients showed a patent bypass in the postoperative as determined by angiography and controlled by Doppler sonography.

The following case history illustrated our method of studying these patients (Fig. 1). A 55-year-old female suffered a stroke in May 1977 with left hemiplegia due to right internal carotid artery occlusion. Within 2 weeks the hemiplegia improved from 0 to 8 points (18 points represents the normal motor power of one side). On admission to our clinic 1 month later she was in a chronic poststroke stage with moderately severe left hemiparesis (neurological score: 8 points). She was given hyperbaric oxygen therapy which resulted in improvement of the left hemiparesis by another 3 points (1, 5). This was considered to be evidence of the partial reversibility of the neurological deficit and was the indication for bypass operation, which was carried out in July 1977. Postoperative angiography showed a functioning bypass with filling of the territory

Edited by H. Dietz, M. Brock, and M. Klinger

of the left middle cerebral artery. In the course of the next 6 months there was further improvement of the left hemiparesis by 3 points and at the end of the second year by another point. The residual hemiparesis involved distal muscles and remained unaltered till the last neurological examination in April 1984. At that time, however, the patient felt well and was able to carry out full household activities.

Computer analysis EEG showed a significant increase of alpha-activity on the affected side during the first year after surgery. There was also a slight increase of beta-activity, with a decrease of theta-activity. With the exception of a transient increase in the postoperative period, the delta-activity showed no essential changes. During the observation period, the original EEG (Fig. 2) showed a reduction of the focus in the right temporoparietal region, with accentuation of alpha waves.

Results

As a result of observation of our 33 operated patients over a period of 6 to 8 years and based on clinical neurological assessment and EEG analysis, we have divided the patients into three groups (Fig. 3):

Group I (three patients) showed essentially no change in the first year after surgery. From the second postoperative year there was aggravation of neurological deficit by 2 points and a slight decrease of alpha-activity. One patient died 5 years after operation as a result of myocardial infarction.

Group II (nine patients) showed no essential change over an 8-year period apart from a slight postoperative increase of theta- and delta-activities.

Group III (21 patients) showed significant improvement of neurological function by 5 points during the first postoperative year. This correlates with an increase of alpha-activity by 15 points. This improvement was maintained over the 8-year observation period. One patient died in the sixth postoperative year due to myocardial infarction and a second patient died as a result of stroke involving the side opposite to that of surgery.

Discussion and Conclusion

These long-term observations of 33 patients in chronic poststroke stage with fixed neurological deficit after EIAB operation showed that in two-thirds of the patients there was a definite improvement of clinical neurological status and EEG findings within the first postoperative year, especially within the first 3 months, and only a slight improvement during the second year. In one-third of the patients there was either no improvement or a slight deterioration after the second postoperative year. Most authors agree that spontaneous recovery of neurological deficit is rarely observed in the chronic poststroke stage beyond the sixth month (2, 4). NEWMAN examined 39 infarct patients and found no significant improvement after the 4th poststroke month. SKILBECK studied 162 stroke patients with spontaneous recovery and found no clinical changes after the third month after stroke. These findings correspond well with our own observations during the first year of recovery. SKILBECK evaluated the arm function, using a score (Fig. 4), and found a highly significant improvement between the first and third month ($p < 0.0001$), a less significant ($p < 0.05$) improvement between the 6th and 12th month, and later no improvement (Wilcoxon test). This trend is similar to our findings in the third patient group within the first 12 months.

In conclusion:

1. One-third of our patients showed no significant changes after EIAB operation.
2. Two-thirds of our patients showed a similar trend of paresis improvement over the first 12 months to that evidenced by the spontaneously recovered patients.
3. These group III patients later showed a slight but nonsignificant improvement between the 12th and 24th month.
4. Return of the neurological function and EEG changes tend to be complete no later than the 24th poststroke month.
5. The 5-year survival rate of 90% in our patient group was significantly better than the 60% in the spontaneous follow-up of 60-year-old stroke victims (3).

Further studies with more sensitive tests could perhaps show whether neurophysiological recovery may continue for years following some forms of acquired brain damage, and if this late recovery is a result of transfer of function to undamaged neurons.

References

1. HOLBACH, K.H., WASSMANN, H., SANCHEZ, F.: EEG analysis for evaluating chronic cerebral ischemia treated by hyperbaric oxygenation and microsurgery. J. Neurol. 219, 227-240 (1978)
2. NEWMAN, M.: The process of recovery after hemiplegia. Stroke 3, 702-710 (1972)
3. SACCO, R.L., WOLF, P.A., KANNEL, W.B.: Survival and recurrence following stroke. The Framingham study. Stroke 13, 290-295 (1982)
4. SKILBECK, C.E., WADE, D.T., HEWER, R.L., WOOD, V.A.: Recovery after stroke. J. Neurol. Neurosurg. Psychiatry 46, 5-8 (1983)
5. WASSMANN, H.: Quantitative Indikatoren des hirnelektrischen Wirkungsverlaufes bei hyperbarer Oxygenierung. Z. EEG-EMG 11, 97-101 (1980)

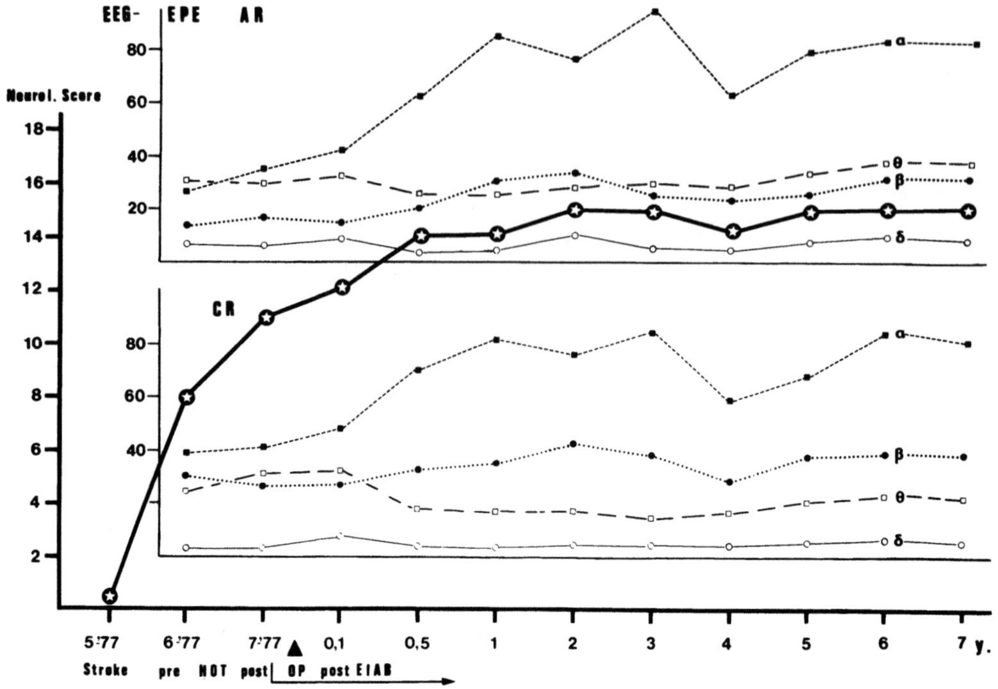

Fig. 1. Neurological (✪) and EEG analytical follow-up examinations of a patient with right internal carotid artery occlusion who underwent hyperbaric oxygen therapy (*HOT*) and EIAB. Electrical power equivalent (*EPE*) values of the affected (*AR*) and contralateral region (*CR*) are divided in the beta, alpha, theta, and delta wave range. The neurological score represents the sum of motor power (6 points represent normal motor power) of the hand, arm and leg

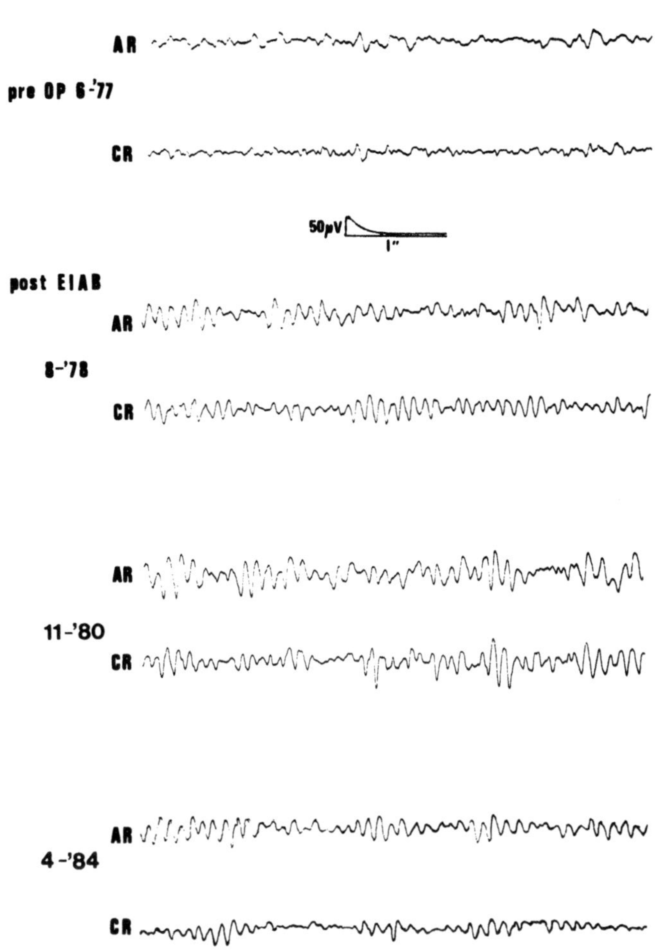

Fig. 2. Follow-up original EEG of the affected (*AR*) and contralateral region (*CR*) in 55-year-old woman with right internal carotid artery occlusion who underwent EIAB

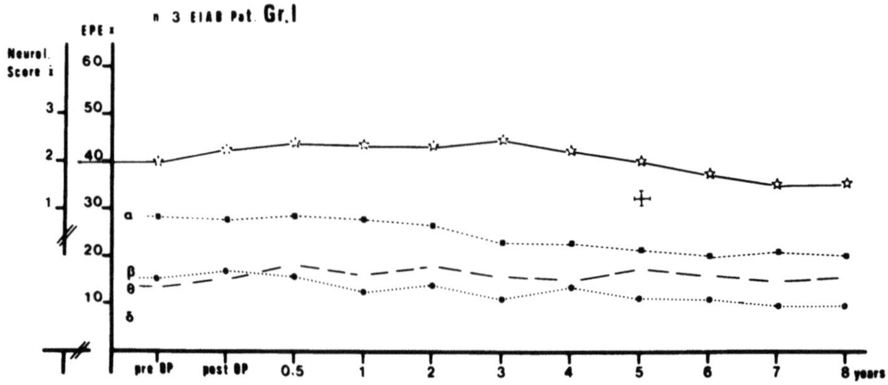
n 3 EIAB Pat. Gr.I
EPE x
Neurol. Score x
60
50
40
30
20
10
3
2
1
α
β
θ
δ
pre OP
post OP
0.5
1
2
3
4
5
6
7
8 years

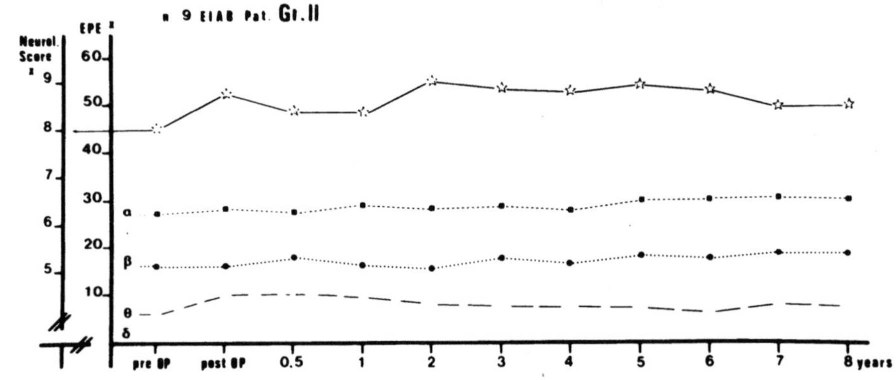
n 9 EIAB Pat. Gr.II
EPE x
Neurol. Score x
60
50
40
30
20
10
9
8
7
6
5
α
β
θ
δ
pre OP
post OP
0.5
1
2
3
4
5
6
7
8 years

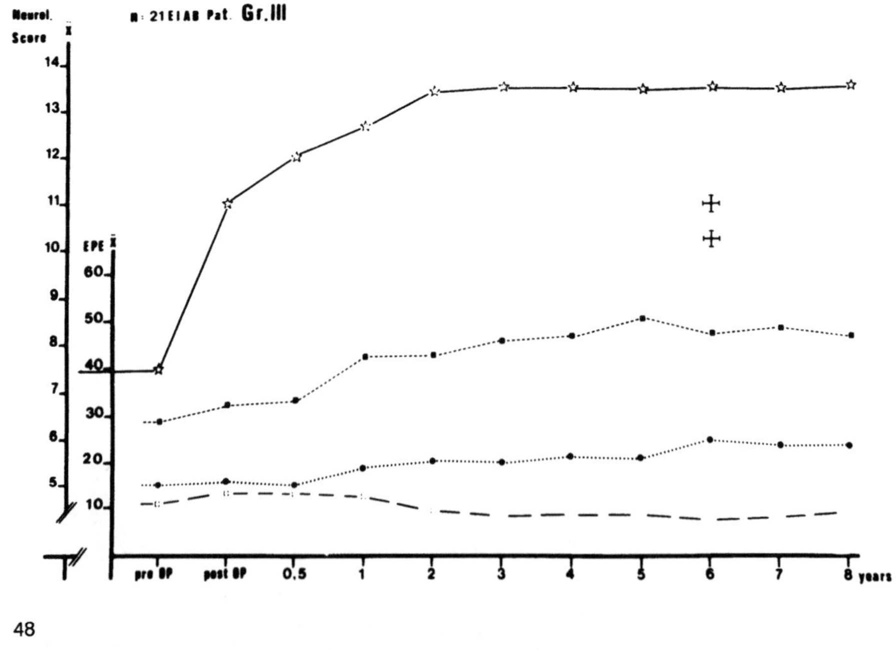
n: 21 EIAB Pat. Gr.III
Neurol. Score x
EPE x
14
13
12
11
10
9
8
7
6
5
60
50
40
30
20
10
pre OP
post OP
0.5
1
2
3
4
5
6
7
8 years

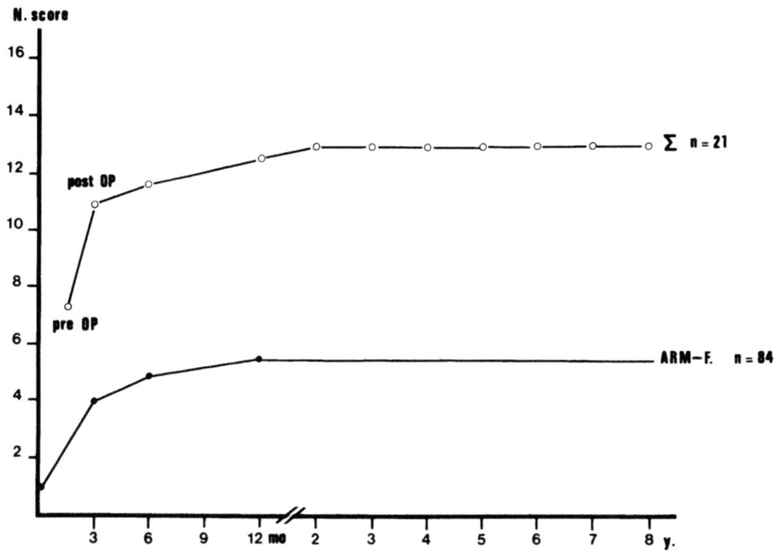

Fig. 4. Neurological recovery of arm function (*ARM-F.*) (●) in 84 post-stroke patients in spontaneous follow-up (SKILBECK et al.), and of hemiparesis (O) in 21 patients (group III) after EIAB. Mean values of neurological score (*N. score*) in the follow-up of 8 years (*y.*)

Fig. 3. Neurological (☆) and EEG analytical follow-up mean values of 33 patients who underwent EIAB in the chronic postapoplectic stage. Patients are divided into three groups according to the extent of their neurological and EEG analytical changes

Rare Indications for EIAB Procedures

H. Friedrich[1], G. Hänsel-Friedrich[1], R. Staffensky[1], and H. Vogelsang[2]

[1] Neurochirurgische Klinik, [2] Neuroradiologische Abteilung, Medizinische Hochschule Hannover, Konstanty-Gutschow-Straße 8, D-3000 Hannover 61

Introduction

Common indications for EIAB surgery are stenosis or occlusion of one internal carotid artery (ICA) or middle cerebral artery (MCA). Prophylactic anastomoses are also carried out to minimize the risk of ischemic complications in patients in whom internal carotid artery ligation is planned for any of a variety of reasons. Among these elective EIAB indications are tumors of the skull base affecting the internal carotid artery and giant aneurysms of the ICA which cannot be attacked by direct approach (1, 2, 4, 5, 7). In addition, a number of cases are known where EIAB has prevented exacerbation of ischemic deficit in patients with certain lesions that are, as yet, untreatable, e.g., Moya-Moya syndrome (8), fibromuscular dysplasia, and Takayasu's syndrome.

Material and Results

Since 1980 we have performed 132 extra-intracranial arterial bypass operations (EIAB) in 114 patients, most of them because of *occlusion* or *stenosis* of the ICA and MCA. Bilateral ICA occlusion occurred in 14 patients (Table 1).

Table 1. Indications for extra-intracranial bypass operations (EIAB)

Indication	Postoperative controls in 98 patients					
	No. of EIABs	Function of EIAB				
		Doppler sonogram		Postop. angiogram		
		+	-	+	-	Not done
Internal carotid artery occlusion (bilateral: 14 pat.)	93	83	10	69	8	16
Internal carotid artery stenosis	7	6	1	5	1	1
Middle cerebral artery occlusion	12	11	1	10	-	2
Middle cerebral artery stenosis	1	1	-	1	-	-
Total	113	101	12	85	9	19

Advances in Neurosurgery, Vol. 13
Edited by H. Dietz, M. Brock, and M. Klinger

In 16 patients, however, the anastomosis was done for different reasons; details regarding these patients are listed in Tables 2 and 3.

In the two patients with *meningiomas of the sphenoid wing*, the ICA and MCA were either stenotic or occluded by the tumor mass. STA-MCA bypass was done in the same operation, providing the possibility to completely ligate the ICA or MCA for radical tumor removal, which could be achieved in our patients. With prophylactic EIAB the development of ischemia as a consequence of radical tumor removal could be prevented (5). Although EIAB was performed in these two patients, there was concern that the carotid artery might have to be sacrificed during surgery, but this turned out to be the case only in one patient. The third case involving a tumor was in an elderly patient with left *frontal meningioma* and occlusion of left ICA and PRINDs.

In three patients with *giant aneurysms* of the ICA, EIAB was performed before surgical occlusion of the ICA by means of the Selverstone clamp. In three patients with giant MCA aneurysms, EIAB was done prophylactically before direct attack of the aneurysm.

Two patients suffered from *multiple vessel occlusion*. Both of them had had several PRINDs but no signs of dementia as mentioned in the literature (9). In one panangiography revealed occlusion of both ICAs and one vertebral artery and stenosis of the other vertebral artery. The other patient had (four vessel) occlusion of both vertebral arteries and one ICA, stenosis of the other ICA, and occlusion of MCA on the same side.

EIABs using venous grafts 32-47 cm long were done in three patients, two of whom were suffering from occlusion of one common carotid artery (CCA) and one from so-called *Takayasu's syndrome*.

Table 2. Extra-intracranial bypass operations: exceptional indications

Indication	Postoperative controls in 16 patients					
	No. of EIABs	Function of EIAB				
		Doppler sonogram		Postop. angiogram		
		+	-	+	-	Not done
Tumor	3	3	-	2	-	1
Aneurysm	7	6	1	5	1	1[a]
Occlusion of 3 arteries with additional stenosis of the fourth	4	4	-	2	-	1[b]
Moya-Moya disease	2	2	-	2	-	-
Common carotid artery occlusion (saphenous bypass, 2 pat.)	2	2	-	2	-	-
Takayasu's disease	1	1	-	1	-	-
Total	19	18	1	14	1	3

a Died of intracerebral hemorrhage between EIAB and aneurysm operation
b Suicide

Table 3. Details regarding the 16 patients who underwent EIAB owing to exceptional indications

Patient	Preoperative symptoms	Preoperative angiography	EIAB	Postoperative angiography	Complications	Results
Tumor						
1 m 72	PRIND Seizures Aphasia Hemiparesis	l ICO Tumor fronto-parietal	l STA-MCA Tumor removal	Patent bypass	None	Normal
2 f 41	PRIND Hemiparesis	r MCO Tumor sphenoid wing	r STA-MCA Tumor removal	Patent bypass	None	Normal
3 f 33	PRIND Hemiparesis	r ICS/MCS Tumor sphenoid wing	r STA-MCA Tumor removal	No angiogram Positive Doppler	12th postop. day rupture of ICA Ligature ICA	Hemiparesis
Aneurysm						
4 m 18	Embolic episodes Completed stroke Hemiplegia Aphasia	8 cm traumatic dissecting aneurysm l IC l MCO	l STA-MCA Selverstone clamp	Patent bypass	None	Hemiplegia Aphasia improved
5 f 58	Progressive visual loss	4 cm aneurysm Infraclinoid	r STA-MCA Selverstone clamp	Patent bypass	None	Full visual function
6 f 67	SAH Palsy N III, IV, VI	4 cm aneurysm Infraclinoid	r STA-MCA Selverstone clamp	Patent bypass	None	Normal
7 f 31	SAH visual loss	3.5 cm carotid ophthalmic aneurysm, infraclinoid	r STA-MCA Selverstone clamp	Patent bypass	None	Normal

8 m 39	PRIND Aphasia	4 cm aneurysm MCA	1 STA-MCA	No angiogram Positive Doppler	Fatal bleeding at 12th postop. day	Died
9 m 21	PRIND Seizures Aphasia	4 cm aneurysm MCA	1 STA-MCA Clipping	Patent bypass	None	Normal
10 m 55	Completed stroke Dementia	3.5 cm aneurysm MCA	1 STA-MCA Clipping	Patent bypass	None	Normal
Multiple occlusions - 3/4 vessels						
11 m 43	Completed stroke	BICO, VO, VS	Bilateral STA-MCA	No angiogram positive Doppler	None	Died, suicide 6 w. postop.
12 m 46	Completed stroke Aphasia Hemiparesis	BVO, ICO r, ICS 1, MCO 1	Bilateral STA-MCA	Patent bypass	None	Aphasia Hemiparesis improved
Moya-Moya disease						
13 f 5	PRIND Aphasia Hemiparesis	1 ICO "Moya Moya", r ICS "Moya Moya"	Bilateral STA-MCA	Patent bypass	None	Aphasia Hemiparesis improved
Saphenous graft						
14 m 55	PRIND Hemiparesis	r CCO	r CC - saphenous graft, MCA	Patent bypass	None	Normal
15 m 60	PRIND Aphasia Hemiparesis	1 CCO	1 CC - saphenous graft, MCA	Patent bypass	None	Normal
16 f 28	TIA Drop attacks	Aortic arch syndrome	aorta - saphenous graft, MCA	Patent bypass	None	Normal

BICO, bilateral internal carotid occlusion; BVO, bilateral vertebral occlusion; CC, common carotid artery; CCO, common carotid occlusion; EIAB, extra-intracranial arterial bypass; IC, internal carotid artery; ICO, internal carotid occlusion; ICS, internal carotid stenosis; l, left; MCA, middle cerebral artery; MCO, middle cerebral occlusion; MCS, middle cerebral stenosis; r, right; SAH, subarachnoid hemorrhage; STA, superficial temporal artery; VO, vertebral occlusion; VS, vertebral stenosis

The clinical presentation of all our patients is documented in Table 3.

Two Case Reports (see Table 3)

Patient No.1. This 72-year-old patient presented with a 4-year history of seizures and repeated PRINDs. Neurological examination revealed slight right hemiparesis and speech disturbance. CT showed a left frontoparietal meningioma with extensive edema. Angiography revealed occlusion of the left ICA and a dilated left STA supplying a large frontoparietal meningioma (Figs. 1, 2). A left STA-MCA anastomosis was performed using the dilated tumor artery, and the tumor was removed during the same operation. A directional Doppler flow study showed the bypass to be patent, as was also proved by postoperative angiography (Fig. 3). So far the patient has no further neurological signs or ischemic attacks, though he still suffers seizures occasionally.

Patient No. 2. This 28-year-old woman presented with drop attacks. She had suffered a PRIND 4 years previously with right hemiparesis. In 1980 vertebrobasilar insufficiency was diagnosed, and in 1982 Takayasu's syndrome. From 1982 onward she was unable to get up and suffered TIA almost every day. Angiography showed the typical aortic arch syndrome with only one stenotic vertebral artery supplying the cerebral circulation (3, 6). An unsuccessful attempt was made to disobliterate the vertebral artery, and subsequent occlusion of this vessel occurred with a left-side hemorrhagic infarction. In April 1983 a saphenous bypass, 47 cm long was performed from the aortic arch to the MCA in cooperation with the thoracic surgeons. Postoperative angiography showed filling of the main branches of right MCA and ACA. The left vertebral artery was filled by collaterals from muscle branches. The patient now lives a normal life and has not suffered any TIA or PRIND since the operation (Figs. 4, 5).

Discussion

For certain aneurysms prophylactic EIAB is an effective treatment, if direct obliteration of the aneurysm proves impossible because of its size or location and if ligation of the vessel proximal to the aneurysm is planned (1, 2, 4, 7).

If preoperative angiography does not show sufficient natural collaterals there is a high risk that proximal ligation will not be tolerated without ischemic deficit. Our limited experience with four aneurysms shows that prophylactic bypass has allowed stepwise occlusion of ICA by a Selverstone clamp without permanent deficit. The value of EIAB patients with MCA aneurysms remains debatable because this operation carries a high risk even with a bypass (7). Since EIAB and irreversible occlusion of the MCA are performed in a one-stage operation, the flow through the anastomosis may not be sufficient to prevent ischemic deficit at once.

On the other hand, retrograde thrombosis may occur at the site of occlusion of MCA. To reduce the complication prophylactic heparinization has been advocated in major vessel occlusion, though this is contraindicated in these patients with intracranial aneurysms.

Moya-Moya disease is a rare chronic occlusive cerebrovascular disease appearing mainly in Japanese patients. While prognosis in adult patients with repeated PRINDs seems to be poor, children apparently profit from STA-MCA anastomosis, as shown by KARASAWA et al. (8). So far we have seen one child, who after several TIAs suffered from a completed stroke which finally led to bilateral STA-MCA anastomoses. Neurological function improved postoperatively and there has not been another TIA or PRIND so far, the follow-up time being 14 months.

Long venous grafts from the saphenous vein have been used for various bypass operations, among them common carotid artery or subclavian artery to MCA bypass (10). We added a new case to these indications by providing a young patient with so-called *Takayasu's syndrome* with an aortic arch to MCA anastomosis via a saphenous graft 47 cm long. Since the etiology of this disease is still unclear and no effective therapy has been found, the otherwise fatal course can only be influenced by construction of anastomotic channels to increase blood supply to the brain (3, 6). The result in this case was encouraging both clinically and angiographically.

Conclusion

EIAB has become a routine operation with low morbidity and mortality for the treatment of cerebrovascular disease. While it is generally accepted that anastomosis is indicated for MCA and ICA occlusion or stenosis, only small series have been reported concerning EIAB for CCA occlusion, multiple vessel occlusion, Moya-Moya disease, and Takayasu's syndrome. Since this minor operation is able to improve markedly the patient's quality of ife by preventing further ischemic attacks or even improving neurological deficit,it should be performed for extraordinary indications even though long-term results are not yet availabe.

References

1. BRAMBILLA, G., PAOLETTI, P., RODRIGUEZ Y BAENA, R.: Extracranial-intracranial arterial bypass in the treatment of inoperable giant aneurysms of the internal carotid artery. Acta Neurochir. 60, 63-69 (1982)
2. BUSHE,K.A., BOCKHORN, J.: Extracranial-intracranial arterial bypass for giant aneurysms. Acta Neurochir. 54, 107-115 (1980)
3. FRAGA, A., et al.: Takayasu's arteriitis: Frequency of systemic manifestations and favourable response to maintenance steroid therapy with adrenocorticosteroids. Arthritis Rheum. 15, 617 (1972)
4. GELBER, B.R., SUNDT, T.M.Jr.: Treatment of intracavernous and giant carotid aneurysms by combined internal carotid ligation and extra- to intracranial bypass. J. Neurosurg. 52, 1-10 (1980)
5. GRATZL, O., SCHMIEDEK, P., STEINHOFF, H.,: Extra-intracranial arterial bypass in patients with occlusion of cerebral arteries due to trauma and tumor. In: HANDA, H. (ed.): Microneurosurgery, pp 68-80, Tokyo, Igaku Shoin, Baltimore, University Park Press, 1975
6. HACHIYA, J.: Current concepts of Takayasu's arteriitis. Seminars Roentgen. 5, 245-259 (1970)
7. HOPKINS, L.N., GRAND, W.: Extracranial-intracranial arterial bypass in the treatment of aneurysms of the carotid and middle cerebral arteries. Neurosurg. 5, 21-31 (1979)
8. KARASAWA, J., KIKUCHI, H., FURUSE, S., KAWAMURA, J., SAKAKI, T.: Treatment of moyamoya disease with STA-MCA anastomois. J. Neurosurg. 49, 679-688 (1978)
9. PEERLESS, S.J., CHATER, N.L., FERGUSON, G.F.: Multiple vessel occlusion in cerebrovascular disease - a further follow-up of the effects of microvascular bypass on the quality of life and the incidence of stroke. In: SCHMIEDEK, P. (ed.): Microsurgery for stroke, pp 251-259, Springer-Verlag, New York, Heidelberg, Berlin, 1977

10. SPETZLER, R.F., RHODES, R.S., ROSKI, R.A.: High flow extracranial to intracranial bypass. 7th Int. Congr. Neurol. Surg., München, July 12-18, 1981

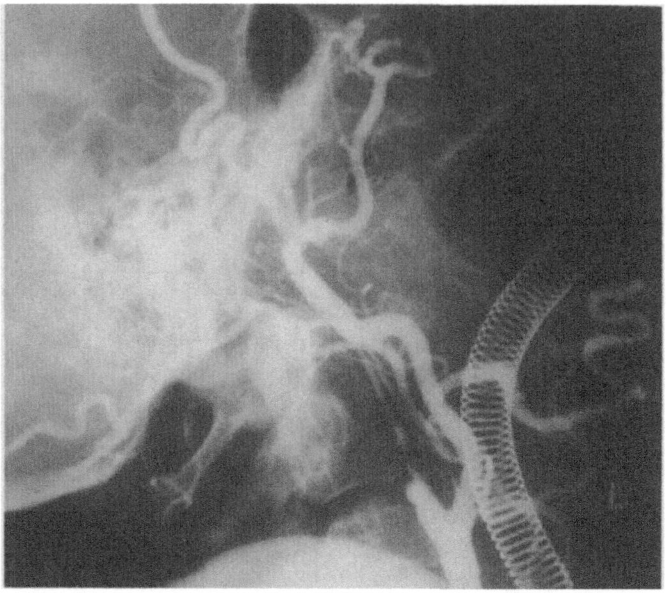

Fig. 1. Left internal carotid artery stenosis with occlusion in the supraclinoidal part. Case 1

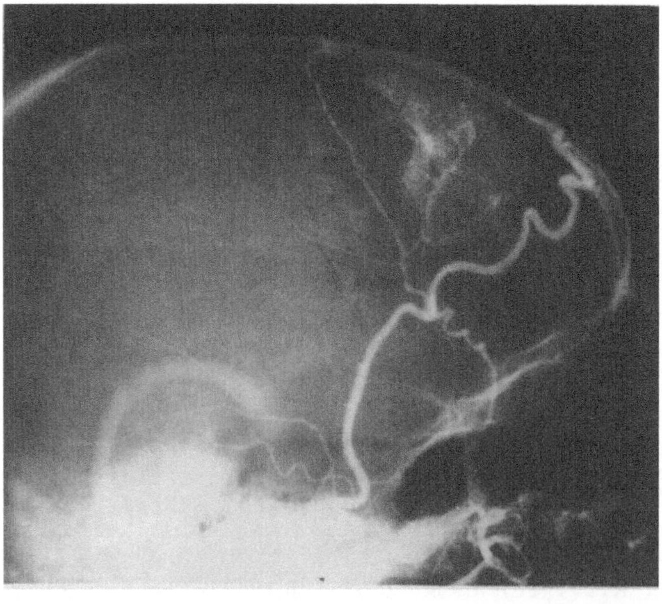

Fig.2. Dilated superficial temporal artery supplying left frontoparietal meningioma. Case 1

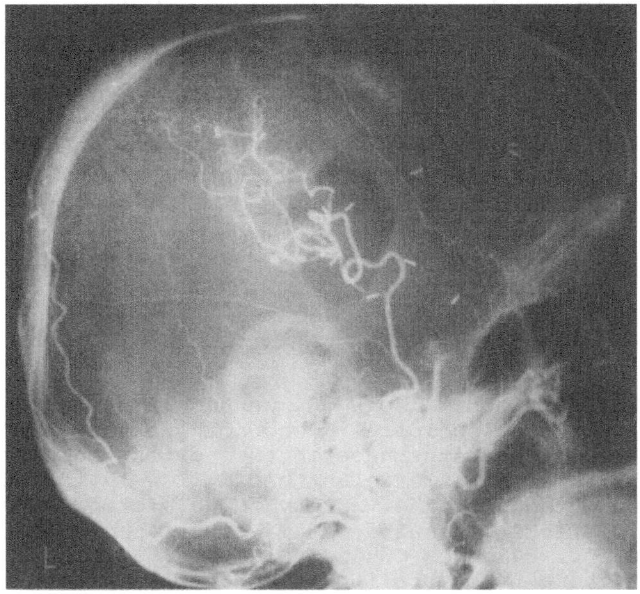

Fig. 3. Postoperative EIAB. Case 1

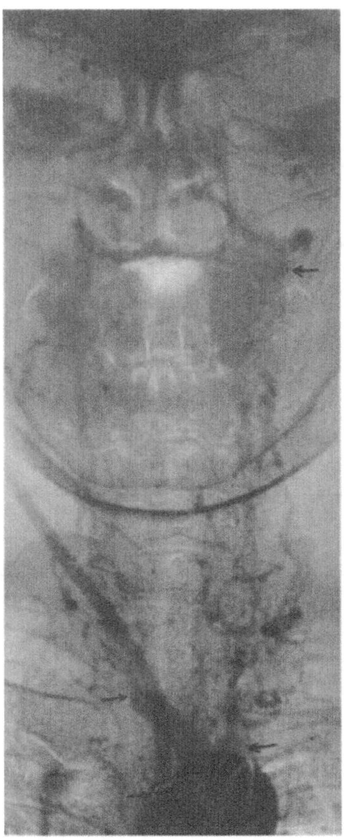

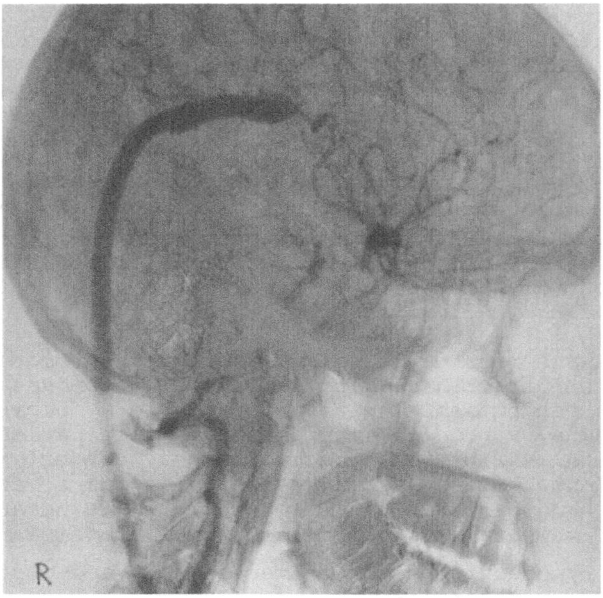

Fig. 4. Takayasu's syndrome. Occlusion of the major branches of the aortic arch with saphenous bypass. Case 16

Fig. 5. Postoperative EIAB; the distal part of vertebral artery is filled by collaterals in the neck. Case 16

Extra-Intracranial Microvascular Anastomosis with the Arteria Occipitalis: Indications and Operative Technique

S. Vogel and R. R. Unger

Neurochirurgische Abteilung der Chirurgischen Klinik im Bereich Medizin (Charité) der Humboldt Universität zu Berlin, Schumannstraße 20/21, DDR-1040 Berlin

There are two reasons why we should perform microvascular anastomosis with the a. occipitalis and not with the a. cerebri media. Firstly there is a disturbance in the vertebrobasilar circulation. Secondly there is an insufficient blood flow in the a. temporalis superficialis and we need another artery for a microvascular anastomosis with the a. cerebri media and/or a. cerebri posterior and the a. cerebelli superior. Evidence of occlusion or stenosis with hemodynamic efficacy in the a. vertebralis, a. cerebelli inferior posterior, a. basilaris, and a. cerebri posterior is an indication for a microvascular anastomosis. This is only possible with the a. occipitalis if strain between the anastomosed arteries is avoided.

In 1973, KHODADAD (4) reported on microvascular anastomosis between the a. lingualis and the a. basilaris and he obtained a sufficient blood flow in the vertebrobasilar circulation. In 1975, PALKOVIC (6) also discussed use of this approach in experiments with dogs. In 1974, SPETZLER (8) described results of anastomoses between the a. occipitalis and the a. cerebelli inferior posterior, and such anastomoses were likewise performed by AUSMAN in 1976 (1). Many variations are possible, e.g., an interposition from a part of the a. radialis between the a. carotis externa and the a. cerebelli inf. post. and a direct anastomosis of the a. carotis externa with the a. cerebelli inf. post. by means of the a. lingualis. Today it is not possible to give a final assessment of these methods because the number of patients is insufficient and the indications vary too greatly.

In a series of 219 microvascular anastomoses we have performed 18 extra-intracranial microvascular anastomoses with the a. occipitalis. In ten patients we anastomosed the a. occipitalis with the branch of the a. cerebelli inf. post.; in four patients we connected the a. occipitalis with the branch of the a. cerebri posterior; and in four patients we used the a. occipitalis for a vascular anastomosis with the r. angularis of the a. cerebri media, because the blood flow in the a. temporalis superficialis was insufficient. Indications were:

- Hypoplasia of the a. vertebralis and occlusion of the contralateral a. vertebralis
- Hypoplasia or occlusion of the a. vertebralis and kinking of the contralateral a. vertebralis
- Occlusion of the a. cerebelli inferior posterior
- Occlusion of the a. cerebelli superior
- Occlusion of the a. cerebri posterior
- Stenosis of the a. basilaris.

Advances in Neurosurgery, Vol. 13
Edited by H. Dietz, M. Brock, and M. Klinger

In all patients there was a clinical syndrome of transient or permanent ischemia with nuclear and/or cerebellar symptoms. At the same time we performed an infarctectomy in three patients.

All patients with ischemia of the brain stem were operated on in the horizontal position since the sitting position is very dangerous for these patients. The operative technique involved the normal osteoclastic trepanation of the fossa posterior or occipital region (Figs. 1-3).

For the bypass with the a. cerebelli inf. post., after incision of the dura mater we prepared a loop of the tonsillar branch beside the lobulus biventer cerebelli. Strain on this loop is extremely dangerous because it may cause malfunction of the nervus glossopharyngeus, n. vagus, and n. accessorius. We dissected the a. occipitalis over a distance of 6 cm and preserved its branches to the musculature, because these arteries are collaterals for the vertebrobasilar circulation.

The operative technique for microvascular anastomoses with supratentorial arteries required another approach. We performed a medial or lateral trepanation without a flap of skin and muscle. It is better to make a longitudinal incision above the a. occipitalis. We never observed intraoperative or postoperative complications. By contrast, in 1978 SUNDT (9) described bleeding in the subarachnoid space and the epidural space, and in 1980 KHODADAD reported a patient with postoperative infarction. We usually observed a typical syndrome, with ataxia, dysdiadochokinesia, dysmetria, and vertigo caused by motion of the head; speech disturbances were rare, whereas diplopia and drop seizures were very common.

Nine out of the ten patients in the group with anastomosis with the a. cerebelli inf. post. have shown an improvement. Two are able to pursue their occupation full time, while seven are able to work for short periods. Only one patient has shown a deterioration. All patients in this group have had a patent anastomosis for between six weeks and three years after operation. In six patients we observed circulation of cerebellar arteries in the periphery. The improvement in two patients is perhaps connected with the infarctectomy in the cerebellum, because there is only a regional circulation through the anastomosis. We performed angiographic control in five of the eight patients in the group with supratentorial anastomosis with the a. occipitalis. In each of the five, this revealed a patent anastomosis, and there was corresponding clinical improvement. The hemodynamic value of the anastomoses, with a mean flow of 15 ml/min, is lower than the blood flow through the anastomoses with the a. temporalis superficialis. We believe that anastomosis with the a. occipitalis is an important addition to the neurosurgical treatment of disturbances of cerebral circulation.

References

1. Ausman, J.C., Lee, M.C., Klassen, A.C., Chon, S.: Stroke: What's new? Cerebral revascularization. Minn. Med. 59, 223-227 (1976)
2. Ausman, J.C., Nicloff, D.M., Chon, S.N.: Posterior fossa revascularization: Anastomosis of vertebral artery to PICA with interposed radial artery graft. Surg. Neurol. 9, 281-286 (1978)
3. Corkill, G., French, B.N., Michas, C., Cobb, C.A., Mims, T.J.: External carotid-vertebral artery anastomosis for vertebrobasilar insufficiency. Surg. Neurol. 7, 109-116 (1977)

4. Khodadad, G.: Sublingual and lingual-basilar artery anastomoses and carotid-basilar bypass grafts. Surg. Neurol. 1, 175-179 (1973)

5. Khodadad, G., Sing, R.S., Oplinger, C.P.: Possible prevention of brainstem stroke by microvascular anastomosis in the vertebrobasilar system. Stroke 8, 316-321 (1977)

6. Palkovic, S.: Contribution of the anastomosis of the lingual artery and basilar artery of the dog to the microsurgery of cerebral vessels. Rozhledy v chirurgii 54, 746-748 (1975)

7. Reichmann, O.H.: Experimental lingual-basilar arterial microanastomosis. J. Neurosurg. 34, 501-505 (1971)

8. Spetzler, R.F., Chater, N.: Occipital middle cerebral artery anastomosis for cerebral arterial occlusive disease. Surg. Neurol. 2, 235-238 (1974)

9. Sundt, M.T., Piepgras, D.G.: Occipital to posterior inferior cerebellar artery bypass surgery. J. Neurosurg. 48, 916-928 (1978)

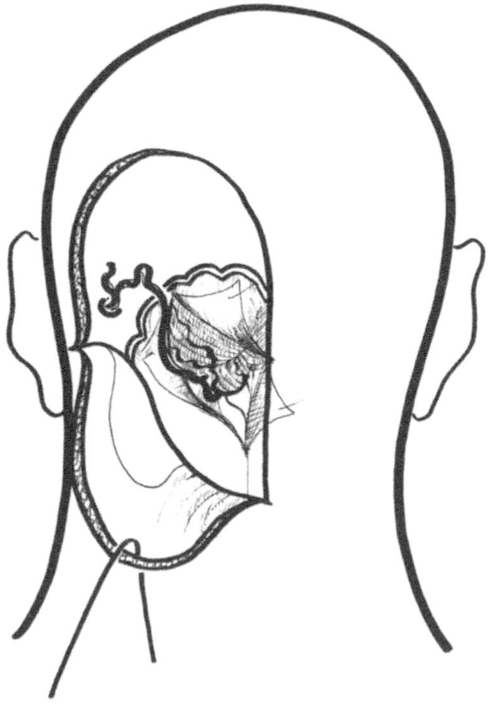

a

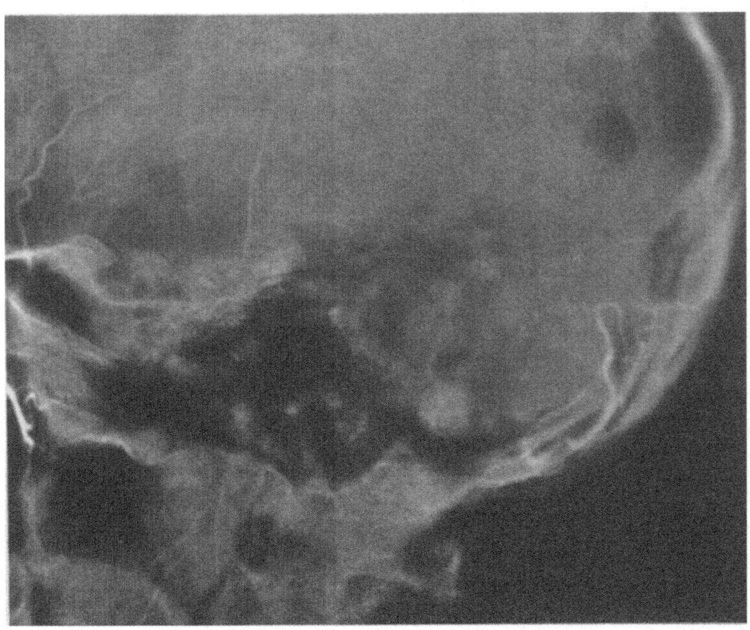

b

Fig. 1. a Microvascular anastomosis with the a. occipitalis and a. cerebelli inferior posterior. b Angiographic control

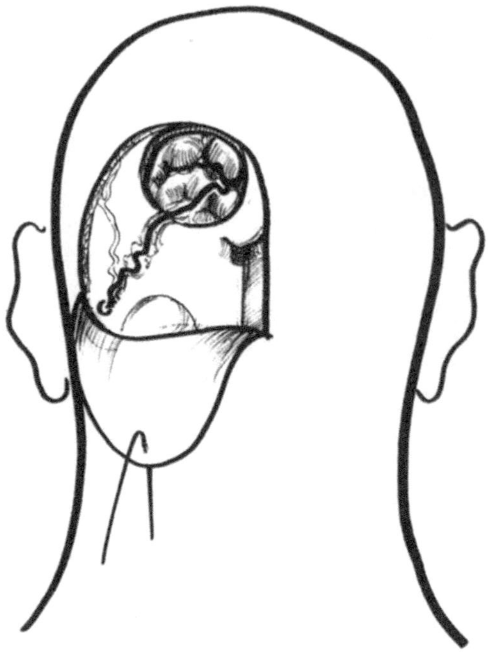

a

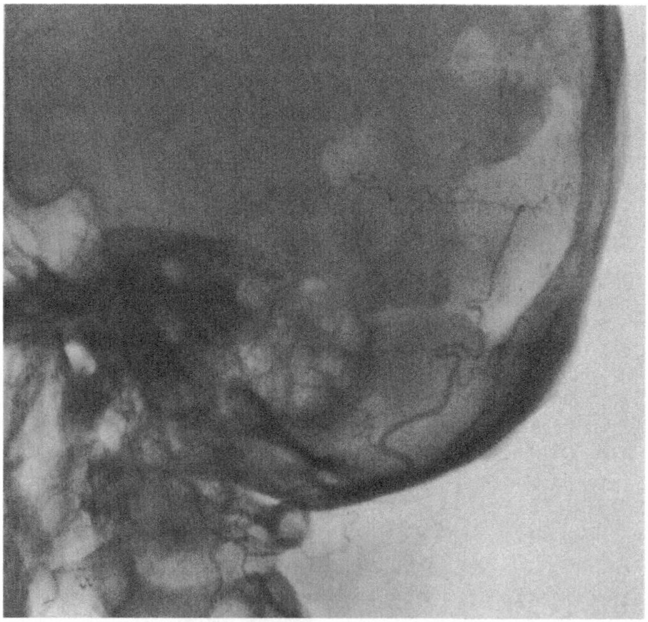

b

Fig. 2. a Microvascular anastomosis with the a. occipitalis and a. cerebri posterior. b Angiographic control

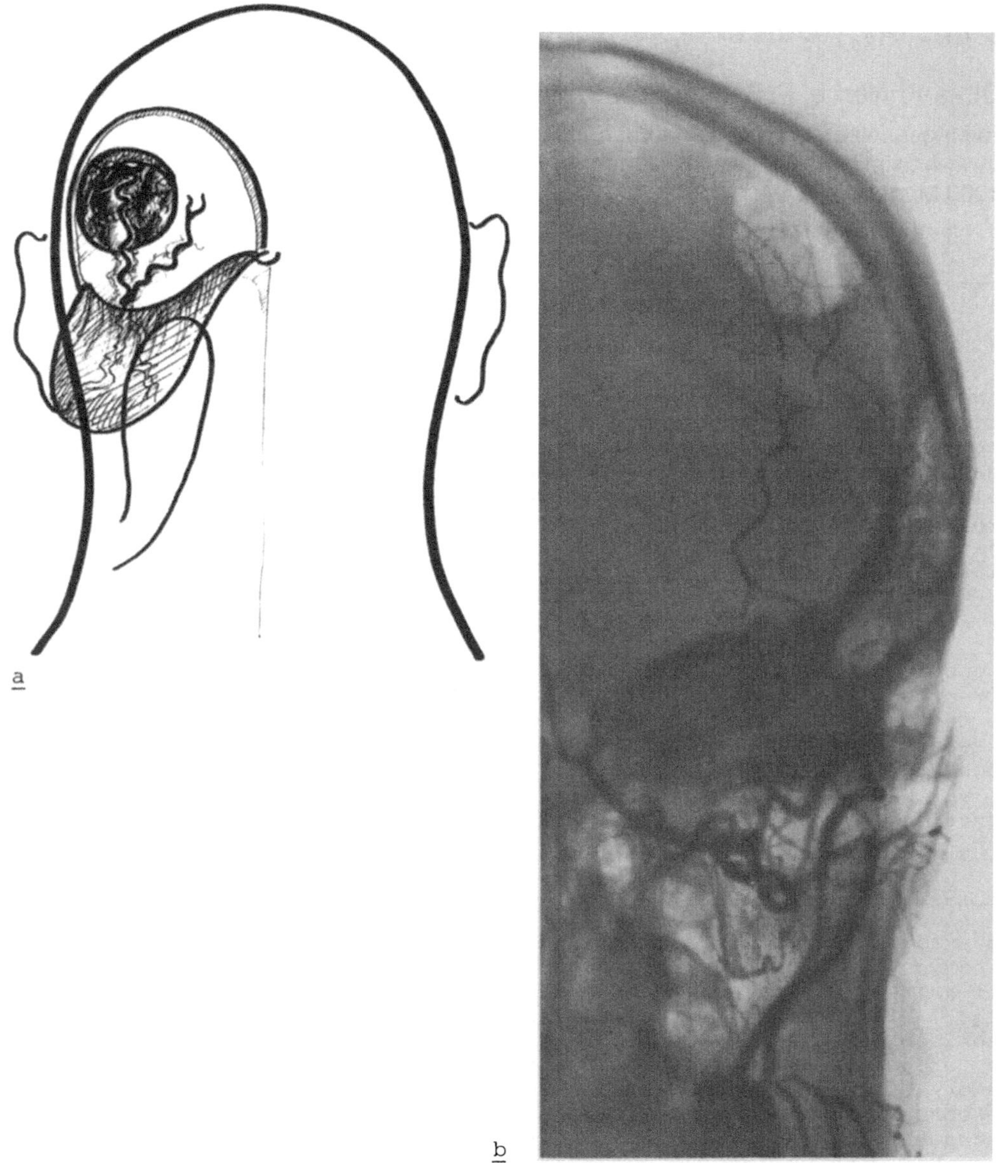

a

b

Fig. 3. a Microvascular anastomosis with the a. occipitalis and a. cerebri media (r. angularis). b Angiographic control

Brain Revascularization Surgery for Vertebrobasilar Insufficiency Due to Obstructive Vertebral Artery Disease

V. Olteanu-Nerbe, P. Schmiedek, and F. Marguth

Abteilung für Neurochirurgie, Institut für Chirurgische Forschung der Ludwig-Maximilians-Universität München, Klinikum Großhadern, Marchioninistraße 15, D-8000 München 70

Although a definitive evaluation of the benefit of brain revascularization surgery of the carotid circulation in patients with cerebrovascular insufficiency is not yet possible, encouraging results of several individual series of patients have been published. As a result, additional indications for brain revascularization procedures have been suggested, among them vertebrobasilar insufficiency (VBI). The first extra-intracranial arterial bypass (EIAB) to the posterior circulation was performed in 1975 by AUSMAN (1). Since then SUNDT and PIEPGRAS (10), KHODADAD (7), ROSKI et al. (9), and OLTEANU-NERBE et al. (8) have presented their experiences with small series of patients.

Depending on the localization of the obstructive lesions within the vertebrobasilar system, various procedures for revascularization of the posterior circulation have been described (2, 3). Our experience is reported with bypass surgery between the occipital artery (OA) and the posterior inferior cerebellar artery (PICA) or the vertebral artery (VA) in a group of 15 patients presenting with VBI due to an obstructive lesion of the VA.

Clinical Material

The study includes six females and nine males with an age range from 31 to 54 years. Clinical and angiographic data, the type of EIAB, as well as the results and the complications of surgery are presented in Table 1. Ten patients revealed clinically neurologic deficits of a minor completed stroke (CS) as a sign of circulatory insufficiency in the cerebellum and/or the brain stem. Four patients presented with a history of several typical transient ischemic attacks (TIAs) of the vertebrobasilar system. Angiographic studies revealed in all cases an obstructive lesion of one or both vertebral arteries. Seven patients presented with unilateral occlusion, four with unilateral, distally localized or long stretched stenoses, and the remaining four with a bilateral obstructive lesion. In 11 cases an OA to PICA anastomosis was performed. In the remaining four patients the EIAB procedure was a direct anastomosis between the OA and the intra- or extradural parts of the VA. Because of the small caliber of the OA in two of these cases, a vein interposition graft was used. In another two cases an additional thromboendarterectomy of the VA at the C-1 level was performed.

Advances in Neurosurgery, Vol. 13
Edited by H. Dietz, M. Brock, and M. Klinger

Table 1. Clinical data and results after EIAB in 15 patients with VBI

Case	Patient, sex, age	Clinical symptoms	Vascular pathology	EIAB	Bypass patent	Complications	Clinical results
1	SA, M, 44 y.	CS	VA-S (L) ICA-O (L)	OA-PICA (L)	Yes	Trans. ataxia Flap necrosis	Good
2	JE, M, 50 y.	TIA	VA-O (R)	OA-PICA (L)	-	Pulm. embolism	Died
3	SK, M, 42 y.	CS	VA-O (L)	OA-PICA (R)	Yes	None	Excellent
4	TG, F, 31 y.	CS	VA-O (L)	OA-VA (L)	Yes	None	Excellent
5	BM, M, 52 y.	CS	VA-O (L)	OA-PICA (L)	Yes	Flap necrosis	Excellent
6	SE, M, 49 y.	CS	VA-O (R/L)	OA-PICA (L)	Yes	None	Excellent
7	SJ, M, 47 y.	CS	VA-S (R/L)	OA-PICA (L)	No	None	Unchanged
8	DA, M, 53 y.	TIA	VA-S (L) ICA-O (R)	OA-PICA (R) STA-MCA (R)	Yes Yes	None None	Excellent
9	HB, F, 51 y.	TIA	VA-O (L) VA-S (R)	OA-PICA (L)	No	CSF collection	Unchanged
10	SW, M, 50 y.	CS	VA-O (R) VA-S (L)	OA-VA (R)	Yes	Trans. ataxia	Excellent
11	KW, F, 36 y.	CS	VA-S (L)	OA-VA (L)	Yes	None	Excellent
12	FR, F, 54 y.	TIA	VA-O (R)	OA-PICA (L)	Yes	None	Unchanged
13	KR, M, 39 y.	TIA	VA-O (R)	OA-PICA (R)	No	None	Good
14	SJ, M, 50 y.	CS	VA-S (L)	OA-VA (L)	-	None	Unchanged
15	KJ, M, 52 y.	CS	VA-O (L)	OA-PICA (L)	-	None	Excellent

EIAB, extra-intracranial arterial bypass; VBI, vertebrobasilar insufficiency; CS, completed stroke; TIA, transient ischemic attacks; VA, vertebral artery; PICA, posterior inferior cerebellar artery; ICA, internal carotid artery; MCA, middle cerebral artery; STA, superficial temporal artery; S, stenosis; O, occlusion; CSF, cerebrospinal fluid

Operative Technique

The first ten cases were operated on using the "hockey stick" skin incision as initially described by AUSMAN et al. (1) (Fig. 1). For the last five cases, however, a modified approach was adopted, using a paramedian "arch"-shaped skin incision. This modification was used in order to avoid an accumulation of cerebrospinal fluid (CSF) and also to decrease the risk of necrotic skin lesions in the flap area. In addition, using the paramedian approach to the OA, which allows an antegrade preparation of the vessel by maintaining the blood flow until just before starting the anastomosis, an increase of the patency rate of the donor artery was expected (Fig. 2). Surgery was performed in 12 of the 15 patients by using the sitting position, whereas in the remaining three the lying prone position was used.

Results

Postoperative angiographic studies were performed in 12 patients. With three exceptions (cases 7, 9, and 13) the angiograms revealed a patent bypass. Additionally, a severe stenotic lesion of the VA (case 11) could not be identified after a thromboendarterectomy had been performed.

Postoperative complications were encountered in five patients. One of them (case 2) died from a massive pulmonary embolism on the first postoperative day, just after he was remobilized. Other complications included transient ataxia in two patients (cases 1 and 10) and a minor flap necrosis in another two (cases 1 and 5). Another patient (case 9) developed a persistent accumulation of CSF under the flap, requiring lumboperitoneal shunt treatment. Clinical results were excellent in eight patients. In none of these cases were new attacks of VBI seen during a postoperative period ranging from one month to four years. In two patients (cases 1 and 12) presenting with multifocal cerebral obstructive vessel disease, however, further attacks of VBI were noted although control angiograms had shown a patent bypass. The clinical results were unchanged in another two patients (cases 7 and 9) in whom bypass patency could not be demonstrated postoperatively, as well as in another patient (14) in whom the control angiogram had not yet been performed. The clinical result was finally good in another patient (case 13) although control angiograms had not shown a patent bypass.

Case Report

A 50-year-old man (case 10) was admitted to the hospital because of a history of multiple minor strokes of the posterior circulation with dizziness, double vision, slurred speech, swallowing disturbances, and cerebellar ataxia. Cerebral angiography revealed distally localized obstructive lesions of both VAs, with occlusion of the right VA and stenosis of the left. Because conservative treatment with aspirin as well as blood pressure monitoring did not influence the rate of his VBI attacks, the indication for brain revascularization surgery to the posterior circulation was given. The patient underwent a right OA to VA anastomosis in the sitting position. Because of the small caliber of the OA, a vein interposition was used. The postoperative follow-up was without major complications, and since then no further attacks of VBI have been reported. In addition, preoperative residual symptoms such as discrete ataxia and dizziness completely disappeared. Postoperative control angiography revealed a patent bypass with excellent filling of the vertebrobasilar system via the donor vessel (Fig. 3).

Discussion

The diagnosis of VBI is based primarily on clinical findings and angiographic results. Blood flow measurements which can be used for the study of cerebral ischemia are less reliable, mainly because of methodological difficulties, for the investigation of cerebellar or brain stem ischemia. In the present series, therefore, only those patients were selected for revascularization procedures who had either a history of multiple reversible VBI attacks or symptoms attributable to posterior circulation ischemia. In contrast to standard superficial temporal artery to middle cerebral artery bypass surgery, which is predominantly used as a prophylactic procedure in patients with reversible symptoms of cerebral ischemia, the majority of patients in this group had completed strokes of varying degrees. In accordance with anatomical and angiographic studies by CASTAIGNE et al. (6) as well as CAPLAN and ROSENBAUM (4) concerning the pathogenesis of VBI, only those patients were included who had hemodynamically significant occlusive or stenotic lesions of the vertebrobasilar system. All patients had arterial lesions localized distally to the neck collaterals of the VA. Additionally, surgery was performed in patients who had further attacks of VBI in spite of a course of conservative treatment with aspirin.

Although one patient died during the first postoperative day, typical complications due to the sitting position such as orthostatic or air embolism-induced hypotensive brain stem stroke, as described by others (7), were not observed in our group of patients. In contrast to OA to the anterior inferior cerebellar artery bypass for treatment of VBI due to obstructive disease of the proximal basilar artery (which was, without exception, performed using the lying position), we preferred the sitting position for bypass surgery to the PICA or the VA.

Although the number of operated cases in which the paramedian "arch"-shaped skin incision was used is too small for a definitive comparison with the standard "hockey stick" flap, we feel that this approach presents certain advantages: In none of the operated patients was skin necrosis or accumulation of CSF under the flap observed. Moreover, the preparation time of the OA could be reduced substantially. However, whether the patency rate of the anastomotic vessels has been increased by using this technique remains to be evaluated.

Although it is too early to assume a definitive therapeutic effect of brain revascularization surgery to the posterior circulation in patients with VBI, our results as well as those reported in the literature are acceptable if compared with the natural history of the disease (5).

References

1. Ausman, J.I., Lee, M.C., Klassen, A.C., Seljeskog, E.L., Chou, S.N.: What's new? Cerebral revascularization. Minn. Med. 58, 223-227 (1976)
2. Ausman, J.I., Diaz, F.G., de los Reyes, R.A., Pak, H., Patel, S., Boulos, R.: Superficial temporal to proximal superior cerebellar artery anastomosis for basilar artery stenosis. Neurosurg. 9, 56-60 (1981)
3. Ausman, J.I., Diaz, F.G., de los Reyes, R.A., Pak, H., Patel, S., Boulos, R.: Anastomosis of occipital artery to anterior inferior cerebellar artery for vertebrobasilar junction stenosis. Surg. Neurol. 16, 99-102 (1981)

4. Caplan, L.R., Rosenbaum, A.E.: Role of cerebral angiography in vertebrobasilar occlusive disease. J. Neurol. Neurosurg. Psychiatry 38, 601-612 (1975)

5. Cartlidge, N.E.F., Whisnant, J.P., Elveback, L.R.: Carotid and vertebral-basilar transient ischemic attacks. A community study. Rochester, Minnesota. Mayo Clin. Proc. 52, 117-120 (1977)

6. Castaigne, P., Lhermitte, F., Gautier, J.C., Escourolle, R., Deouresne, C., Agopian, P.D., Popa, C.: Arterial occlusions in the vertebrobasilar system. A study of 44 patients with post-mortem data. Brain 96, 133-154 (1973)

7. Khodadad, G.: Short- and long-term results of microvascular anastomosis in the vertebrobasilar system. A critical analysis. Neurol. Res. 3, 33-35 (1981)

8. Olteanu-Nerbe, V., Schmiedek, P., Marguth, F.: Die A. occipitalis-A. cerebellaris inferior posterior-Anastomose zur Behandlung der vertebrobasilären Insuffizienz. Akt. Neurol. 10, 203-207 (1983)

9. Roski, R.A., Spetzler, R.F., Hopkins, L.N.: Occipital artery to posterior inferior cerebellar artery bypass for vertebrobasilar ischemia. Neurosurg. 10, 44-48 (1982)

10. Sundt, T.M. Jr, Piepgras, D.G.: Occipital to posterior inferior cerebellar artery bypass surgery. J. Neurosurg. 48, 916-928 (1978)

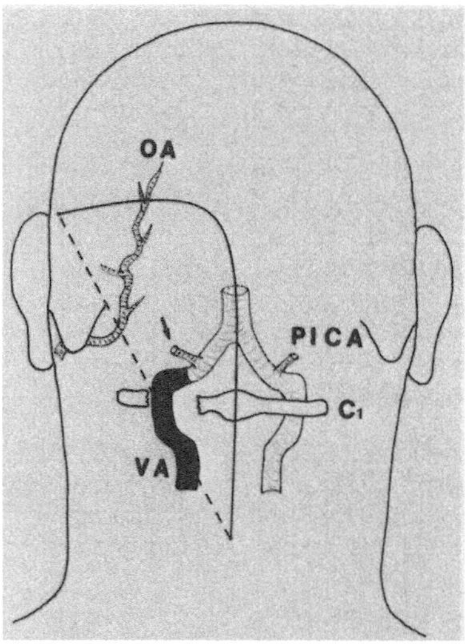

Fig. 1

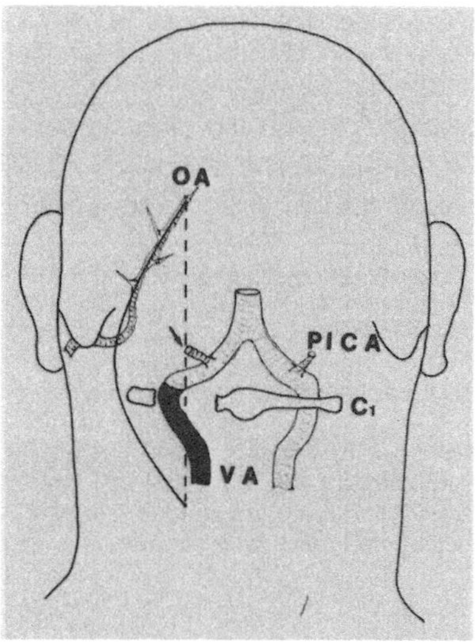

Fig. 2

Fig. 1. Operative technique for OA-PICA anastomosis; median approach

Fig. 2. Operative technique for OA-PICA anastomosis; lateral approach

a

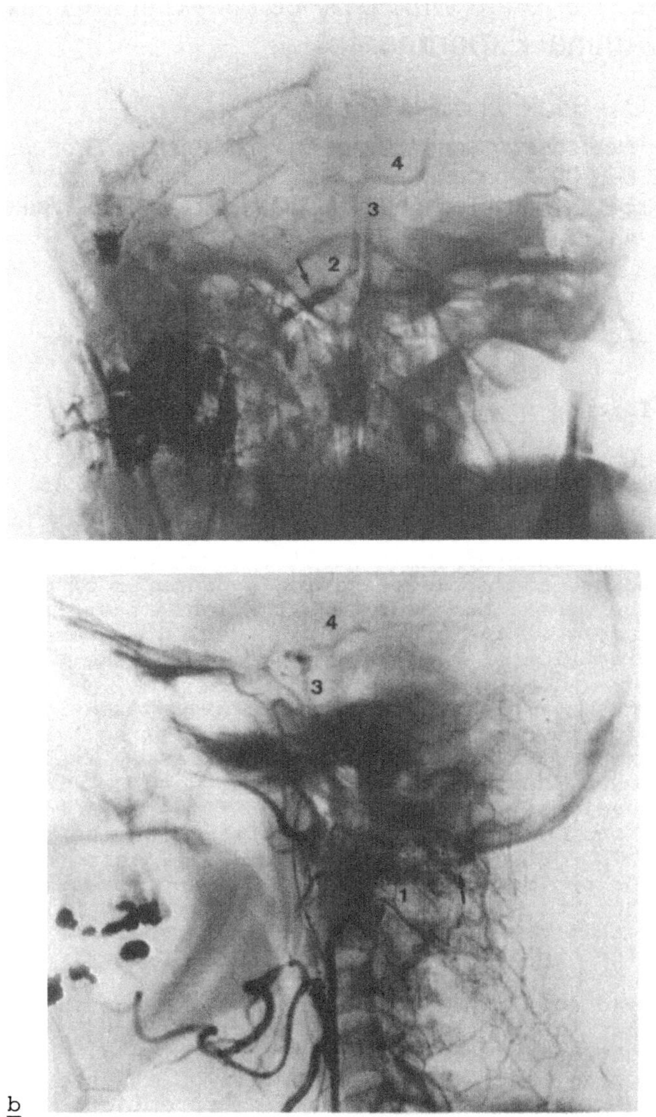

b

Fig. 3a,b. Case report. 50-year-old patient with VBI due to an occlusion of the right and a stenosis of the left VA at the C-1 level. Control angiograms by selective catheterization of the OA after right OA-VA anastomosis, by using a vein interponate *(arrow)*, show a good filling of the vertebrobasilar system via the donor vessel. a Frontal view; b lateral view. *1*, OA; *2*, VA; *3*, basilar artery; *4*, posterior cerebral artery

Experience with CO_2-Laser-Assisted Anastomosis in Animal Experiments

O. J. Beck[1] and J. R. Morris[2]

[1] Neurochirurgische Universitätsklinik, Klinikum Großhadern, Marchioninistraße 15, D-8000 München 70

[2] Bio Quantum Technologies, 4543 Post Oak Place, Suite 114, Houston, TX 77027, USA

Introduction

Comparative observations of longitudinal sections performed with the CO_2 and Nd-YAG lasers on lumbar vessels of the rat (1) have demonstrated the smaller necrotizing zone of the CO_2 laser. Thus following complete coagulation with the CO_2 laser, veins having a diameter of 1 mm achieved their initial lumen with full patency after several weeks, and arteries having a diameter of 0.3 mm recanalized in 50% of the cases. Follow-up examinations after treatment with the Nd-YAG laser, on the other hand, revealed successive transformation and degradation of vascular connective tissue.

Thus by selecting a suitable beam geometry and exposure time, the possibility presented itself of utilizing the smaller necrotizing zone of the CO_2 laser to produce an extremely shallow, superficial coagulation zone. The necessary conditions were met in the low-power CO_2 laser developed by MORRIS and NEBLETT (4). In terms of its outside dimensions, operation, compatibility with the operation microscope, and power output range of 0.01-1 Watt, this laser is specially designed for performing microsurgical anastomoses.

Our initial goal is not sutureless microvascular anastomosis as practiced by JAIN (3) with the Nd-YAG laser, which is time consuming and not yet reliably reproducible. The aim of our efforts is, rather, to lend support to conventional microvascular anastomosis, thus making fewer sutures necessary. In concrete terms, only three conventional sutures are needed for a vessel with a 1 mm diameter and four sutures for, an end-to-side anastomosis of a vessel having the same diameter (Fig. 1). Moving the beam in appropriate sinuous movements, it is possible to fuse the coapted severed vessel walls in a matter of seconds using a power level of about 0.1 Watt (Fig. 2),

Materials and Methods

NEBLETT and co-workers (4) compared conventional microvascular suture anastomosis (CMSA) with laser-assisted microvascular anastomosis (LAMA) on adult male Sprague-Dawley rats weighing 250-300 g. To this end the right femoral artery was severed and provided with conventional microvascular sutures. With the right femoral artery the vessel wall between two or three conventional sutures was fused with the help of the new laser (Fig. 2).

Advances in Neurosurgery, Vol. 13
Edited by H. Dietz, M. Brock, and M. Klinger

Results

The animals were sacrificed at various postoperative intervals, upon which the arteries were excised and examined histologically. Figure 3 shows that the severed ends of the media are fused without loss of the structural integrity of the elastin scaffolding. The thermally altered collagen of the adventitia forms a brown to black zone of necrosis which is readily distinguishable from the light red of the fibrillar normal collagen. Three days post-LAMA, fibrin-filled anastomotic gaps and adventitial plugs are evident. As compared to CMSA, a marked reduction in tissue reaction is apparent. Five weeks after the operation the difference is even more striking.

As shown by electron microscopy, the suture area is completely covered by endothelium three weeks post-LAMA. After six weeks the conventional microvascular suture is thinly covered by endothelium, but a considerable difference is seen in the vascular wall thickness at the anastomotic site as compared with the laser-assisted bypass. The tensile strength of the LAMA was tested by COLEN et al. (2) after disarticulation of the hip joint. The values determined were the same as, or only marginally poorer than, those for CMSA. All LAMAs were completely functional.

Discussion and Conclusion

The advantage of this new technique is that the time needed to perform a bypass operation is reduced by more than half. Thus, with the temporary clamps in position for a shorter period, the ischemia time can be correspondingly shortened. In the future all surgeons should be able to perform their bypass operations themselves after a short period of training. As an example, I would like to cite my first LAMA performed last year on the femoral artery of the rat, pointing out that I am no anastomosis expert. KEIDITSCH, chief physician of the Pathology Department of the Bogenhausen Clinic in Munich, was able to verify the complete patency of the bypass three weeks postoperatively and, like NEBLETT et al. (4), found complete endothelial healing. After a three-day period of anastomosis training in Houston, I had no difficulty in performing three end-to-end and three end-to-side anastomoses, including arteriovenous shunts, on rat carotid and femoral vessels within just a few hours. Like NEBLETT et al. (4), we were also able to show unimpaired functioning of the bypass after LAMA.

Finally, I should like to mention that we have anastomosed not only vessels with the new laser, but also nerves. The precise fusion of the perineurium can be achieved with a power output of about 0.06 Watt. Of course, the results require an extended verification period. The low-power CO_2 laser will not restrict the indications for the Nd-YAG laser and the conventional CO_2 laser in tumor surgery, but will open up a new field of anastomosis.

In the reconstruction of traumatized vessels, in the shrinkage of aneurysms - and perhaps also in the surgical removal of brainstem tumors - the low-power CO_2 laser holds promise as a valuable new tool in the surgeon's armamentarium.

References

1. Beck, O.J.: Comparative studies on the use of lasers in neurosurgery. MBB-AT, Munich, information 4/81
2. Colen, L.B., Gonzales, G.P., Buncke, H.: The relationship between the number of sutures and the strength of microvascular anastomoses. Plastic and Reconstructive Surgery, p. 325, September 1979
3. Jain, K.K.: Sutureless microvascular anastomosis using a Nd-YAG laser. J. Microsurg. 1, 436-439 (1980)
4. Neblett, C., Morris, J.R., Withers, M.D.: A study of CO_2 laser assisted microsurgical anastomosis of small vessels. 7th European Congress of Neurosurgery, Brussels, Belgium, August 28 - September 3, 1983

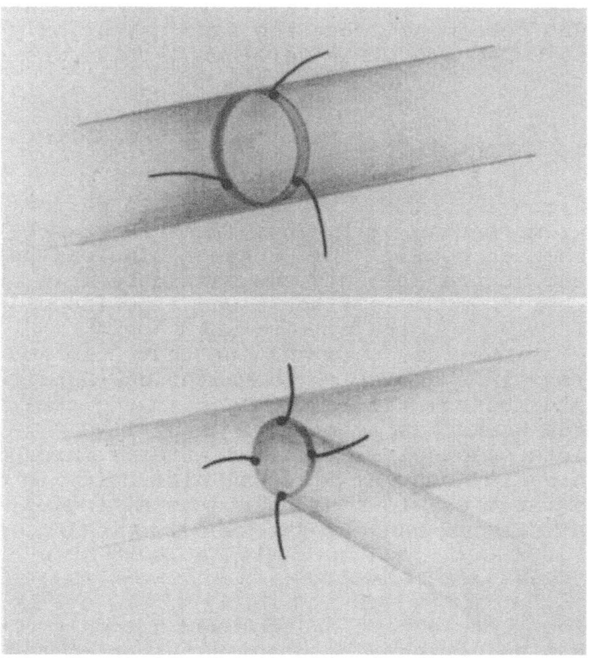

Fig. 1. *Top:* End-to-end anastomosis with three stay sutures at an angle of 120° to each other. *Bottom:* End-to-side anastomosis with four stay sutures at an angle of 90° to each other

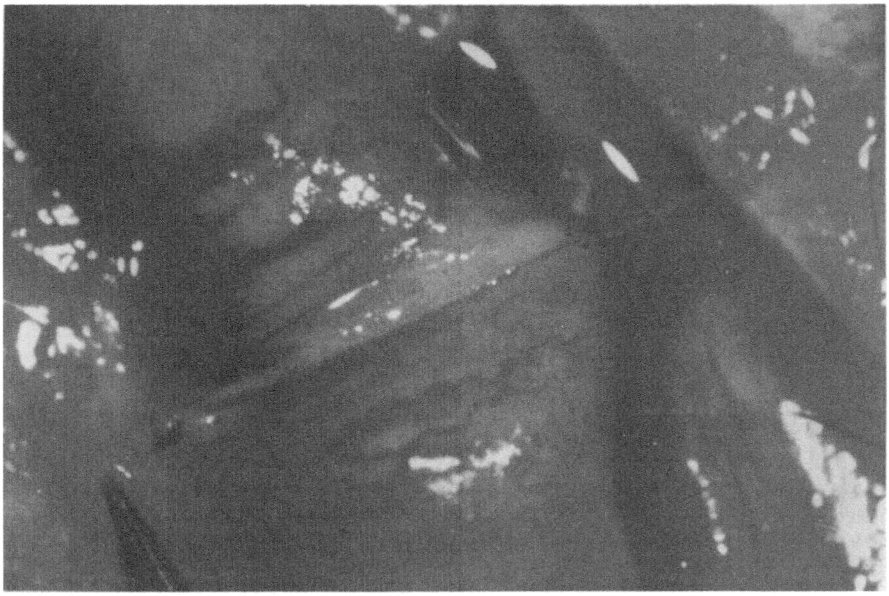

Fig. 2. Following low-power CO_2-laser exposure, the severed vessel ends are fused together between two conventional stay sutures

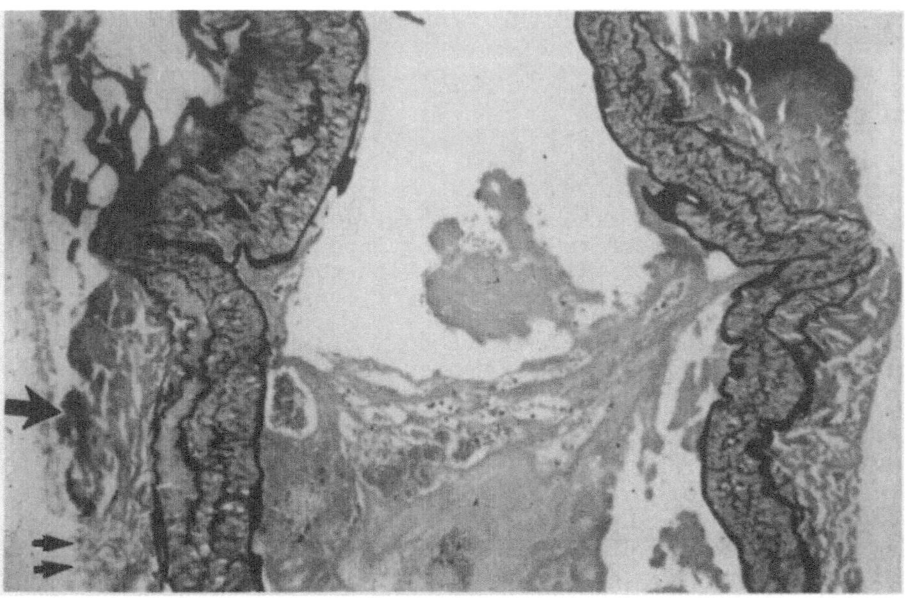

Fig. 3. Primary bond as seen immediately after LAMA. The severed ends of the media are fused without loss of the structural integrity of the elastin scaffolding. The thermally altered collagen of the adventitia *(single arrow)* forms a homogeneous black coagulum as compared with the light red, fibrillar normal collagen *(double arrows)*. (Orig. mag. 100×, Wiegert-van-Geison's stain)

Microsurgical Vascular Anastomoses with Resorbable Suture Material

R. Firsching[1], P. D. Terhaag[1], and W. Müller[2]

[1] Neurochirurgische Universitätsklinik Köln, [2] Pathologisches Institut der Universität Köln, Josef-Stelzmann-Straße 9, D-5000 Köln 41

Introduction

In spite of 20 years of experience with reconstructive surgery of vessels smaller than 2 mm in diameter, microsurgical anastomosis remains a time-consuming procedure. The purpose of this report is to compare the commonly used interrupted suture technique with the time-saving continuous suture technique. Since the continuous suture can only dilate when resorbable suture material is used, resorbable Polyglactin is compared with non-resorbable nylon. Two hundred and ninety-eight end-to-end and end-to-side anastomoses were performed on the carotid arteries of rabbits and rats. Evaluation of the anastomoses was done by measuring the flow rate electromagnetically 1 h and 1-3 months postoperatively.

Twenty end-to-end anastomoses with nylon and 20 with Polyglactin were examined histologically.

Materials and Method

End-to-End Anastomoses (see Fig. 1)

1. Only one carotid artery in each of 40 rabbits and rats was divided. Anastomoses were performed with the interrupted suture technique using nylon. The flow rate was compared with that of the non-operated carotid artery.

2. In 10 rats one artery was cut at a right angle, the other artery at an oblique angle. Anastomoses on each side were performed with the interrupted suture technique using nylon.

3. On 156 arteries anastomoses were performed either with the interrupted or with the simple continuous suture technique using nylon. The outer diameter of the vessels varied from 0.5 mm to 2.0 mm.

4. In 20 rats the interrupted suture technique was used with nylon on one side, while on the other side a locked continuous suture technique was carried out with Polyglactin.

End-to-Side Anastomoses (see Fig. 2)

1. Ninety anastomoses were performed with either a 45°, a 90°, or a 135° angle between the donor and the recipient vessel. The interrupted

Advances in Neurosurgery, Vol. 13
Edited by H. Dietz, M. Brock, and M. Klinger

suture technique with nylon was applied. The outer diameter of the vessels ranged from 0.7 mm to 2.0 mm.

2. At a consistent angle of 45°, 15 anastomoses with the interrupted suture technique were compared with 15 with the locked continuous suture technique. For all 30 sutures Polyglactin was used. Outer vessel diameter ranged from 1.0 mm to 1.4 mm.

Results

End-to-End Anastomoses (see Fig. 1)

1. The interrupted suture technique did not reduce the flow rate as compared with non-operated vessels. The patency rate was 80% for vessels smaller than 0.5 mm, and 100% for vessels wider than 0.5 mm.

2. Patency rate and flow rate were the same, no matter whether the artery had been divided at a right or at an oblique angle.

3. The smaller the diameter, the lower the patency rate and flow rate of the simple continuous suture technique as compared with the interrupted suture technique. At 0.5 mm outer diameter, the patency rate of the continuous suture was 0% as compared against 80% with the interrupted suture technique.

4. With a patency rate of 100% and equal flow rates, the locked continuous suture anastomosis had the same results as the interrupted suture technique.

End-to-Side Anastomoses (see Fig. 2)

1. The patency rate was 100% for the 90 anastomoses. One hour postoperatively, the greater the angle, the lower the flow rate of the donor vessel as compared with the recipient vessel. Between one and three months later, this difference had decreased. Macroscopically the 90° and 135° angle was reduced to 45° preferentially in the younger rats.

2. The locked continuous suture technique was clearly inferior in end-to-side anastomoses, with a patency rate of 50% as compared with 100% with the interrupted suture technique.

Histology of Resorbable and Non-resorbable Suture Material

Between one and three months postoperatively, the resorbable Polyglactin thread was no longer detectable, while the nylon thread showed signs of a foreign body reaction (Fig. 3). On the other hand, Polyglactin is somewhat more difficult to handle because the thread is stiffer.

Discussion

Various suggestions have been made about suture technique and suture material in microsurgical end-to-end and end-to-side anastomoses (1-9).

With the *end-to-end* anastomoses our findings were that an oblique suture had no advantages over a right angle suture. The simple continuous suture was inferior to the commonly used interrupted suture, while the locked continuous suture was equivalent to the latter, having a comparable patency rate and equal flow rates. The difficulty consists in avoiding narrowing at the anastomotic site with the final knot. Some stricture is inevitable with the simple continuous suture to prevent leakage. The smaller the vessel, however, the more serious the effect on the inner diameter of the anastomosis. With the locked continuous suture the final knot cannot cause narrowing of the entire suture. Its inadequacy in the *end-to-side* anastomoses can be attributed to the difficulty of keeping a consistent tension of stay sutures while repairing the back wall. This problem is not relevant with the end-to-end anastomoses, as a suture holding frame could be used.

The angle of the end-to-side anastomoses did not have a major effect on the flow rate.

Conclusion

While the locked continuous suture technique showed good results in microsurgical end-to-end anastomoses, the interrupted suture technique was superior in end-to-side anastomoses. Non-resorbable nylon was easier to handle, but the long-term histocompatibility of resorbable Polyglactin was better.

References

1. Chase, M.D., Schwartz, S.I.: Consistent patency of 1.5 mm arterial anastomosis. Surg. Forum 13, 220-222 (1962)
2. Cobbett, J.R.: Microvascular surgery. Surg. Clin. N. Am. 47(2), 521-542 (1962)
3. Duspiva, W., Ippisch, A., Wriedt-Lübbe, I., Blümel, G.: Mikrochirurgische Nerven- und Gefäßnähte mit resorbierbarem Nahtmaterial. Zentralbl. Chir. 107(7), 392-399 (1982)
4. Hamilton, R.B., O'Brian, B.: An experimental study of microvascular patency using a continuous suture technique. Br. J. Plast. Surg. 32, 153-154 (1979)
5. Harashina, T.: Use of a continuous suture for back wall repair of end-to-end or end-to-side anastomoses. Plast. Reconstr. Surg. (69) 1, 139-144 (1982)
6. Lee, B.Y., Thoden, W.R., Brancato, R.F., Kavner, D., Shaw, W., Madden, J.L.: Comparison of continuous and interrupted suture techniques in microvascular anastomosis. Surg. Gynecol. Obstet. 155(3), 353-357 (1982)
7. Man, D., Acland, D.: Continuous-suture technique in microvascular end-to-end anastomosis. J. Microsurg. 2, 238-243 (1981)
8. Thiede, A., Lütjohann, K., Beck. C., Blunck, F.: Absorbable and non-absorbable sutures in microsurgery: standardized comparable studies in rats. J. Microsurg. 1, 216-222 (1979)
9. Yasargil, M.G.: Suturing techniques. In: Yasargil, M.G. (ed.) Microsurgery applied to neurosurgery. pp. 60-81, Stuttgart, Thieme 1969

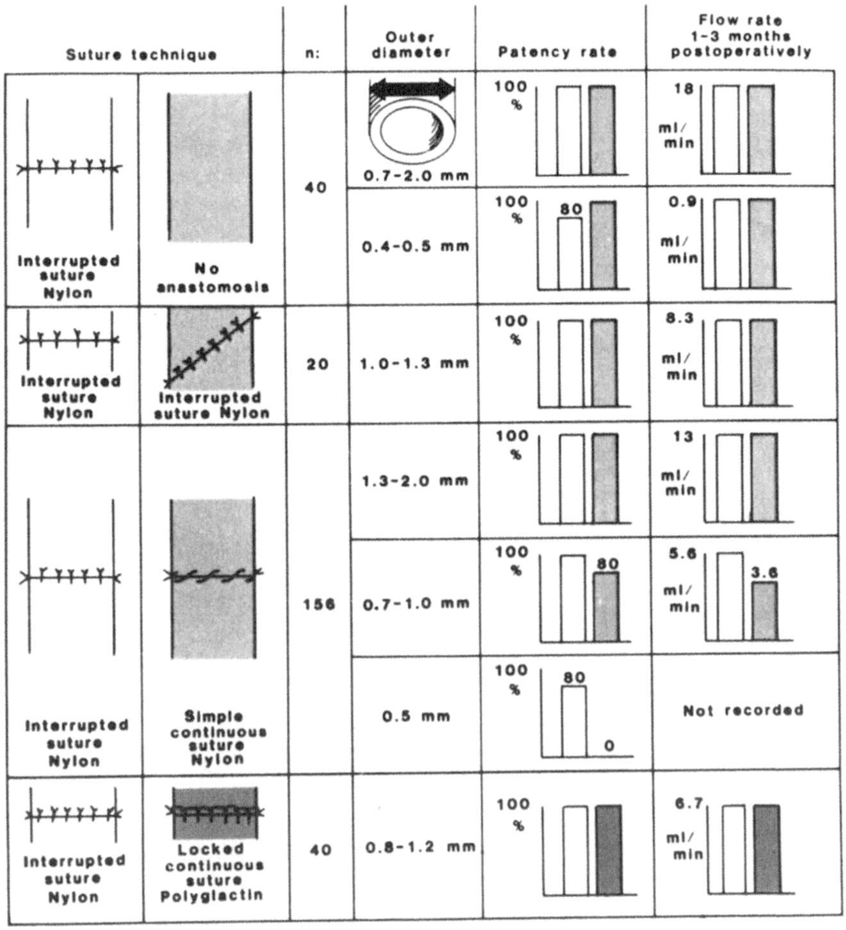

Fig. 1. Experimental end-to-end anastomoses

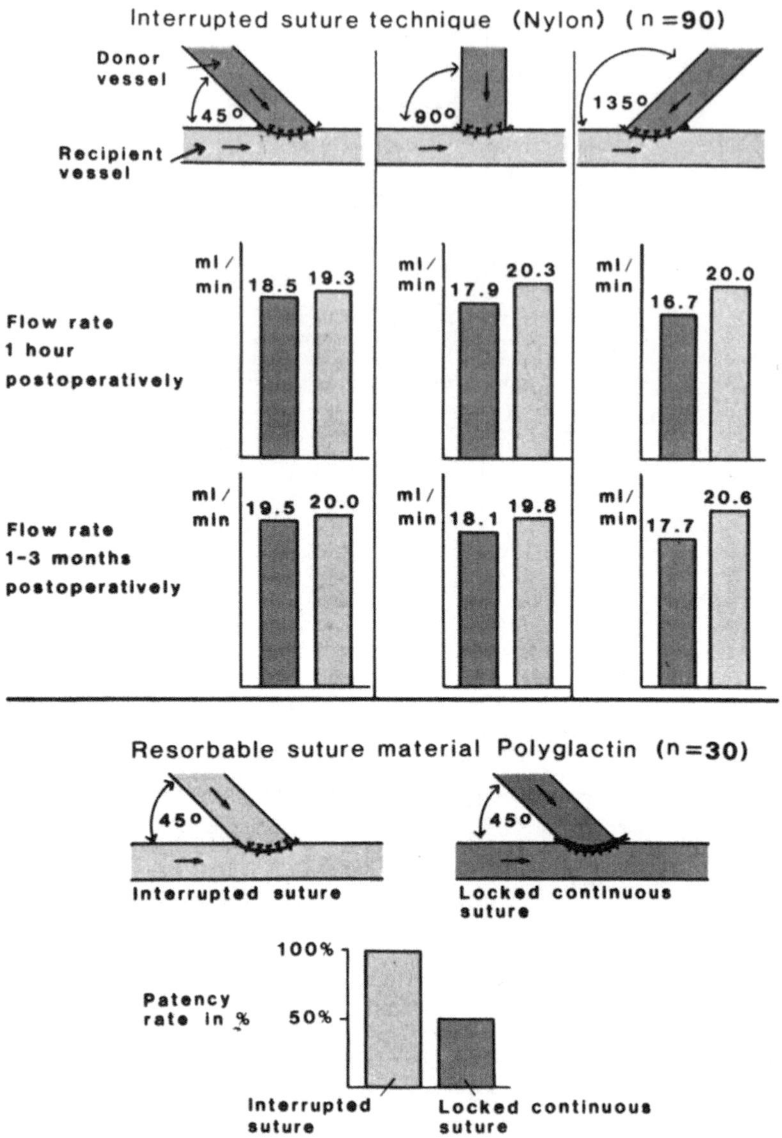

Fig. 2. Experimental end-to-side anastomoses

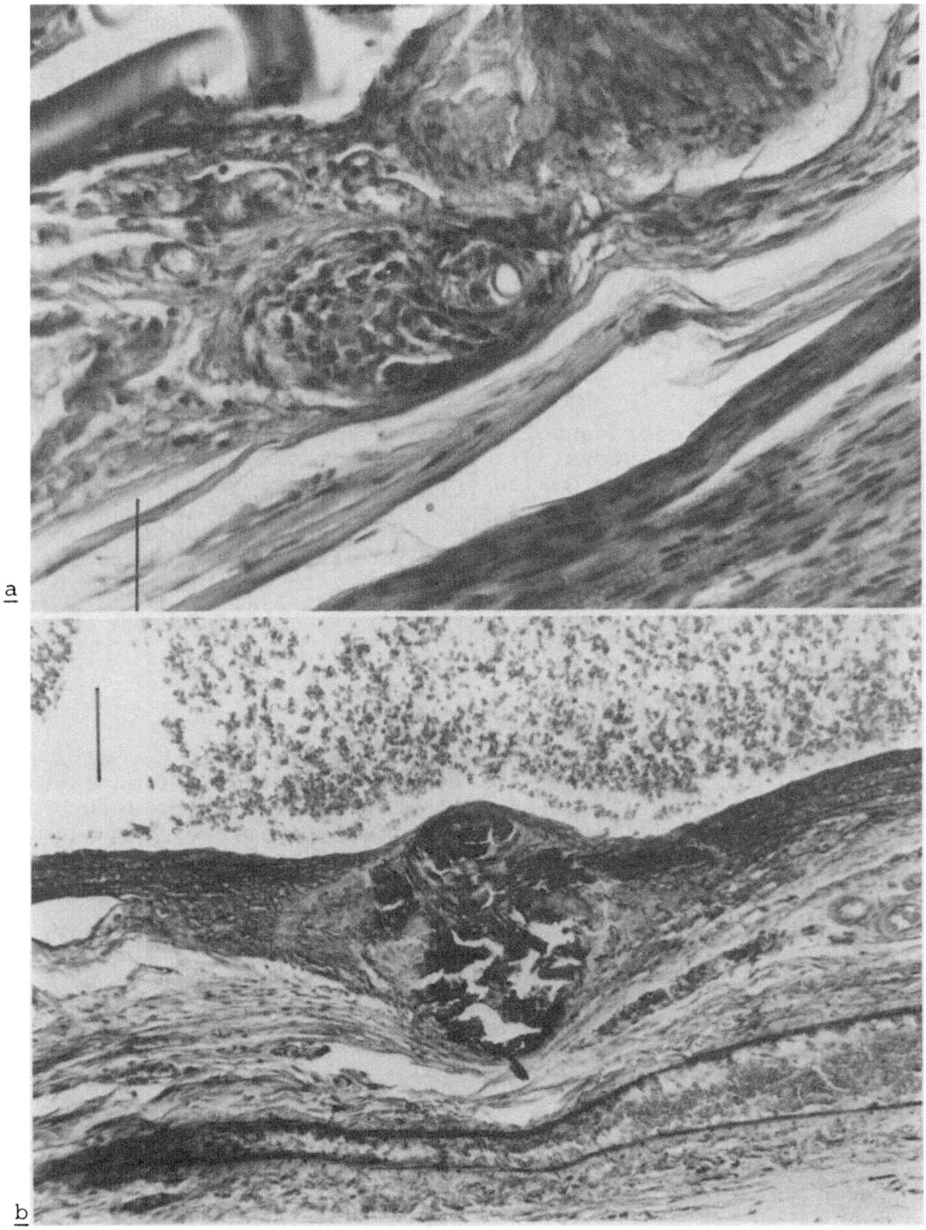

Fig. 3. a Non-resorbable nylon causing some granulomatous reaction (*bar* = 50 μm). b Resorbable Polyglactin cannot be traced. No granulomatous tissue (*bar* = 100 μm)

Microvascular End-to-Side Anastomoses: The Double Patch Technique

A. Harders and J. Gilsbach

Neurochirurgische Universitätsklinik, Klinikum der Albert-Ludwigs-Universität, Hugstetter Straße 55, D-7800 Freiburg

Introduction

The quality of a microvascular end-to-side anastomosis depends mainly on the area of the suture (4). Enlarging methods are thus used, e.g., an obliquely cut (6) or a fish mouth-like incised side branch (5). However, if a donor artery is sutured obliquely on a recipient vessel, the hemodynamic conditions on the acute angle of the anastomosis are not ideal, especially if there is flow division. We therefore developed a technique which produces a wide and smooth area from the donor artery in both recipient branches, similar to the T-anastomosis (3) but without using a pre-existing bifurcation.

Materials and Methods

The rat model that we used was originally described by Collice et al. in 1977 (1) to simulate the hemodynamic conditions of an intra-extracranial bypass with a bilateral flow in the recipient artery (Figs. 1, 3, 4). The hemodynamics in the different parts of the anastomosis were measured intraoperatively by a microvascular Doppler system (2) about 20 min after the temporary clips had been released.

The operative technique is quite simple: The recipient artery is incised longitudinally (length 6 times the diameter of the donor artery) with short transverse cuts at the end of the incision. Both walls of the donor artery are then cut longitudinally (3 times the diameter). The anastomosis is completed as shown in Fig. 2.

Results

Compared with the classic patch anastomosis, the double patch variation showed a higher total flow, less acceleration in the region of the acute angle of the anastomosis, and nearly no disturbances of the laminar flow in the region of the anastomosis (Fig. 4).

Discussion and Conclusions

The patch anastomosis is conducive to end-to-side anastomoses with a lateral side branch which receives a part of the mainstream (2, 4, 5). However, in cases of a total division of the donor artery flow in a bilateral recipient artery flow – such as in extra-intracranial bypass – a patch anastomosis leaves a critical transition zone in the anastomosis. This is the acute angled part which may be a source of stenoses

Advances in Neurosurgery, Vol. 13
Edited by H. Dietz, M. Brock, and M. Klinger

and flow irregularities. For this flow type, the double patch proves to be a better method, since it offers a smooth transition in both directions.

References

1. Collice, E.M., Fornari, M., Porta, M.: End-to-side anastomosis between carotid arteries and serial angiographic controls in rats. In: Schmiedek, P. (ed.) Microsurgery for stroke, pp. 159-162. Springer, Berlin Heidelberg New York 1977

2. Gilsbach, J.: Intraoperative Doppler sonography in neurosurgery. Springer, Wien New York 1983

3. Kletter, G.: The extra-intracranial bypass operation for prevention and treatment of stroke. Springer, Wien New York 1979

4. Robertson, J.H., Robertson, J.T.: The relationship between suture number and quality of anastomoses in microvascular procedures. Surg. Neurol. 10, 241-245 (1978)

5. Rosenbaum, T.J., Sundt, T.M.,Jr.: Thrombus formation and endothelial alterations in microarterial anastomoses. J. Neurosurg. 47, 430-441 (1977)

6. Yasargil, M.G.: Microsurgery applied to neurosurgery. Thieme, Stuttgart 1969

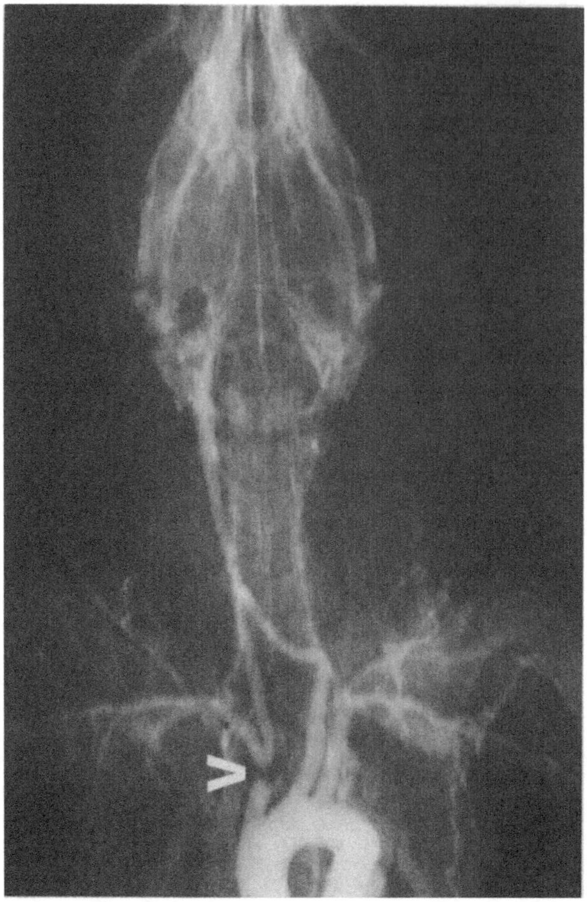

Fig. 1. Animal (rat) model for simulation of the hemodynamics and end-to-side anastomosis for an extra-intracranial bypass. The brachiocephalic trunk is cut *(arrow)* on the right side. The left common carotid artery (donor artery) is sutured to the right (recipient artery), where a bilateral flow distribution occurs: orthograde to the brain and retrograde to the upper extremities

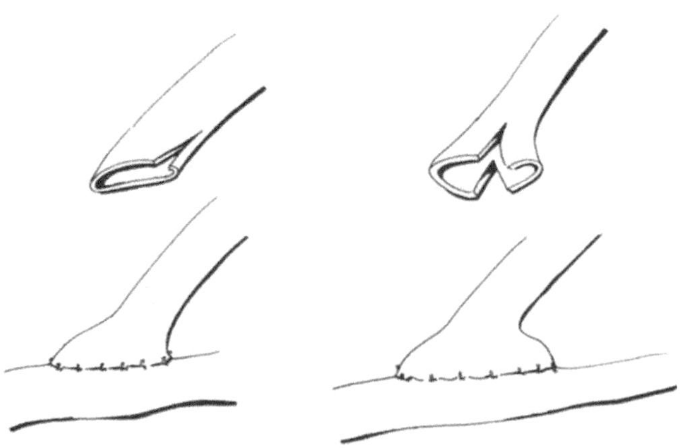

Fig. 2. Type of incision of the donor artery in a patch *(left)* and a double patch *(right)* anastomosis. The recipient vessel is cut longitudinally in both types

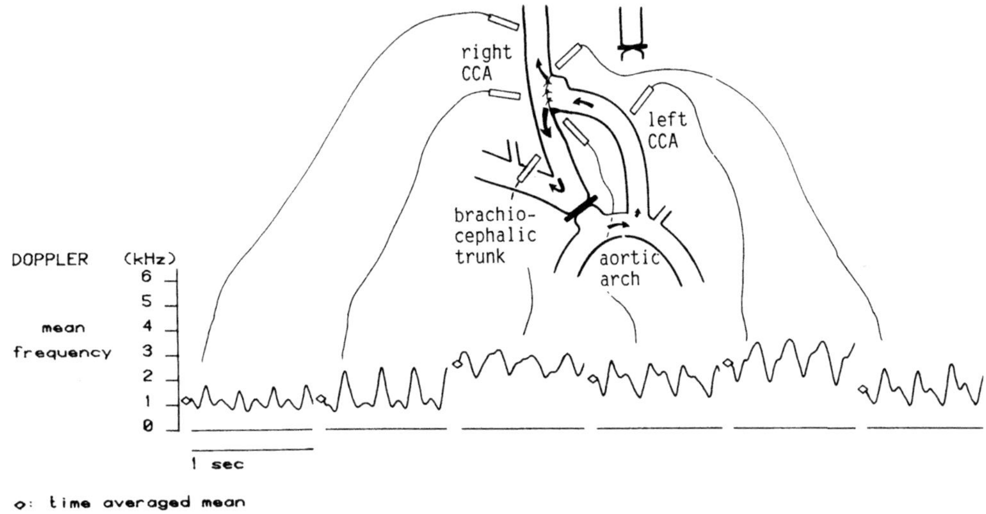

Fig. 3. Doppler flow pattern of a normal patch anastomosis

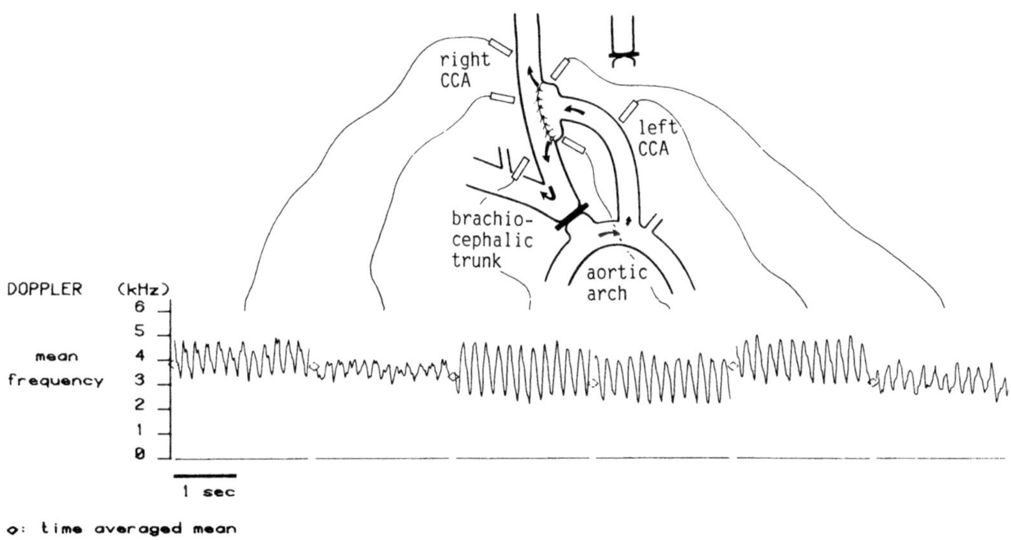

Fig. 4. Doppler flow pattern of a double patch anastomosis

A New Sutureless Microvascular Anastomosis Procedure for Bypass Operations

A. Fantis

Neurochirurgische Abteilung, Niedersächsisches Krankenhaus, Maulbeerallee 2, D-3280 Bad Pyrmont

Six years ago we began using a dense vascular suture method for bypass operations in our hospital. Having standardized the microvascular suture procedure, we tried to reduce the duration of the operation and the amount of suture material employed. In 50 patients with cerebral vascular insufficiency of various degrees, we partially glued the vessels at the anastomosis (1, 3). We preferred a small osteoplastic flap and an intracutaneous suture to minimize ischemia of the tissues.

During the last two years, we have developed an original sutureless gluing method for STA-MCA anastomosis, which may be summarized as follows: In an isolated side branch of the STA, a fine catheter or a mandrin of the Vygon catheter 1.2 mm to 1.8 mm in diameter is introduced and pushed through the main trunk of the STA, approximately 2 mm to 3 mm outwards (Fig. 1a). A small arteriotomy is made on the exposed cortical branch of the MCA and the mandrin further introduced into the lumen to control the caliber of the anastomosing vessels during the gluing procedure (Fig. 1b). The fibrin glue "Tissucoll human Immuno" is used for gluing the anastomosing vessels and furthermore clots with the solution of thrombin, calcium chloride and aprotinin (5), which serves as the local antifibrinolytic factor (Fig. 1c). The margins of the end-to-side attached vessels are only held together with two micropincettes for about 2 min; once the clot forms a solid connection with the anastomosing vessels, the mandrin can be withdrawn from the vessel. The side branch of the STA is used for peroperative angiography if necessary, for a double bypass anastomosis, or is simply clipped. If the proper side branch is not suitable, the mandrin is introduced in the lumen of the STA through the microincision in the vessel wall. The leakage after the arteriotomy is subsequently closed by gluing a small adventitial flap over it.

Postoperatively, the patients receive 500 ml of 10% Rheomacrodex and intravenous Aspisol 1 g for the first two days; afterwards Colfarit and nicotinic acid preparations are administered for about three weeks.

There has been no incidence of complications, such as leakage, thrombosis, or evidence of hematoma formation. No cases of hepatitis have been recorded in our series either.

In the 23 cases in which we have used the above-described method, the entire operative procedure has not taken more than 3-3.5 h and postoperative follow-up has revealed satisfactory results in more than 80% of the patients. Our results display no disadvantages as compared with those achieved in other groups of patients operated on with the classical microvascular suture method. Further possible refinement of the sutureless microvascular anastomosis procedure (2) is currently under investigation.

Advances in Neurosurgery, Vol. 13
Edited by H. Dietz, M. Brock, and M. Klinger

References

1. Fantis, A.: Microvascular bypass operation by means of fibrin gluing method. 7th Europ. Congress of Neurosurgery, Brussels, Abstracts: 268 (1983)
2. Hatanaka, M.: Nonsuture small vessels replacement with vascular prosthesis using microballoon catheter. 7th Europ. Congress of Neurosurgery, Brussels, Abstacts: 309 (1983)
3. Kletter, G., Matras, H., Dinges, H.P.: Zur partiellen Klebung von Mikrogefäßanastomosen im intrakraniellen Bereich. Wr. Klin. Wschr. 90, 415-419 (1978)
4. Rickling, B.: Zur Verwendung humanen Fibrinklebers in der Technik extra-intrakranieller bypass-Operation. Acta chir. Austriaca 1, 10-12 (1981)
5. Schimpf, K.: Fibrinogen, Fibrin und Fibrinkleber. Stuttgart (1980)

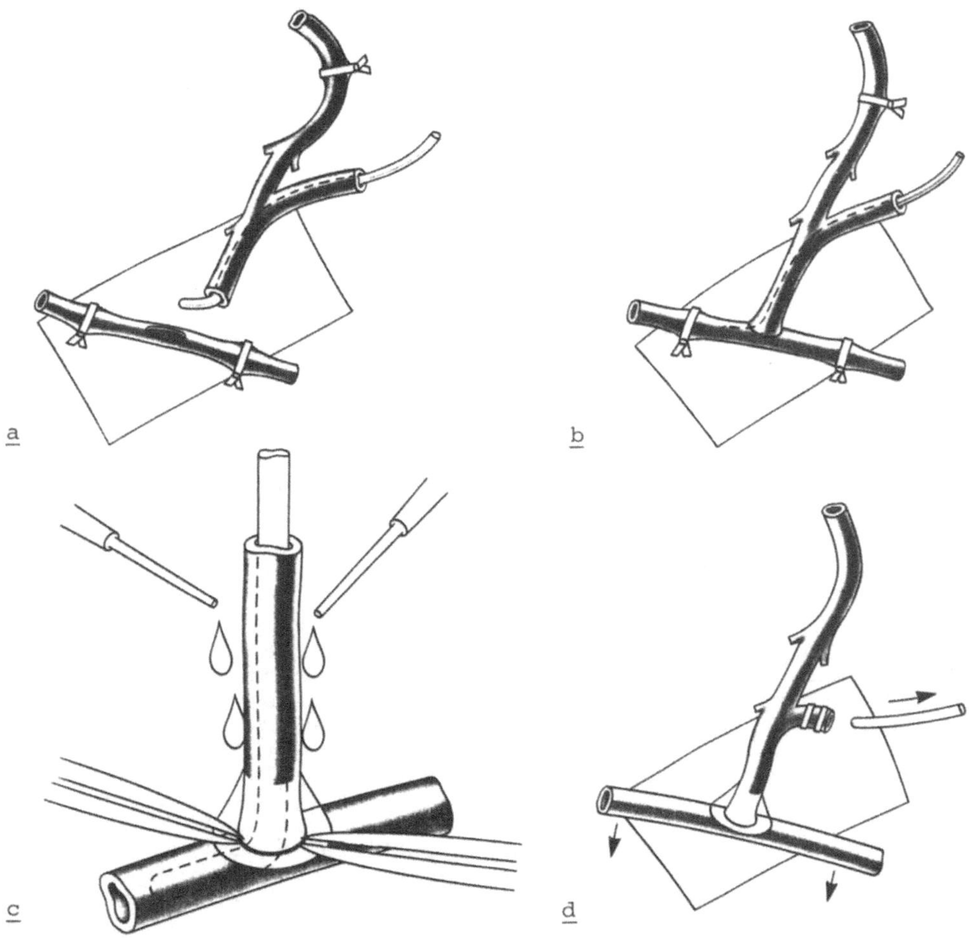

Fig. 1. The sutureless microvascular anastomosis procedure by means of the fibrin gluing method. a Introduction of the mandrin in the STA. b Introduction of the mandrin in the MCA branch. c Gluing of the anastomosing vessels. d Withdrawal of the mandrin and clipping of the side branch

Aneurysm Formation After Suturing or Gluing the Common Carotid Artery in the Rat

H.-U. Thal*

Neurochirurgische Klinik, Medizinische Einrichtungen der Universität Düsseldorf, Moorenstraße 5, D-4000 Düsseldorf

The duration of ischemia in the recipient area during an extra-intracranial arterial bypass operation is a limiting factor, and in order to shorten it, many modifications of the suture line have been suggested (2, 5, 6). In this investigation long-term results with a partial gluing method are compared against those with a modified suture procedure.

Method

In 30 Wistar rats of either sex and weighing 250-400 g, the common carotid artery was cut transversely and repaired microsurgically. In one series, after two holding sutures a modified technique with only six or seven stitches in this 1-mm vessel was performed using 10 × 0 nylon. In another series, the arteries were fixed with two to three stitches and glued with microdrops of human fibrin glue (Tissucol Immuno) (6).

Results

Sixteen vessels were investigated and stained. The mean survival time was two months, ranging from one day up to more than one year. The patency rate in both series was about 85%, this figure including those animals killed early. The histological stages of repair mechanisms[1] as described by KLETTER and MEYERMANN were well seen up to 12 days postoperatively (7).

Depending on their surgical technique involving 8 to 12 stitches, they saw necroses in the anastomosed site more often and more extensively. In the first few days after the operation one sees the glue inside the arteries, trapping the lumen partly or totally (Fig. 1). In the long-term experiments the anastomosed vessels were without exception patent in both groups. The most striking effect in the long surviving animals of both series was aneurysm formation in the suture line. These pseudoaneurysms were found in one-third (three out of eight) of the rats with sutured arteries and in more than half of the animals with glued arteries when they were examined more than four weeks after operation. However, after more than 100 days survival time, all animals developed pseudoaneurysms in the glued series. This aneurysm formation, proven macro- and microphotographically, starts after the first month, with

* The help of Professors Hort and Frenzel and the staff of the Department of Pathology is gratefully acknowledged.

Advances in Neurosurgery, Vol. 13
Edited by H. Dietz, M. Brock, and M. Klinger

a "bulging" of the connective tissue. Despite the rich formation of elastic neomembranes, the bulging develops into large aneurysms up to 5 mm in diameter after three to four months (Figs. 2, 3). At this stage vasa vasorum necroses can also be seen in the wall of the aneurysm, which so far have not led to "aneurysm in the aneurysm" or a rupture (Fig. 4).

Discussion

Only a few investigators have reported true aneurysms and pseudoaneurysms related to STA-MCA anastomoses (3, 4, 9, 10). In one out of 20 rats in which end-to-end laser welding was performed, JAIN described a dilatation after six months which he called aneurysmatic (5). FANTIS operated on 50 patients with a fibrin gluing method without complications (2). KLETTER reported one case of severe bleeding in 375 partially sutured and glued patients (8). STEINBOK investigated two pathological cases with vessel wall abnormalities, and LECLERCQ saw one case of fatal bleeding from a pseudoaneurysm of the donor artery and collected eight more cases out of 411 patients in the literature (11, 10). The development from a tiny "bulging" after one month to a large 5-mm pseudoaneurysm after three to four months is a progression which has been described by SUZUKI for growing aneurysms, and CROMPTON stated that when aneurysms reach 5 mm they are likely to rupture (12, 1).

Conclusion

In conclusion, one has to state that in microsurgical anastomoses of the common carotid artery in the rat using less sutures than usual, pseudoaneurysms occur in more than one-third of the animals if they live long enough, i.e., for more than one or two months. This is related to the surgical technique with only six to seven stitches instead of eight to twelve. A pseudoaneurysm rate of more than 50% in long-term experiments after gluing end-to-end carotid anastomoses tells us not to glue arterial microanastomoses solely but rather to suture at short intervals. At best a sealing of the suture line with human fibrin glue can be helpful.

The death, from a severe hemorrhage in the anastomosed site, of a patient nine days postoperatively who had not been operated on by the author but had received a partially glued STA-MCA bypass, illustrates the pertinence of this warning.

References

1. Crompton, M.R.: Mechanism of growth and rupture in cerebral aneurysms. Br. Med. J. 1, 1138-1142 (1966)
2. Fantis, A.: Microvascular bypass operation by means of fibrin gluing method. Abstracts of the 7th European Congress of Neurosurgery, Brussels 1983
3. Fein, J.M., Dujovny, M., Kossovsky, N.: Angiographic demonstration of postoperative cortical artery stenosis induced by Biemer temporary clips. Neurosurgery 13, 520-522 (1983)
4. Fleischer, A.S., Faria, M.A., Jr., Hoffman, J.C., Jr.: Pseudoaneurysm complicating superficial temporal artery-middle cerebral artery bypass. Surg. Neurol. 12, 305-306 (1979)
5. Jain, K.K.: Sutureless microvascular anastomosis using a Neodymium-YAG laser. J. Microsurg. 1, 436-439 (1980)

6. Kletter, G., Matras, H., Dinges, H.P.: Zur partiellen Klebung von Mikrogefäßanastomosen im intrakraniellen Bereich. Wien. klin. Wschr. 12, 2-6 (1978)

7. Kletter, G., Meyermann, R.: Histological case control of microanastomoses, In: Koos, W.T., Böck. F.W., Spetzler, R.F. (eds.) Clinical microneurosurgery, pp. 234-238. Thieme, Stuttgart 1976

8. Kletter, G., Stula, D., Horaczek, A.: The use of fibrin sealant in neurosurgery. In: Skioldborg, H. (ed.) Immuno scientific workshop 1982, pp. 83-89. Immuno, Aarhus 1982

9. Lantos, G., Fein, J.M., Knep, S.: Cortical artery aneurysm formation after extracranial to intracranial bypass surgery. J. Neurosurg. 60, 636-639 (1984)

10. Leclercq, T.A., Ambler, M.W.: Fatal subdural bleeding following superficial temporal-middle cerebral artery anastomosis. J. Neurosurg. 52, 392-394 (1980)

11. Steinbok, P., Berry, K., Dolman, C.: Superficial temporal artery-middle cerebral artery (STA-MCA) anastomosis. Pathological study of two cases. J. Neurosurg. 50, 377-381 (1979)

12. Suzuki, J., Ohara, H.: Origin, rupture and growth of cerebral aneurysms: A clinicopathological study. In: Pia, H.W., Langmaid, C., Zierski, J. (eds.) Cerebral aneurysms, pp. 28-41. Springer, Berlin Heidelberg New York 1979

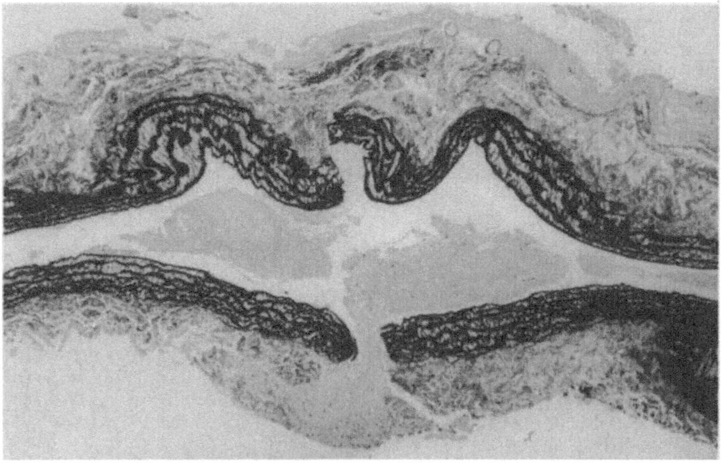

Fig. 1. Longitudinal section of a glued end-to-end anastomosis two days postoperatively. The lumen is filled with fibrin glue. van Gieson, × 80

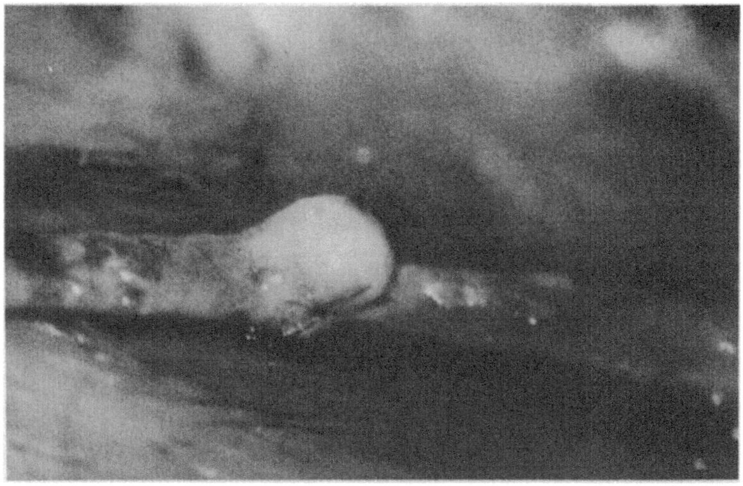

Fig. 2. Macroscopic aneurysm formation 115 days after suturing a dissected common carotid artery. The vessel is patent. Operating microscope, × 10

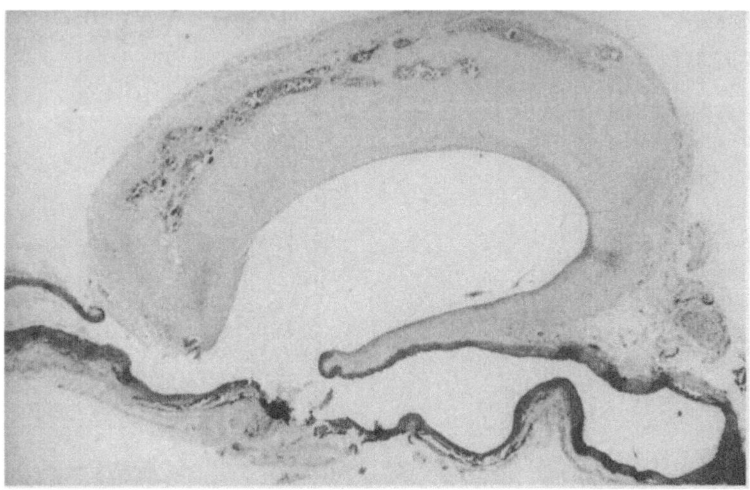

Fig. 3. Longitudinal microphotograph of a large pseudoaneurysm 110 days after gluing. Hematoxylin-eosin, × 22.5

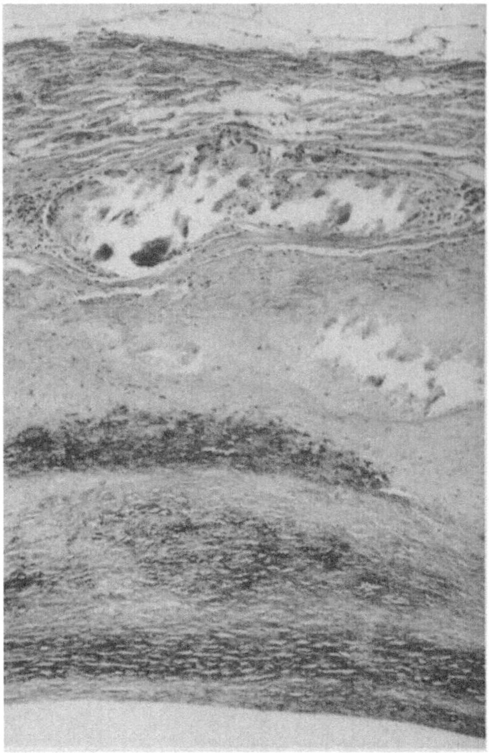

Fig. 4. Section of the vessel wall of Fig. 3 with vasa vasorum necroses and hemorrhages. van Gieson, × 100.8

Morphology of Vessel Wall Changes After Microsurgical End- to-Side Anastomosis and Their Pharmacological Prevention

H. M. Mehdorn[1], S. Hickler[2], K. Venjakob[3], V. Reinhardt[2], and W. Grote[1]

[1] Abteilung für Neurochirurgie, [2] Institut für Neuropathologie, [3] Anatomisches Institut, Universitätsklinikum der Gesamthochschule Essen, Hufelandstraße 55, D-4300 Essen 1

Introduction

Morphological alterations in the arteries which are involved in extracranial-intracranial (EC/IC) anastomoses may be harmful to EC/IC bypass function. Only a limited number of human specimens of EC/IC anastomoses have been evaluated, by STEINBOK and co-workers (15) and BODOSI and MEREI (3). They described development of arteriosclerotic changes such as interruption of the internal elastic membrane (IEM) and (myo-)-intimal hyperplasia (MIH) which, in some instances, led to a marked stenosis of the lumen of the arteries. However, arteriosclerosis occurs frequently in the superficial temporal arteries of EC/IC bypass patients (12), and therefore the finding of arteriosclerosis cannot necessarily be considered as postoperative development.

In order to study the long-term development of vessel wall changes in an animal model which simulates the high flow situation found in a well functioning EC/IC bypass and their possible pharmacological prevention, an arteriovenous end-to-side anastomosis (ESA) on the rat femoral vessels was used.

Methods

In 120 male Wistar rats of 200-250 g body weight (b.w.), a microsurgical ESA was performed between the femoral artery [internal diameter (ID) 0.7 mm] and the femoral vein (ID 1 mm). The femoral vessels were dissected over their course from the inguinal ligament to the branching of the profound femoral vessels. The artery was closed temporarily using Mehdorn clips (Aesculap, Tuttlingen, FR Germany) with a closing force of 15-20 g which were applied 4-6 mm apart, the artery was cut just proximally to the distal clip, and the adventitia was stripped close to the end of the artery. The vein was closed with temporary Mehdorn clips, 3-5 mm apart, incised over 1 mm length, and both vessels were irrigated with 0.9% saline. The ESA was performed using 10-0 monofilament nylon (22 μm) on an 80-μm needle (Ethicon, Norderstedt, FR Germany), with eight interrupted sutures. Upon completion of the anastomosis, the clips were removed and the skin closed.

Besides free access to standard pellets, half of the animals received tap water, while the other half had access to water in which acetylsalicylic acid (ASA, Aspirin, Bayer, Leverkusen, FR Germany) had been diluted in a concentration to ensure a daily ASA uptake of 20-30 mg/kg b.w. At intervals ranging from 30 min to 25 mos postop., animals were killed by transaortic in vivo perfusion fixation using glutaraldehyde (2.5%) in phosphate buffer (pH 7.4) at physiological pressure. Speci-

Advances in Neurosurgery, Vol. 13
Edited by H. Dietz, M. Brock, and M. Klinger

mens were removed en bloc and prepared for light microscopy (LM) and scanning electron microscopy (SEM). LM specimens were sectioned serially and stained with hematoxylin-eosin, elastica-van Gieson, and sudan III stain for lipids; SEM specimens were critical point dried, mounted with silver stain, coated with gold, and observed in a Cambridge Stereoscan 180 at a beam voltage of 20 keV.

Results

Animals Operated Without ASA

Subsequent to release of blood flow in the ESA, endothelial denudation occurred in the dissected area of the artery and in the funnel-shaped area in the vein underneath the anastomosis. Endothelium remained intact at the clip sites. Platelets adhered rapidly to the subendothelial structures.

In the artery, re-endothelialization began two to three days postoperatively. Flat endothelial lining cells progressed from the intact endothelium towards the damaged areas more rapidly along the inner side of the curvature than on its outer side. After four to six weeks, endothelial lining cells orientated in a whirlpool fashion produced intimal cushions which could be found, in the entrance area to the curvature, on the outer part of the curvature, and, further downstream, in the inner part of the curvature (Figs. 1, 2). Later, they were covered by polygonal cells with a rough surface (Fig. 3). In about half of all specimens observed 17 to 25 mos postoperatively, these cushions led to a marked narrowing of the distal arterial lumen. In no instance could lipid deposits be seen in the cushions. The internal elastic membrane (IEM) underneath these cushions was interrupted, and media-myocytes migrated through the gaps into the cushions. Only rarely could calcification be seen in the arterial wall.

The arterial lumen distant from the curvature was covered by smooth endothelial cells. The IEM was intact, the media formed by stretched myocytes. This stretching corresponded to the dilatation of the proximal artery.

Endothelialization of the artery was not always complete after 25 mos. Particularly the most distal part of the artery was still covered by a few flat cells, platelets, and fibrin thrombi.

In the vein, endothelial lining cells started to grow toward the anastomosis at the end of the first week. Similarly to what had been seen in the artery, these cells showed varying responses to blood flow perturbations: cell orientation in a whirlpool fashion, and the appearance of (myo-)intimal cushions which were either flat, longitudinal, or formed like polyps (Figs. 3, 4). These areas of focal (myo-)intimal hyperplasia (MIH) were mainly located underneath the anastomosis. On LM (Fig. 4), they consisted of (myo-)intimal cells on a thickened IEM which was occasionally split in two layers. In contrast to the cushions on the arterial side, fine lipid granules were visible in the (myo-)-intimal cells and in the interstices. Occasionally, capillaries penetrated these cushions. Besides these areas of MIH opposite to the anastomosis, another type of hyperplasia developed close to the anastomosis itself, originating in the angle formed by artery and vein. This type of endothelial hyperplasia produced polyps (Fig. 3) which joined occasionally with the MIH from the other side of the vein and led to a labyrinth-like appearance of the venous lumen (Fig. 1). It consisted of focal areas of curled (myo-)intimal cells, areas of platelet accumulations, and calcium deposits. Lipid staining revealed prominent lipid deposits mainly in the vicinity of the calcium deposits. The vein wall distant from the anastomosis showed no major changes as compared with a normal femoral vein. Also, the clip sites showed no abnormality.

Animals Operated While Under ASA Medication

Endothelial denudation related to surgical trauma and restoration of blood flow occurred similarly to that observed in the unmedicated group. However, it appeared that the denuded areas were smaller. Endothelial regeneration started two to three days later and proceeded slower than in the unmedicated group.

Although it was impossible to quantify the degree of MIH in the artery, it could clearly be seen that MIH was less pronounced in the rats which were under ASA treatment than in the unmedicated animals. MIH never caused a marked stenosis of the arterial lumen. The arterial dilatation extended over the entire length of the vessel down to the anastomosis. Endothelial hyperplasia in the vein opposite to the anastomosis was less pronounced than in the unmedicated animals.

Discussion

So far, experimental evaluation of the microsurgical end-to-side anastomosis (1, 9, 11, 17) has mainly been directed towards the phase of endothelialization, that is the first few weeks following surgery. In contrast, this study had been undertaken to evaluate long-term changes which may occur in both vessels involved in the ESA in order to provide useful information about long-term changes in the arteries involved in EC/IC bypass. Surgical techniques and changes in hemodynamics have been shown to lead to vessel wall damage. Endothelial damage caused by surgical techniques can be minimized by "atraumatic" microsurgical handling of the vessels and by using soft-pressure clips particularly developed for these fine vessels, such as those used in the present experiment.

The first step of repair is platelet adhesion to denuded subendothelium. The process of vessel wall damage and repair depends upon three factors:

- hemodynamic situation
- extent of endothelial denudation
- adhesiveness of platelets

1. The hemodynamic situation of the model ESA can be explained by the boundary layer separation theory (7, 10) to understand localization of areas of focal MIH (a) in a curvature and (b) in the ESA itself. Obviously, the hemodynamic situation does not change drastically some time after completion of the anastomosis, and thus it can be assumed that the hemodynamic stress continues to influence the development of MIH. This can be well demonstrated by the results obtained in the experiments presented here: in the specimens removed after the maximum length of time, that is 25 mos postoperatively, MIH had reached its maximum and had led to a marked stenosis of the distal part of the artery.

2. It is known that the extent of endothelial denudation depends mainly on the hemodynamic stress situation (8), and that the endothelial cell orientation is flow-dependent as well (6).

The localization of the different (myo-)intimal cushions in the arterial curvature and the cushions and polyps on the venous side corresponds well with the localization of areas of hemodynamic stasis as suggested by FOX and HUGH (7) and HOULE and ROACH (10). Because endothelialization was not yet always complete 25 mos postoperatively, it appears logical to assume a continuous wear-and-tear mechanism that affects the inner surface of the vessel wall and may lead to the development of atherosclerosis.

Development of atherosclerosis is due to release of a platelet-derived growth factor which stimulates smooth muscle cell proliferation (14) and the development of MIH. This theory explains the close relationship between the areas of platelet aggregation and (myo-)intimal cell proliferation.

Because the experimental data presented here are able to confirm the relation between hemodynamics of the ESA and the development of focal areas of MIH, they also confirm the suggestion of STEINBOK and co-workers (15) and of BODOSI and MEREI (3) that focal MIH may represent a vessel wall response to the alteration of blood flow characteristics.

3. The primary importance of platelet aggregation in the development of MIH as a form of atherosclerosis has been stressed. Platelet aggregation can be reduced by ASA. Although the value of high doses of ASA in the suppression of platelet aggregation has been questioned (2, 13), the results presented here clearly show that it is possible, by giving such a high dosis – which is similar to that given in man for the prevention of stroke (4) – to reduce the development of MIH.

Because of the continuous wear-and-tear vessel wall damage and the fact that, in the high-flow system of arteriovenous anastomosis thought to resemble the hemodynamic situation in an EC/IC anastomosis, endothelialization was not yet always complete after 25 mos postoperatively, it appears logical that ASA should be given for ever. This is in contrast to the assumption related to mechanical denudation of longitudinal arteries (5) and microsurgical end-to-end anastomosis (16). In these instances, it can be assumed that endothelialization is complete after two weeks, and that it is not necessary to continue ASA medication for a longer period.

As has also been shown by FISHMAN and co-workers (5), MIH is most pronounced in those surface areas which are last covered by endothelium. Endothelialization of both artery and vein was slower in the group of animals treated with ASA than in the untreated group. This side-effect of ASA could counteract its beneficial effect in the prevention of MIH. However, in the given experimental situation, no adverse effect could be noted.

Conclusion

The experimental end-to-side anastomosis between the rat femoral artery and vein leads to the development of (myo-)intimal cushions, interruption of the internal elastic membrane, and thickening of the muscular media in hemodynamically stressed areas that are the curvature of the artery and the funnel-shaped area in the vein located underneath the anastomosis. These wall changes resemble atherosclerosis. In rats receiving a daily dosis of acetylsalicylic acid (ASA) of approximately 20 mg/kg b.w. these wall changes occur only in a mild form. It is suggested that ASA should be given as a long-term routine medication following EC/IC in order to reduce the risk of late bypass occlusion or stenosis.

References

1. Albanese, V., Spadaro, A., Tomasello, F., et al.: Dynamics of endothelial repair in end-to-side microsurgical carotid anastomoses in rats: A scanning electron microscopic study. Neurol. Res. 3, 267-287 (1981)
2. Amezcua, J.L., O'Grady, J., Salmon, J.A., Moncada, S.: Prolonged paradoxical effect of aspirin on platelet behaviour and bleeding time in man. Thromb. Res. 16, 69-79 (1979)
3. Bodosi, M., Merei, F.T.: Development of histological structure of microanastomosis. Presented at the 5th Int. Symp. on Microvasc. Anastomoses for Cerebral Ischemia, Vienna, Sept. 14-17, 1980 (Abstr. No. 24a)
4. Canadian Cooperative Study Group: A randomized trial of aspirin and sulfinpyrazone in threatened stroke. New Engl. J. Med. 299, 53-59 (1979)
5. Fishman, J.A., Ryan, G.B., Karnovsky, M.J.: Endothelial regeneration in the rat carotid artery and the significance of endothelial denudation in the pathogenesis of myointimal thickening. Lab. Invest. 32, 339-351 (1975)
6. Flaherty, J.T., Pierce, J.E., Ferrans, V.J., et al.: Endothelial nuclear patterns in the canine arterial tree with particular reference to hemodynamic events. Circ. Res. 30, 23-33 (1972)
7. Fox, J.A., Hugh, A.E.: Localisation of atheroma: Theory based on boundary layer separation. Br. Heart J. 28, 388-399 (1966)
8. Fry, D.L.: Acute vascular endothelial changes associated with increased blood velocity gradients. Circ. Res. 22, 165-197 (1968)
9. Gelderman, P.W., Berendsen, W.: Re-endothelialization of microvascular carotid end-to-side anastomoses in the rat – a scanning electron microscope study. J. Neurosurg. 51, 785-795 (1979)
10. Houle, S., Roach, M.R.: Flow studies in a rigid model of an aorto-renal junction. Atherosclerosis 40, 231-244 (1981)
11. Mehdorn, H.M., Weinstein, P.R., Chater, N.L.: Vessel wall response to the end-to-side anastomosis. Stroke 9, 10 (1978)
12. Mehdorn, H.M., Wiedemeyer, H., Reinhardt, V., et al.: Histologische Veränderungen der A. temporalis superficialis und ihre Bedeutung für die extra-intrakranielle Bypass-Operation. Neurochirurgia 26, 181-186 (1983)
13. O'Grady, J., Moncada, S.: Aspirin: a paradoxical effect on bleeding-time (Letter to the editor). Lancet Oct 7, 780 (1978)
14. Ross, R., Glomset, J.A.: The pathogenesis of atherosclerosis. New Engl. J. Med. 295, 396-377, 420-425 (1976)
15. Steinbok, P., Berry, K., Dolman, C.L.: Superficial temporal artery middle cerebral artery (STA-MCA) anastomosis. J. Neurosurg. 50, 377-381 (1979)
16. Weinstein, P.R., Mehdorn, H.M., Szabo, Z.: Microsurgical anastomosis. Vessel injury, regeneration and repair. In: Serafin, D., Buncke, H.J., Jr. (eds.) Microsurgical composite tissue transplantation, pp. 111-144. Mosby, St. Louis Toronto London 1979
17. Young, P.H., Imhoff, H.G., Chu, H.L.: Scanning electron microscopic evaluation of variably angled end-to-side microvascular anastomoses. Neurosurgery 12, 306-312 (1983)

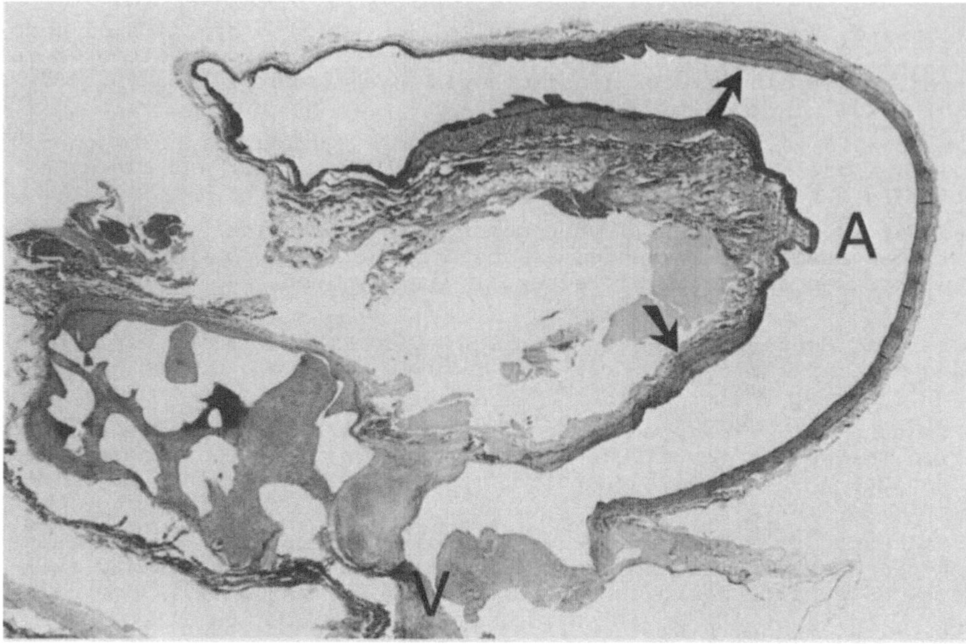

Fig. 1. Longitudinal section through anastomosed artery and vein 3 mos postoperatively. Note focal (myo-)intimal hyperplasia (→) in certain areas of the artery (*A*); *V* = vein. × 20

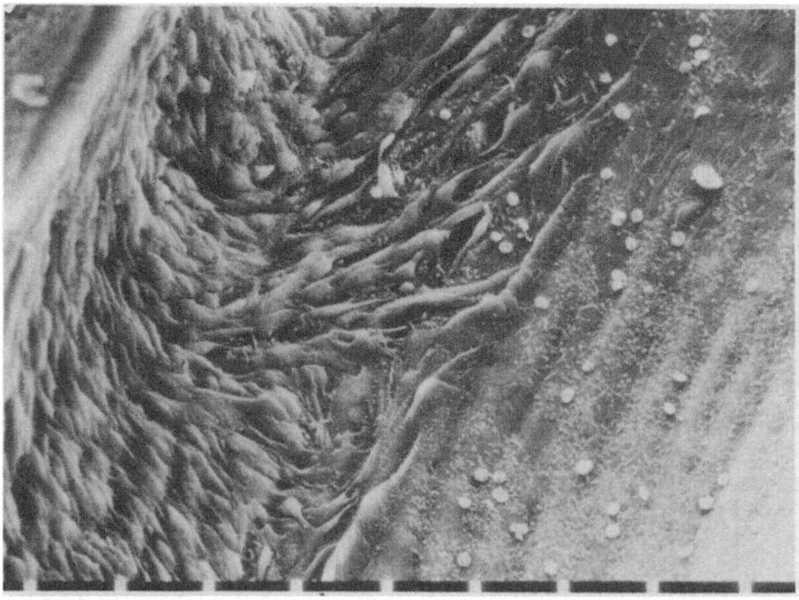

Fig. 2. Artery, distal part, 1 month postoperatively; ---- = 30 μm. On the *left*, the inner part of the curvature is already covered with advancing cells; the outer part of the curvature (on the *right*) is still void of cells

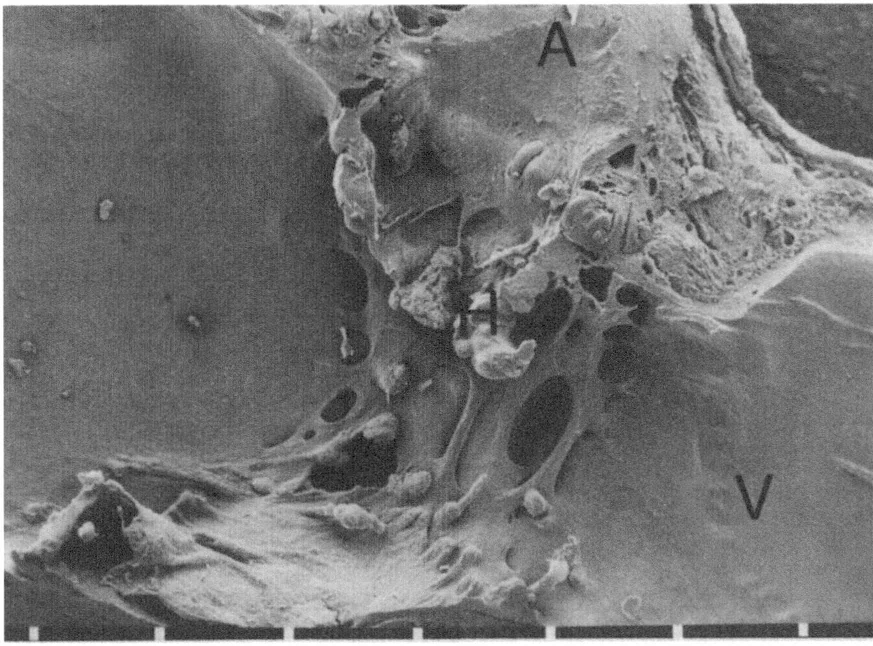

Fig. 3. ESA 3 mos postoperatively. Note marked MIH in the distal part of the artery (*A*), and areas of focal MIH (*H*) in the angle between artery and vein (*V*) and in the vein itself. ---- = 300 μm

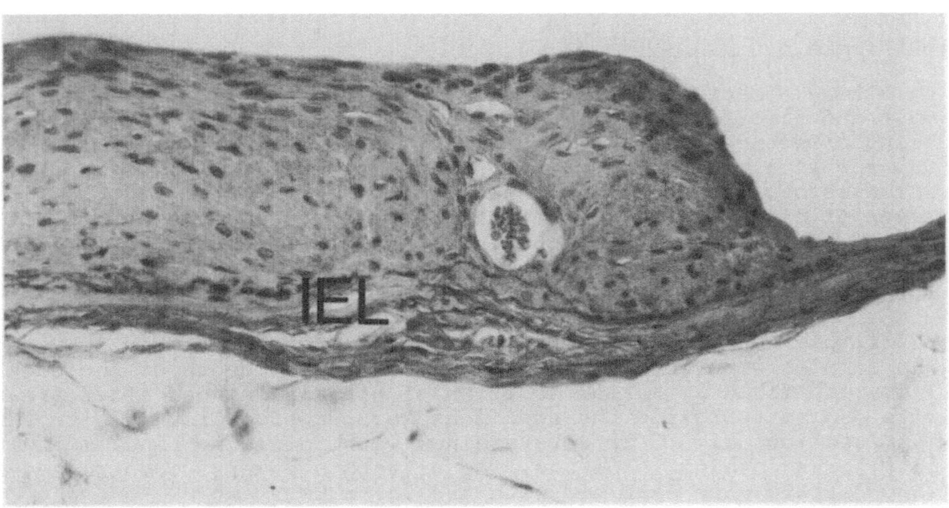

Fig. 4. Vein underneath the anastomosis, 7 1/2 mos postoperatively. Note: Myointimal hyperplasia over interrupted internal elastic lamina (*IEL*). × 625

The Ultrastructure of the Superficial Temporal Artery in Extra-Intracranial Bypass Surgery*

G. Ebhardt[1], Th. Rommel[2], and D. Eymer[2]

[1] Pathologisches Institut, [2] Neurochirurgische Klinik, Krankenhaus Merheim, Ostmerheimer Straße 200, D-5000 Köln 91

Introduction

Extra-intracranial arterial bypass surgery has been well known for several years. Systematic morphological investigations of the superficial temporal artery (STA) used as a graft, however, have only been carried out by DIAZ and co-workers (2) and by MEHDORN et al. (11). To our knowledge, findings concerning the ultrastructure of the graft vessel have not been published.

In patients selected for arterial bypass surgery, a disease of the extracerebral and the intracranial arteries is usually present. It may therefore be safely assumed that the STA is involved in the disease, too. Knowledge about the changes in the vessel wall existing at the time the anastomosis is created is essential for the evaluation of the effect of bypass surgery. By no means all changes in the condition of the vessel walls can be demonstrated via angiography. Examination of the tissue by light microscopy may be sufficient to recognize changes in the vessel wall. Investigations of the ultrastructure, however, yield more information on the alterations of the intracellular structures.

Materials and Methods

An extra-intracranial anastomosis was placed into 15 patients – ten male and five female. The age of the men ranged from 41 to 70 years, being close to 55 years in the majority. Except for one patient aged 59, the females were between 66 and 70 years old. In two men bilateral anastomoses were placed, permitting the investigation of 17 segments of blood vessels. Patients requiring craniotomy due to a tumor in the brain or for an arachnoidal cyst served as controls. In these patients the STA was prepared as in the patients undergoing bypass surgery.

The samples obtained via biopsy ranged in length between 4 mm and 6 mm. The samples were cut into blocks of which the length of the edges was 1 mm, and fixed in a 2.5% solution of glutaraldehyde. After treatment with osmium tetroxide the specimens were embedded in Araldite. Semithin sections of 0.5 μm were stained with toluidine blue, methylene blue, or according to Giemsa. The ultrathin layers recontrasted with lead citrate were examined with the Zeiss EM 9 and EM 109.

---

* Dedicated to Prof. Dr. Dr. Rolf Wüllenweber on the occasion of his 60th birthday.

Advances in Neurosurgery, Vol. 13
Edited by H. Dietz, M. Brock, and M. Klinger

Results

Light Microscope Findings

In all vessels the tunica intima was enlarged to a varying degree, sometimes up to ten times the regular thickness. The cells of the endothelial layer were partly damaged or destroyed by the surgical intervention. In other places the endothelial cells were flat, extended lengthwise, or hyperplastic, protruding into the lumen, which was restricted in all cases. The intima appeared to be rich in cells due to the smooth muscle cells arranged in groups or distributed diffusely. In most cases these cells were smaller than those seen in the tunica media. Complexes of collagenous connective tissue, amorphous material, and fractions of elastic lamellae were located between the cells. The lamina elastica interna no longer formed a continuous ribbon, but was split into numerous lamellae which extended below the endothelium and had disintegrated into fractions. In three cases the lamina elastica interna had separated from the tunica media due to the surgical procedure and blood had accumulated within the defect. The tunica media was enlarged in all cases. The cells were grouped lengthwise in the lower levels only. Predominantly the cells had separated from the integral cell structure and were rounded. Below the lamina elastica interna, the cells were positioned perpendicular to the lumen of the vessel and could be demonstrated between the fragments of elastic lamellae. The tunica adventitia consisted of densely packed collagenous fibers and individual elastic lamellae (Fig. 1).

Ultrastructural Findings

The endothelial cells were partly flat, extended lengthwise, and formed a continuous layer. Mostly the cells were large and rich in organelles. Between these cells defects of varying size were visible in which smooth muscle cells had penetrated. In other places blood clots had been deposited on the intima denuded of endothelial cells. In the subendothelial layer, there were bundles of collagenous fibers of varying width, partly appearing to be swollen. The structure was frequently dissolved, the material granulated and opaque against electrons. A continuous lamina elastica interna was no longer recognizable. Numerous lamellae as well as bundles of elastic fibrils with and without elastin could be demonstrated, reaching below the endothelial lining.

In all samples partly single, partly grouped cells were observed which were shown to be smooth muscle cells due to the surrounding basal membrane (Fig. 2). Groups of the cells were frequently located perpendicular to the lumen between the fragments of the lowest lamellae of the lamina elastica interna. These cells were predominantly atrophic, exhibiting a narrow profile extended lengthwise and sparse cytoplasm only (Fig. 3). In the tunica media smooth muscle cells were positioned lengthwise only in the layer adjacent to the tunica adventitia as well as in the normal media. They were predominantly arranged irregularly, in the form of knots, or located perpendicular to the lumen. Some of the cells correspond in shape and size to the elements found in the undisturbed tunica media. In addition, hyperplastic, atrophic, and degeneratively altered muscle cells were seen. The hyperplastic elements were sometimes star-shaped or were rounded. Besides densely packed myofibrils, they frequently featured a strongly developed, rough endoplasmatic reticulum which sometimes penetrated the entire cytoplasm. Shrinking of the cysterns of the endoplasmatic reticulum marked the transition to degenerative forms. In most cases the process started in the vicinity of the nucleus and was accompanied by an increasing loss of the ribosomes. The mitochondria were frequently enlarged, swollen, and showed fragmentation and disintegration of the cristae. This should, however, be considered as an artifact due to surgery. Dissolution of the myofilaments started in the perinuclear zone; it sometimes continued and could affect the entire cell. In all cells lysosomes occurred to a varying frequency. Lipid droplets were usually confined to a circumscribed area within the cell body. Frequently the basal membrane was present in parts only, often being separated from the plasma membrane and extending parallel to that membrane (Fig. 4). Differentiation of the cell sections in which a basal membrane was no longer recognizable and which demonstrated a grossly developed rough endoplasmatic reticulum against fibroblasts was difficult, particularly if the myofilaments had also dissolved. Probably, smooth muscle cells were present here also. The intercellular space varied in width and was interspersed with bundles of collagenous fibers. Remnants of basal membranes and loose material of varying density, opaque against electrons, were located in between.

Discussion

The advantage of investigating the distal segment of the STA ultrastructurally is based on the assumption that degenerative changes will manifest approximately uniformly along the entire extension of the blood vessel. Additionally, it has to be considered that the damage resulting from surgical intervention will not be limited to the distal segment, but will continue in the part of the vessel to be anastomosed. Defects between the intima and the media, filled with blood, have to be organized and accordingly can intensify alterations within the vessel wall, including the constriction of the lumen. Even during careful surgery, the endothelial cells are partly destroyed (up to 70%). During entirely atraumatic preparation only, i.e., if the vessel is touched neither by instruments nor by tampons, the endothelium can be preserved almost completely (6). If the endothelium is desquamated, the subendothelial connective tissue will be exposed, and soon agglomerated by thrombi (14, 15). Within the next days, the endothelial cells regenerate and may grow across the thrombus. Additional stenosis of the lumen which is already reduced due to the widening of the intima, or even occlusion, may result, however.

It was possible to demonstrate regeneration of the endothelial cells via mitotic division in animal experiments (5). Based on results obtained via scanning electron microscopy, MEHDORN (10) supported the opinion that smooth muscle cells immigrating into the subendothelial zone are able to form a surface of endothelial cells.

Morphological investigations of anastomoses at different postsurgical intervals have been performed predominantly in models using animals (8, 9, 16). After anastomotic operation, a proliferation of the intimal cells takes place which is more pronounced downstream. Widening of the intima is caused by immigration of smooth muscle cells from the media and by enlargement of the subendothelial space (16). These results correlate with our findings and those reported by DIAZ et al. (2) and MEHDORN et al. (11), except that they existed in the human arteries even before the operation. It can therefore be assumed that the hyperplasia of the intima will still increase in both segments of the arteries. MEYERMANN et al. (12) investigated the anastomoses in two patients who had died as a consequence of bypass surgery. Not only in the STA but particularly in the intracranial artery a proliferation of intimal cells occurs. Widening of the vessel wall is not only due to the hyperplasia of the intima, but also of the media. According to MEHDORN et al. (11), the media is 200 μm thick in patients 60 years old, as compared with a thickness of 30-80 μm in juveniles. The thickening of the media is due to an increase of the intercellular space with a proliferation of collagenous fibers, and also to hyperplasia of the smooth muscle cells. This hyperplasia appears always to develop in the same pattern, regardless of whether the changes are due to hypertension, arteriosclerosis, malformation, or inflammation. Hyperplastic, rounded, or star-shaped as well as degeneratively modified muscle cells as observed in the STA were seen in intracranial aneurysms (3), in intracranial angiomas (4), and in temporal arteritis (1). If morphologically such changes are seen in the vessel walls, preceding and following anastomotic operation, the question remains open of how to correlate this with the numerous clinical reports about a significant improvement in the neurological symptoms and an increase of blood supply following arterial bypass surgery. It has been speculated that the STA will be expanded passively as a result of the increased blood flow and that the restriction of the lumen will be compensated for accordingly (12, 2, 11), though corresponding morphological investigations have not yet been performed. It may, however, be assumed that the leptomeningeal collateral circulation reserve may be enhanced by surgery (8, 2, 7). This hypothesis is also supported by an observation by SPETZLER et al. (13), who did not find a suitable cortical branch for a direct arterial anastomosis. The STA was therefore sutured to the arachnoid. The postoperative carotid angiogram demonstrated an impressive number of collaterals from the STA to the cortex and the middle cerebral artery.

Acknowledgment. The technical assistance of Mr. Hoffmann of the Department for Electron Microscopy of the University of Cologne (FRG), (Director Prof. G. Addicks, M. D.) is gratefully acknowledged.

References

1. Cervós-Navarro, J., Ebhardt, G., Stoltenburg-Didinger, G.: Die Degenerationsformen der glatten Muskelzellen bei zerebralen Gefäßkrankheiten. Zbl. allg. Path. 124, 173 (1980)

2. Diaz, F.G., Chason, J., Shrontz, C., Ausman, J.I., Dujovny, M.: Histological structural abnormalities of superficial temporal arteries used for extracranial-intracranial anastomosis. J. Neurosurg. 57, 328-333 (1982)

3. Ebhardt, G., Wüllenweber, R., Cervós-Navarro, J.: The ultrastructure of the aneurysmatic vessel wall. In: Cervós-Navarro, J., Betz, E., Matakas, F., Wüllenweber, R. (eds.) The cerebral vessel wall, pp. 67-74. Raven Press, New York 1976

4. Ebhardt, G., Cervós-Navarro, J., Wüllenweber, R.: Ultrastruktur der Wand intrakranieller arteriovenöser Rankenangiome. Zbl. allg. Path. 121, 567 (1977)

5. Freudenberg, N., Riese, K.H.: Standortunterschiede des normalen Gefäßendothels und Veränderungen durch Endotoxinschock. In: Fischer, H., Betz, E. (eds.) Das Gefäßendothel, pp. 31-41. Wiss. Verlagsgesellschaft, Stuttgart 1981

6. Gottlob, R.: Regeneration der Gefäßendothelien nach verschiedenartigen Traumata. In: Fischer, H., Betz, E. (eds.) Das Gefäßendothel, pp. 42-53. Wiss. Verlagsgesellschaft, Stuttgart 1981

7. Halsey, J.H. Jr., Morawetz, R.B., Blauenstein, U.W.: The hemodynamic effect of STA-MCA bypass. Stroke 13, 163-167 (1982)

8. Hitchon, P.W., Kassell, N.F., Gross, C.E.: Influence of superficial temporal artery to middle cerebral artery bypass on cerebral blood flow in dogs with middle cerebral artery occlusion. Stroke 12, 224-228 (1981)

9. Iglesias-Rozas, J.R., Gutierrez, J.A., Córdoba, A., Enriquez de Salamanca, C.L.: Strukturelle Veränderungen der venösen Patchs bei kleinen extrazerebralen Arterien. Zbl. all. Path. 124, 173 (1980)

10. Mehdorn, H.M.: Rasterelektronenmikroskopische Untersuchungen zur Endothelialisierung von Mikrogefäßprothesen in der Neurochirurgie. In: Fischer, H., Betz, E. (eds.) Das Gefäßendothel, pp. 54-63. Wiss. Verlagsgesellschaft, Stuttgart 1981

11. Mehdorn, H.M., Wiedemeyer, H., Reinhardt, V., Gerhard, L., Zais, E.: Histologische Veränderungen der A. temporalis superficialis und ihre Bedeutung für die extra-intrakranielle Bypass-Operation. Neurochirurgia 26, 181-186 (1983)

12. Meyermann, R., Kletter, G., Koos, W., Wismann, H.: Zur operativen Behandlung zerebraler Ischämien: Morphologische Veränderungen an mikrochirurgischen Anastomosen zwischen Arteria superficialis und Arteria gyri angularis. Zbl. allg. Path. 121, 563-564 (1977)

13. Spetzler, R.F., Roski, R.A., Kopaniky, D.R.: Alternative superficial temporal artery to middle cerebral artery revascularization procedure. Neurosurgery 7, 484-487 (1980)

14. Staubesand, J., Seydewitz, V.: Endotheldefekte mit Plättchenadhäsion in fehlbelasteten Arterien der Ratte; experimentelle elektronenmikroskopische und ultracytochemische Untersuchungen. In: Fischer, H., Betz, E. (eds.) Das Gefäßendothel, pp. 110-119. Wiss. Verlagsgesellschaft, Stuttgart 1981

15. Thilo, D.G.S., Heinrich, D.: Die Endothelzelle – eine pluripotente Kontrollzelle der Gefäßwand. In: Fischer, H., Betz, E. (eds.) Das Gefäßendothel, pp. 5-30. Wiss. Verlagsgesellschaft, Stuttgart 1981

16. Wismann, H., Meyermann, R.: Early morphological changes in microvascular anastomoses. In: Driesen, W., Brock, M., Klinger, M. (eds.) Advances in neurosurgery, Vol. 10, pp. 340-343. Springer, Berlin Heidelberg New York 1982

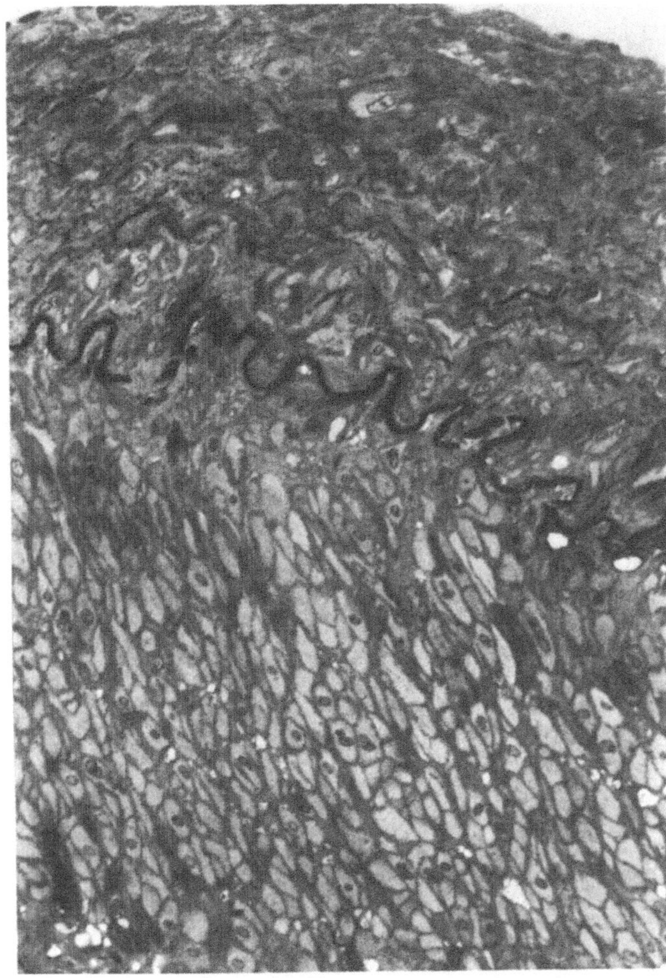

Fig. 1. The tunica intima is rich in cells due to smooth muscle cells. Endothelial cells are damaged. The lamina elastica interna is split in numerous lamellae. In the tunica media smooth muscle cells are arranged irregularly, with collagenous fibers in between. Giemsa, × 400

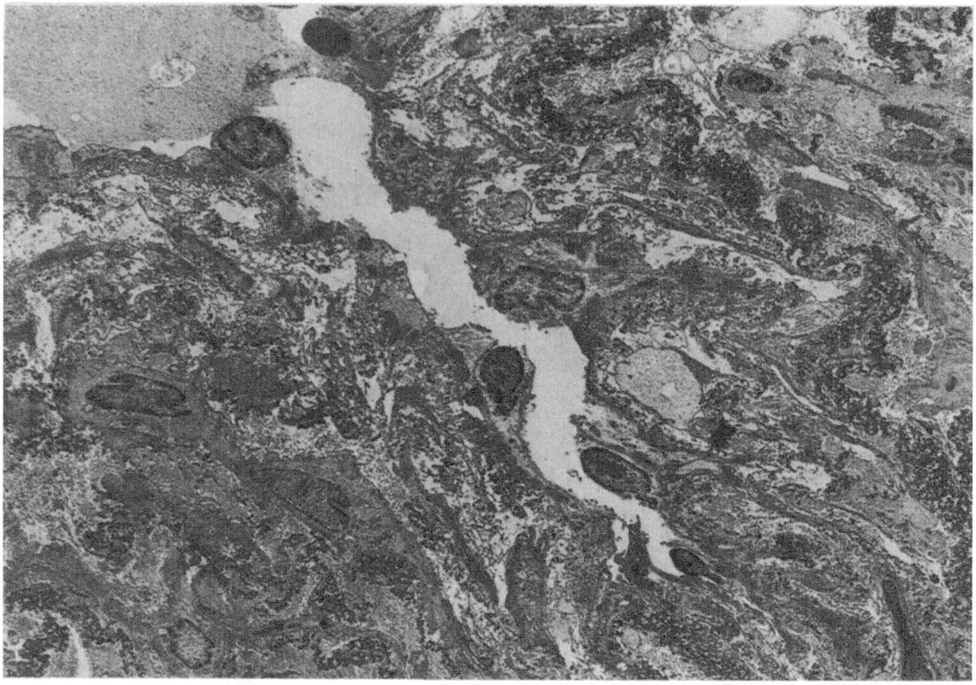

Fig. 2

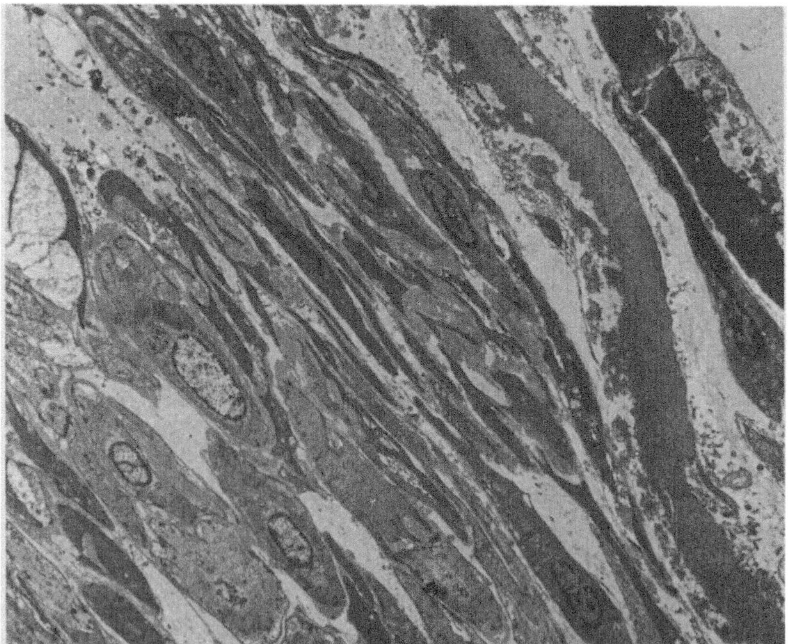

Fig. 3

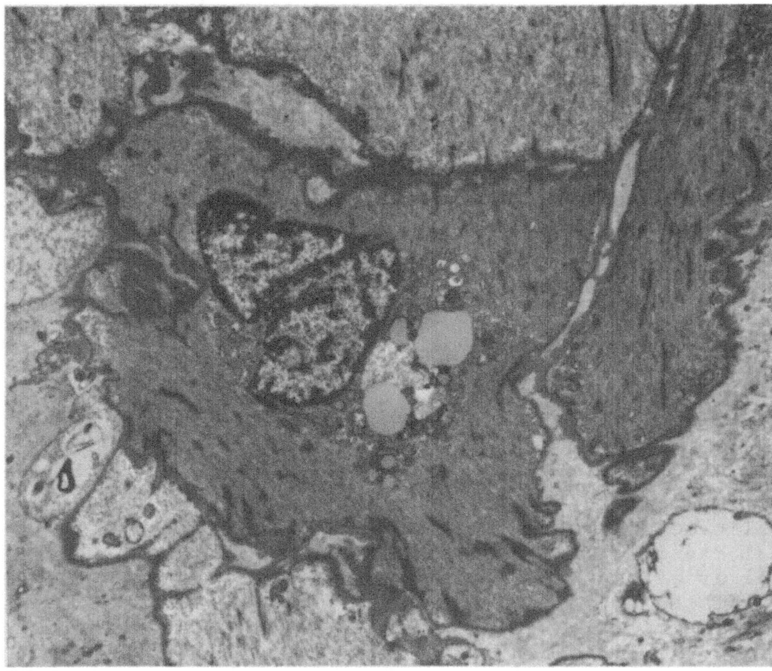

Fig. 4. Hypertrophic star-shaped smooth muscle cell of the tunica media. The organelles are grouped around the nucleus, with some lysosomes and lipid droplets. The basal membrane around the muscle cell is destroyed in parts. × 8000

Fig. 2. The endothelial cells of the tunica intima are large and rich in organelles or they are flat. Within the thickened intima, smooth muscle cells are visible. The intercellular space is markedly enlarged, with bundles of elastin and of collagen as well as with amorphous material. × 2750

Fig. 3. Atrophic smooth muscle cells with a narrow profile and sparse cytoplasm are located perpendicular to the lumen, between fragments of the lamina elastica interna. × 4300

The Functional Defect of Surgically Injured Endothelial Cells and Its Influence on Extra-Intracranial Arterial Bypass Surgery

R. Meyermann[1] and J. Wickboldt[2]

[1] Max-Planck-Gesellschaft, Klinische Forschungsgruppe für Multiple Sklerose, Josef-Schneider-Straße 11, D-8700 Würzburg

[2] Neurochirurgische Abteilung, Fachkrankenhaus Klinik Schildautal, Karl-Herold-Straße 1, D-3370 Seesen/Harz

Different disturbances of the cerebrovascular system can be treated successfully by extra-intracranial arterial bypass (EIAB) surgery. Most of these disturbances are caused not by a localized nonpatent blood vessel but by a general disease of the circulatory system. This implies that the pathologically changed blood vessel causing the cerebral blood flow disturbances is not the only one exhibiting pathological changes. Thus it must be assumed that those extra- and intracranial arteries which come under consideration for EIAB surgery might be affected, too. This has been demonstrated in the case of the superficial temporal artery, which most often demonstrates a severe fibrosis of the tunica intima (3). However, these pathological changes do not prevent the use of this blood vessel for EIAB surgery.

The intracranial artery which is connected with the superficial temporal artery (STA) has never been studied with regard to preexistent pathological changes. So the first part of this study demonstrates the changes which can be found at the light microscopic as well as the electron microscopic level in the vessel wall of the angular artery of the cerebral cortex.

The second part of this study examines experimentally whether or not there are functional changes of the endothelial cells after microsurgical interventions. In this way we gain knowledge of the damage preexisting in the operated blood vessel, and of that which is added by the microsurgical procedure.

Material and Methods

I. During EIAB surgery on 35 patients a sample of the arterial wall was excised from the angular artery. The excision extended 5-8 mm along the blood vessel and had a width of less than 1 mm. After removal, the tissue was immediately fixed in a buffered 3% glutaraldehyde solution. General transmission electron microscopic methods were applied to study the morphology of the specimens light and electron microscopically. Specimens of the STA were gained by similar methods.

II. Twenty two-month-old rats were anesthetized with ether, and end-to-end anastomoses of the left common carotid artery were performed by microsurgical methods. The operative technique has been described by MEYERMANN and colleagues (6). In order to study the entry of blood plasma into the vessel wall, the KARNOVSKY method was applied (2, 9). 200 mg/kg horseradish peroxidase was injected into the venous system. The animals were killed after the horseradish peroxidase had circulated for 15 min. The right and left common carotid arteries were removed

Advances in Neurosurgery, Vol. 13
Edited by H. Dietz, M. Brock, and M. Klinger

and immediately incubated in a 2.5% glutaraldehyde solution. The horseradish peroxidase was then developed by the KARNOVSKY medium (110 mg 3,3-diaminobenzidine dissolved in 100 ml 50 mM TRIS buffer; 0.1 ml 30% H_2O_2 is added immediately before the incubation of the specimens). The incubation lasted 60 min and was carried out in the dark. In order to identify endogenous peroxidase, corresponding specimens of animals which had not been injected with horseradish peroxidase before killing were tested using the same procedure.

The identification of horseradish peroxidase was followed by general electron microscopic methods as described above. However, any kind of counterstaining whatsoever was omitted.

The presence of lysosomes was demonstrated by identifying acid phosphatase in the vessel walls of animals which had not been injected with horseradish peroxidase, using the technique published in 1966 by KREUTZBERG and HAGER (4). After both the common carotid arteries had been removed, they were fixed in glutaraldehyde for half an hour. Small pieces of the fixed specimens were washed in cacodylate-saccharose wash buffer at 37°C for 10 min. This procedure was followed by incubation for 15 min in a medium containing 95 mg sodium glycerophosphate, 65 mg lead nitrate, and 2.94 mg saccharose which were dissolved in 50 ml 0.05 M acetate acetic buffer (pH 5.0). After washing in an isotonic acetic wash buffer, the general electron microscopic methods were applied.

Results

Morphology of the Specimens Obtained from the Human Angular Artery

The undulated internal elastic lamina, as well as the protrusion of the endothelial cells into the lumen (Fig. 1a), indicate the vasospasm of the vessel wall. The endothelial cells bear cytoplasmin processes and microvilli. Their cytoplasm contains large amounts of filaments. The cell-to-cell contacts are intact (Fig. 1b). However, the endothelial cell layer is not closed. Several cells are necrotic, and large areas of the widened subendothelial space are naked. Other endothelial cells display a light cytoplasm which indicates swelling. Processes of smooth muscle cells penetrate the internal elastic lamina (Fig. 2b) and partially invade the subendothelial space. Throughout the whole length of the studied vessel wall, the elastic material incorporates collagen fibrils and cell debris (Fig. 2a).

Within the tunica media the number of collagen fibrils seems to be increased. The smooth muscle cells have a thickened basement membrane in some areas and their cytoplasm contains amorphous material within large vacuoles which resembles the invagination of necrotic smooth muscle cells described by JORIS and MAJNO (1) (Fig. 2c).

Although the Schwann cells are swollen due to the preparative procedure, nerve fibers with tubules can be detected regularly within the arachnoidal tissue (Fig. 2d).

The specimens gained from the STA demonstrate those changes discussed extensively by KLETTER et al. (3) and MEHDORN et al. (5).

Results of the Animal Models

Horseradish Peroxidase. Ten days after the operation, the injected horseradish peroxidase can be observed penetrating the inner layers of the intima and the tunica media. Penetration happens at the site of anastomosis and in parts of the vessel that had been occluded by clips during the operation (Fig. 3a).

The concentration of horseradish peroxidase was highest in the innermost layers of the vessel walls and decreased progressively in an outward direction; the differences in concentration probably correspond to differences in the rate of diffusion (Fig. 3a,b). Horseradish peroxidase moved out of the blood plasma by means of intercellular diffusion and transcellular transport.

A normal endothelium completely protects the inner layer from penetration of horseradish peroxidase.

The findings in the damaged endothelium can be observed unchanged several weeks to six months after the operation. The concentration of horseradish peroxidase in the anastomosed ends of the vessel was unchanged. However, the amount of horseradish peroxidase penetrating seems to depend on the degree of proliferation of the cell coat of the inner part of the vessel wall. A monolayer seems to prevent tracer penetration much less than does a cell coat consisting of several cell layers. Less horseradish peroxidase diffused into sites of clipping than into the site of anastomosis, but extracellular pathways were still open at these areas of the surgically treated vessels (Fig. 3b,c).

Acid Phosphatase. Reactive products of acid phosphatase were seen in the extracellular space three days after operation and for as long as eight weeks to six months later (Fig. 4). Slight accumulation of reaction products was observed inside the cytoplasm of smooth muscle cells. Reactive products were not seen in the intimal cell coat and the Weibel-Palade bodies were free of acid phosphatase.

Discussion

The morphological changes of the human angular artery used for intracranial anastomosis can clearly be divided into an acute one and another which is clearly of a chronic type. Vasospasm of the vessel wall is surely induced mechanically by the manipulation at the vessel wall and occurred during this procedure. Additionally, the loss of endothelial cells as well as the occurrence of microvilli at the endothelial cytoplasm membrane is a finding which can be termed an acute change. However, the invasion by the smooth muscle cells cannot be explained mechanically alone, because it is accompanied by fibrotic changes within the internal elastic lamina. Both findings cannot be judged exactly, but might be considered an indication of starting fibrotic changes. The increase of collagen fibers observed within the tunica media supports this supposition. However, even in the tunica media acute changes occur. These correlate with the necrotic changes within smooth muscle cells probably induced by the initial vasospasm.

The results can confirm the opinion that the cortical artery is affected by the disease which causes the cerebral blood flow disturbances. Due to the fact that sclerotic areas of the cortical vessel wall are avoided for use in the EIAB, only fibrotic changes could be demonstrated.

This fibrosis differs from that which is described within the STA by KLETTER et al. (3), which is satisfactorily explained by the different construction of the extracranial blood vessels on the one side and the cortical arteries on the other (11).

Many authors have claimed that blood plasma passes into the walls of vessels even though they were not able to provide strong evidence that such diffusion occurs after different mechanical injuries (10). We have demonstrated that this phenomenon occurs with the horseradish peroxidase method. During the first few days after operation, diffusion occurs because the cell layer that coats such vessels is incomplete. WEBSTER et al. (10) have reported that the intimal cell coat, which has all the structural features of normal endothelium, including intercellular contacts, is unable to protect the walls of such vessels against inward flow of blood plasma for six to eight weeks after operation. In our studies this lack of protection was seen up to six months after operation. However, it was previously unknown that active proliferation of intimal cells provides better protection for a vessel wall than does restoration of a complete monolayer.

Diffusion of blood plasma into the wall of the vessel at the sites of clipping indicates that endothelial cells show the same functional disturbances after clipping as they do after other mechanical injuries that occur during surgical intervention. The incomplete protection of the vessel wall by the intimal cell coat a long time after the operation demonstrates that the endothelial cells are unable to recover from injury. The demonstration of acid phosphatase inside the cytoplasm of smooth muscle cells and endothelial cells and in extracellular lysosomes indicates that enzymatic activity has increased. This increase in enzymatic activity has been described by POTT and STAUBESAND (8), who used the same methods as described in this report. However, the increase in enzymatic activity of lysosomes is not limited to the walls of mechanically damaged vessels; rather it is observed in the walls of vessels having hemodynamic or metabolic disturbances. Thus the lack of a major difference in enzymatic activity between operated and nonoperated vessels can be explained.

However, the presence of acid phosphatase remaining even after a long period of time in the extracellular space and in smooth muscle cells confirms the functional changes in the vessel wall. Both demonstration of enzymatic activity and demonstration of the decreased protection of the vessel wall by the tracer method indicate that the microsurgically treated blood vessel remains a metabolically and hemodynamically imbalanced part of the intracranial circulation system.

The clinical results and the findings in experimental studies, including those presented here, seem to be a contradiction. Microsurgical procedures cause longlasting damage to the vessel wall. However, this obviously has no influence on the clinical result when the operative treatment of the cerebrovascular disease is chosen with strict regard to the hemodynamic situation. This means that the increased risk of thrombotic occlusion of the EIAB can be reduced by a high blood flow within the site of anastomosis. This supposition is supported by several observations. One of them is the fact that EIAB have a reduced patency rate in the case of small focal strokes, which induce a low flow rate. Additionally, in autopsied cases of EIAB fresh adherent thrombotic material was found exclusively at the site of the anastomosis (7). This phenomenon can be explained by the increased penetration of blood plasma which results in blood clotting at this area when the circulation system stops.

Regarding the pathological changes in the human angular artery, the preexistent pathological changes in the vessel wall do not increase the risk of occlusion of microsurgical anastomoses. The extensive proliferation of myointimal cells, which was described in autoptic material of EIAB, probably prevents that penetration of blood plasma which encourages the occurrence of thrombosis. This study underlines the fact that the increase in cerebral blood flow, which is the aim of the extra-intracranial anastomosis, is most important for this microsurgical anastomosis itself.

Conclusion

The present morphological investigations into the healing process of microsurgical anastomoses between the extra- and intracranial blood circulation system are completed by two different studies:

1. Biopsies of the vessel wall of the human angular artery of 35 patients treated by EIAB were studied light and electron microscopically. The aim of this study was to gain knowledge of the preexistent pathological changes in the intracranial artery. The morphological changes of the extracranial artery and their significance for bypass surgery have been described previously (3).
2. In animal models the functional deficit of intimal cell coat after microsurgical procedure was visualized. This intimal coat cannot protect the vessel wall against penetration of blood plasma over a long time, and displays an increased enzymatic activity.

This reduced function of the intimal coat does not contradict the excellent clinical results, but indicates the importance of the hemodynamics at the site of anastomosis. The preexisting damage in the vessel wall resulting from the disease of the circulation system probably induces an increased myointimal proliferation after microsurgical procedures, but does not increase the risk of thrombosis at the site of the anastomosis.

References

1. Joris, I., Manjo, G.: Cell-to-cell herniae in the arterial wall. 1. The pathogenesis of vacuoles in the normal media. Am. J. Pathol. 87, 378-387 (1977)
2. Karnovsky, M.J.: The ultrastructural basis of capillary permeability studied with peroxidase as a tracer. J. Cell Biol. 35, 213-236 (1967)
3. Kletter, G., Meyermann, R., Feigl, W., Sinzinger, H.: Importance of the histological structure of the superficial temporal artery for the function of extra-intracranial bypass. In: Schmiedek, P. (ed.) Microsurgery for stroke. Springer, New York 1977
4. Kreutzberg, G.W., Hager, H.: Electron microscopical demonstration of acid phosphatase activity in the central nervous system. Histochemie 6, 254-259 (1966)
5. Mehdorn, H.M., Wiedemeyer, H., Reinhardt, V., Gerhard, L., Zais, E.: Histologische Veränderungen der A. temporalis superficialis und ihre Bedeutung für die extra-intrakranielle Bypass-Operation. Neurochirurgia 26, 181-186 (1983)
6. Meyermann, R., Ahyai, A., Kletter, G., Pini, C.: Ultrastructural control of small vessels following microsurgical intervention by tissue adhesion with fibrin. In: Peerless, S.J., McCormick, C.W.

(eds.) Microsurgery for cerebral ischemia, pp. 190-197. Springer, New York Heidelberg Berlin 1980

7. Meyermann, R., Kletter, G.: Histologische und ultrastrukturelle Befunde nach extraintrakraniellen Gefäßanastomosen. In: Lechner, H., Ladurner, G. (eds.) Die zerebralen transitorisch-ischämischen Attacken. Hans Huber, Bern Stuttgart Wien 1979

8. Pott, G., Staubesand, J.: Lysosomen and lysosomale Enzyme in der Wand fehlbelasteter Arterien der Ratte. Res. Exp. Med. 170, 271-281 (1977)

9. Reese, T.S., Karnovsky, M.J.: Fine structural localization of a blood brain barrier to exogenous peroxidase. J. Cell Biol. 34, 207-217 (1967)

10. Webster, W.S., Bishop, S.P., Geer, J.C.: Experimental aortic intimal thickening. Am. J. Pathol. 76, 265-274 (1974)

11. Wilkinson, I.M.S.: The vertebral artery. Extracranial and intracranial structure. Arch. Neurol. 27, 392-396

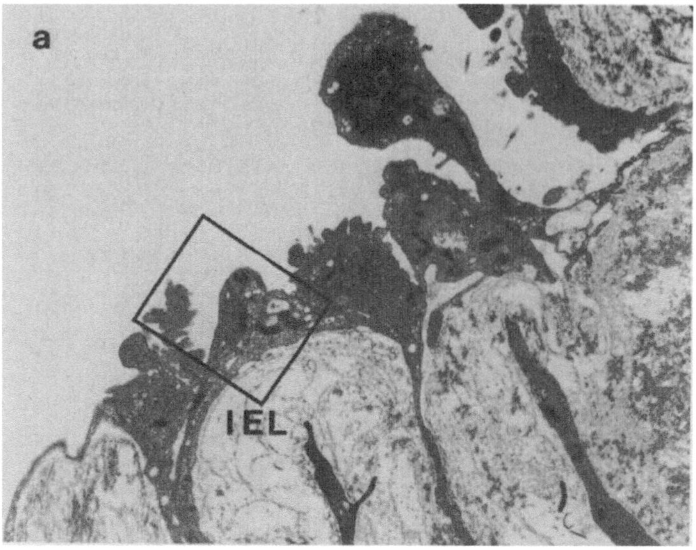

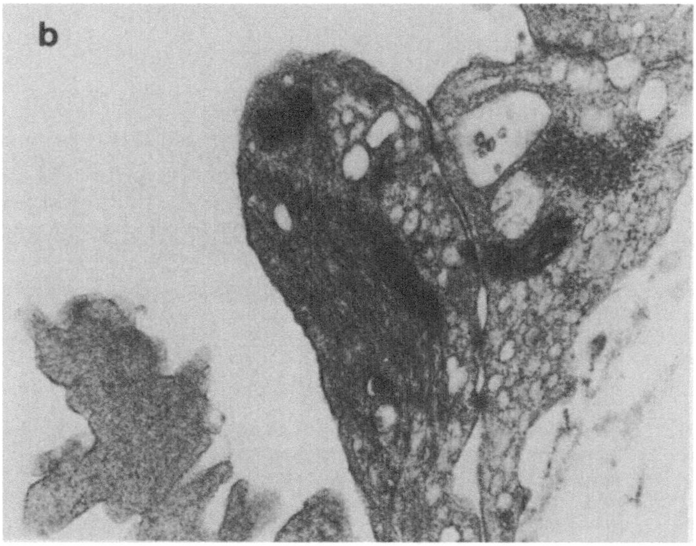

Fig. 1. Angular artery of a 63-year-old male patient. a The vessel wall displays a clear undulating internal elastic lamina *(IEL)* which causes the endothelial cells to protrude into the lumen of the vessel. These morphological changes are caused by contraction of the vessel wall. × 9650. b Higher magnification of the framed area within Fig. 1a. The endothelial cytoplasm contains an increased number of light vesicles and many filaments. The tight junctions are intact. × 42,500

Fig. 2. a,b Angular artery of an 85-year-old male, tunica intima. a The endothelial cell covers an internal elastic lamina which contains high amounts of extracellular vesicles and collagen fibrils *(arrowheads)*. × 14,580. b The dark cytoplasm of a smooth muscle cell has invaded the subendothelial space and partially replaced the light cytoplasm of the endothelial cell. Parts of the smooth muscle cytoplasmic process are still situated within the internal elastic lamina. × 31,680. c,d Same angular artery as in Fig. 1. c The smooth muscle cells within the tunica media which are surrounded by a thickened basement membrane contain large vacuoles which are filled by amorphous material and which are separated by a double membrane. × 9300. d Within the arachnoidal tissue, indicated by collagen fibrils, a swollen Schwann cell ensheaths a nerve fiber *(NF)*, which contains neurotubules and neurofilaments. × 25,040

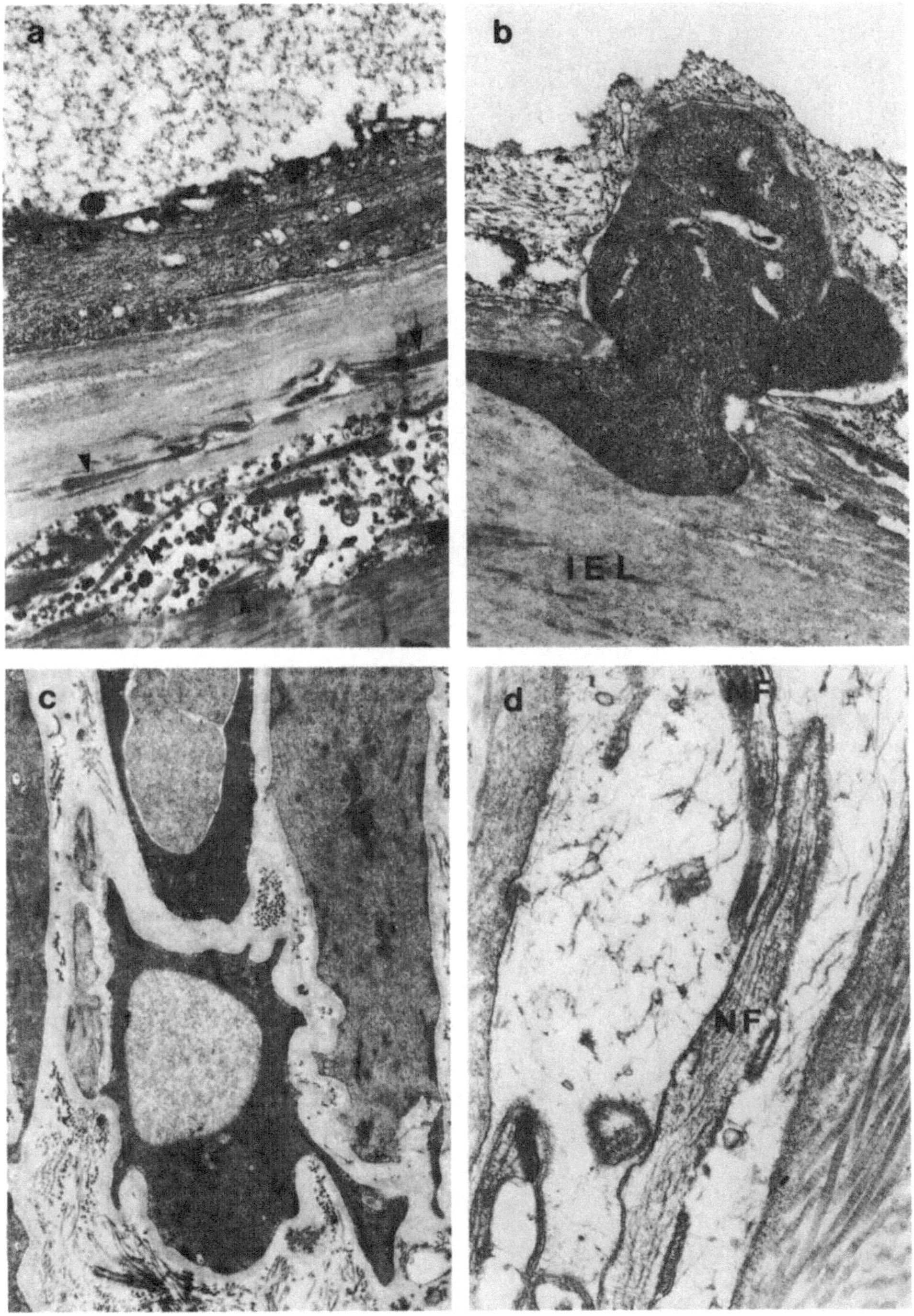
a
b
IEL
c
d
NF
NF

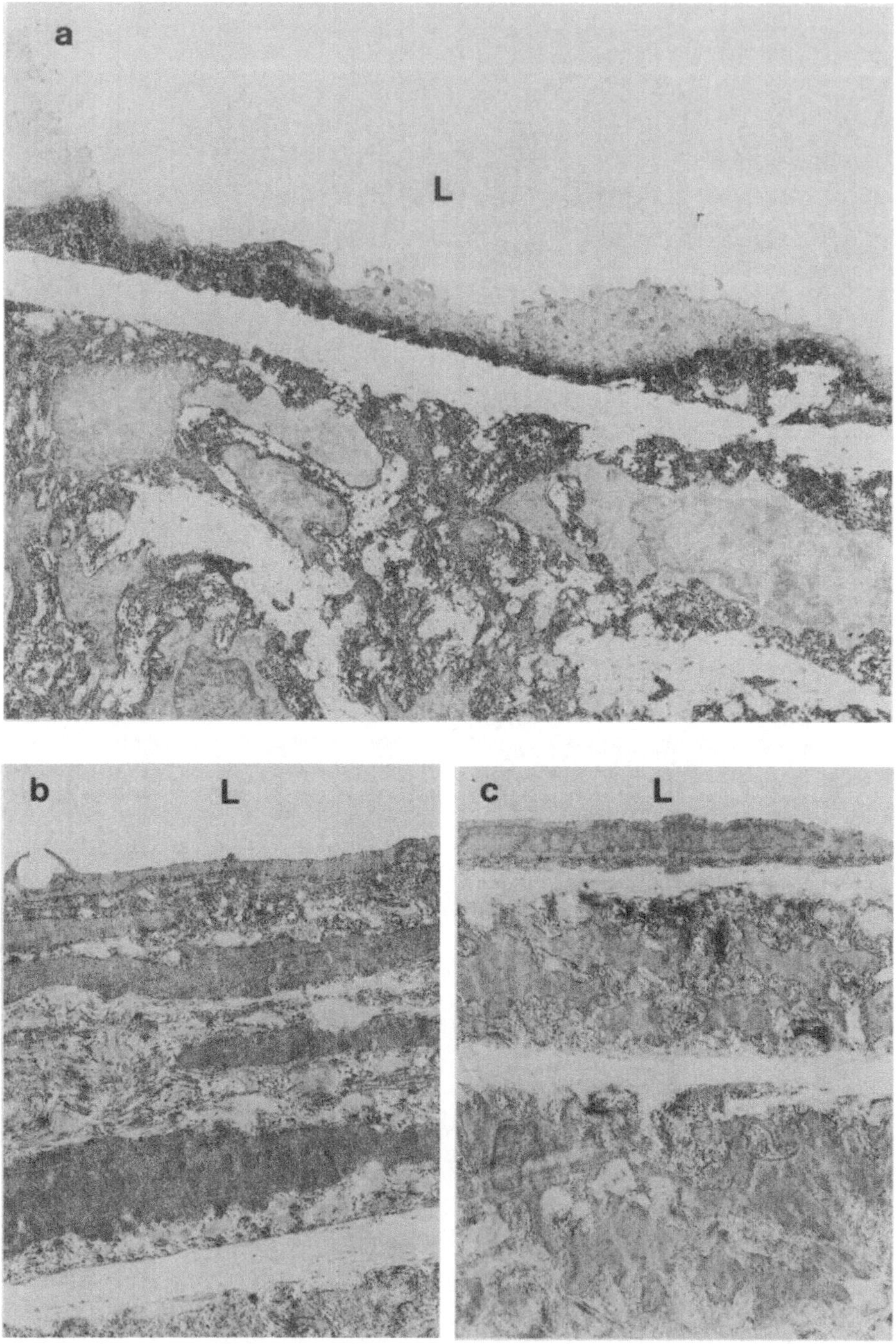

Fig. 3a-c. Legend see page 116

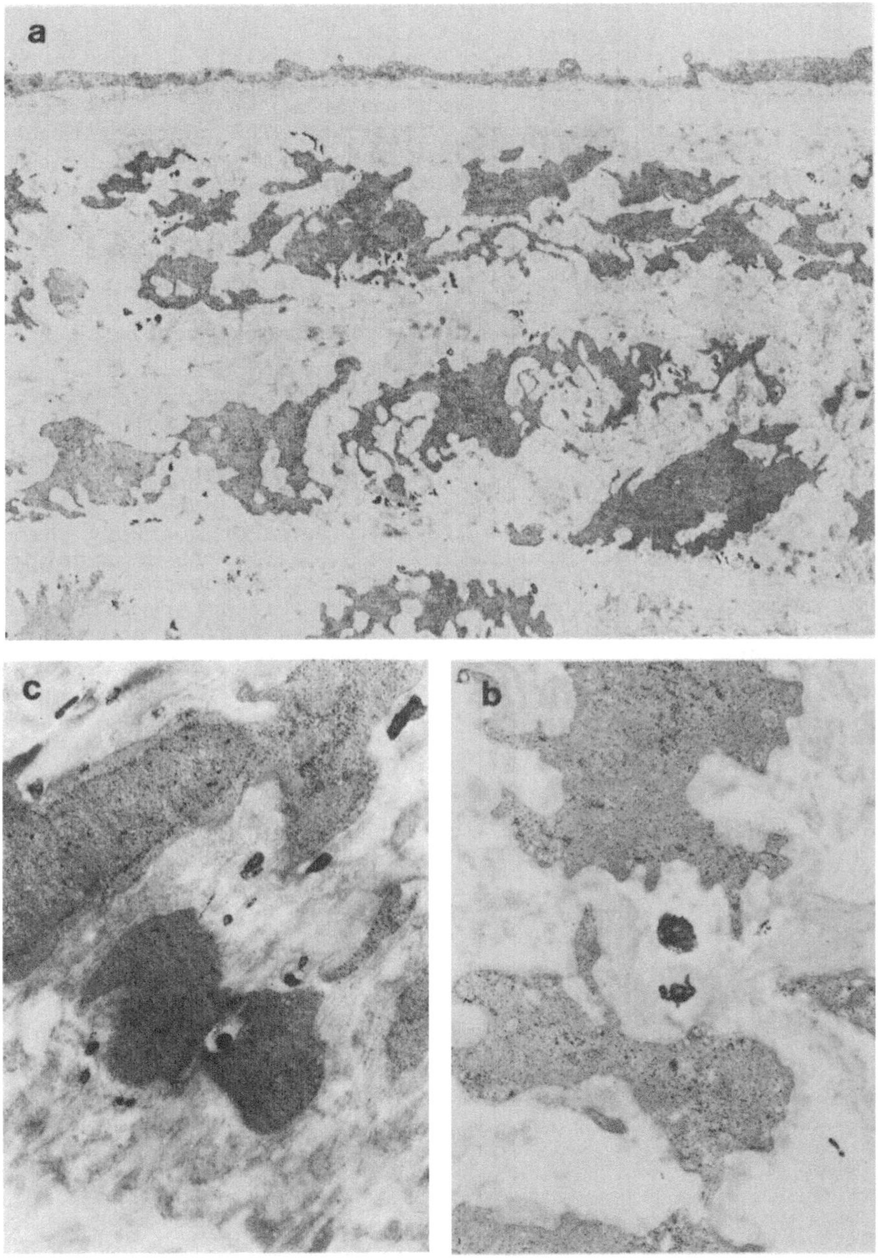

Fig. 4a-c. Legend see page 116

Figs. 3 and 4 see pages 114 and 115

Fig. 3a-c. Horseradish peroxidase study. a Proximal clipped area of an anastomosed left common carotid artery three days after operation. The subendothelial space and the extracellular space of the tunica media are filled with horseradish peroxidase. The concentration of horseradish peroxidase decreases from the intimal layer (*L* = lumen) toward the outer layers. × 6460. b Microsurgical anastomosis of the left common carotid artery six weeks after operation. Horseradish peroxidase had penetrated the intimal cell layer. However, it can be demonstrated only between the two internal intimal cell layers. × 19,200. c Proximal clipped area of the anastomosed left common carotid artery six weeks after operation. Horseradish peroxidase can be seen in the extracellular space of the first and second smooth muscle cell layers. Compare with Fig. 3b. × 18,400

Fig. 4a-c. Acid phosphatase study. a Distal clipped area of the anastomosed left common carotid artery six weeks after operation. The extracellular space is filled with matrix vesicles, which are labeled with lead phosphate, the reaction product of acid phosphatase. × 6460. b Microsurgical anastomosis of the left common carotid artery three days after operation. The lead phosphate label seen in the extracellular matrix vesicle demonstrates the presence of acid phosphatase. × 57,000. c Distal clipped area of the left common carotid artery six weeks after operation. Structures similar to those seen in Fig. 4b are labeled with lead phosphate. × 57,000

Is the Extra-Intracranial Bypass Patent and Supplying the Brain with Additional Blood?

H. M. Keller[1], H.-G. Imhof[2], and A. Valavanis[3]

[1]Departement für Neurologie, [2]Departement für Neurochirurgie, [3]Departement für Diagnostische Radiologie, Universitätsspital, Rämistraße 100, CH-8091 Zürich

Examinations of the extracranial cerebral arteries based on direct and indirect criteria measured by continuous-wave Doppler equipment is an accepted and reliable method in the diagnostic work-up and follow-up of cerebrovascular patients with major extracranial arterial lesions (2, 7). Thus, the natural history of such lesions, their course with specific medical treatment, and the efficacy of direct surgery can be evaluated by noninvasive means. Furthermore, the patency of an extra-intracranial bypass (EC-IC bypass) can be documented by directly recording with Doppler from the vessel (3, 5, 11, 12, 15, 16). Blood flow measurements combined with inhalation techniques, e.g., with 100% O_2 and 5% CO_2 have been used to evaluate vasomotor reactivity and thus the functional reserve of the brain vessels (4, 9, 12).

Direct Doppler recordings from the EC-IC bypass with additional "natural" alternation of blood pCO_2 by means of hyperventilation and apnea were applied to evaluate EC-IC bypass patency and its functional connection to the brain vasculature in our patients.

Patients and Method

EC-IC bypass surgery between the superficial temporal artery (STA) and the middle cerebral artery (MCA) was performed in 42 patients with symptomatic occlusion or non-accessible high-grade stenosis of the carotid or middle cerebral artery. Sixteen patients had a history of transient ischemic attacks (TIA) and 26 patients had infarction with no or only minor disability. The posterior branch of the STA was used as the donor artery if collateral blood to the ophthalmic artery was demonstrated by angiography and/or Doppler, and the more prominent branch of the STA was used if no such collateral blood flow existed. Prior to operation all patients had a complete neurovascular diagnostic work-up, including routine cerebrovascular Doppler examination, Doppler recordings from the STA as the possible donor artery, and selective angiography of both carotid arteries and at least one vertebral artery. Regular clinical examinations combined with routine Doppler examination and Doppler recordings from the EC-IC bypass and the contralateral STA have been performed every 3-6 months for 1-6 years after the operation (mean, 2.9 years). With one exception, no patient has suffered another TIA or stroke on the operated side. Twenty-two patients had postoperative angiography, usually 3-12 months after the operation.

Blood flow registrations from the site of the EC-IC bypass and the STA were performed with the Doppler probe held over the zygomatic portion of the arteries with the patient at rest, after hyperventilation (20-30 quickly and deeply performed breaths), as well as after apnea of

Advances in Neurosurgery, Vol. 13
Edited by H. Dietz, M. Brock, and M. Klinger

varying duration, depending on the patient's condition. With the patient at rest, bypass patency was assumed if the Doppler recordings showed increased diastolic blood flow, since peripheral resistance of the brain vasculature is lower than the resistance of a "normal" STA territory (11, 12). Blood flow signals of the STA before bypass surgery, as well as of the contralateral STA before and after surgery, were used for comparison. A functional connection of the bypass to the brain vasculature was assumed if the hyperventilation-apnea test was positive, i.e., a decrease of diastolic blood flow signals occurred after hyperventilation, and an increase after apnea. The former corresponds to a decrease in arterial pCO_2 during hyperventilation, the latter to an increase in arterial pCO_2 and to lesser extent in pCO_2 during apnea (8). An occluded or functionally insufficient bypass was assumed if the hyperventilation-apnea test had a very weak or no effect on blood flow recordings from the vessel. Since arterial pCO_2 is a more potent vasoregulator for cerebral arteries than for the extracranial arteries of the skull, a markedly weaker effect on blood flow recordings from a "normal" STA during the hyperventilation-apnea test can be expected (8).

Results (Table 1)

A permanent increase in diastolic blood flow signals from the EC-IC bypass was observed in 24 patients, indicating a patent bypass. Additional hyperventilation-apnea testing demonstrated a major decrease in diastolic blood flow after hyperventilation and an increase at the end of the apnea phase compared to the blood flow recordings with the patient at rest. Angiography was performed in 12 of these patients and major filling of intracranial arteries through the bypass was demonstrated. Additional Doppler recordings from the external or common carotid artery near the carotid bifurcation showed a marked decrease of blood flow when the EC-IC bypass was compressed digitally over two to three cardiac cycles (Figs. 1, 2a). Furthermore, a "long-distance" effect of bypass blood flow could be demonstrated by Doppler recordings from the periorbital branches of the ophthalmic artery in four of these patients. Hereby, reserved blood flow in the ophthalmic artery before the operation reinverted to normal intra-extracranial ophthalmic artery blood flow after the operation (6, 15). This "long-distance" effect of the bypass indicating major collateral blood flow through this vessel to the brain was real, since the posterior branch of the STA was used as the donor artery in these patients. Thus, a possible feeding vessel of the "natural" ophthalmic artery collateral pathway, i.e., the anterior branch of the STA, was not influenced directly during the operation. This interpretation was further supported by the follow-up angiograms of these patients. On these, no collateral blood flow through the ophthalmic artery could be demonstrated, contrary to the preoperative angiograms (Fig. 1).

Table 1. Long-term "Doppler" patency of the EC-IC bypass in 42 patients

No. of patients		42
Localization of obstruction	Extracranial	36
	Intracranial	6
Angiography performed	Preop.	42
	Postop.	22
"Doppler"patency of EC-IC bypass		
- Diastolic blood flow increased	Permanent	24
	Transient	18
- Hyperventilation-apnea test	Normal	37
	Pathol.	5

Diastolic blood flow in the EC-IC bypass was markedly increased immediately and during 2 weeks to 12 months after the operation in the other 18 patients. During further follow-up examinations, however, a minor decrease in increased diastolic blood flow signals from the bypass was observed in nine patients and a major decrease in another nine patients. The hyperventilation-apnea test remained normal in 13 patients, indicating a weaker but still patent bypass functionally connected to the brain vasculature (Fig. 2b). In four of these patients with a markedly decreased diastolic blood flow in their bypass 2 weeks to 12 months after surgery, an increase in blood flow was observed 3-9 months later, indicating only a transient "malfunction" of the iatrogenic brain vessels (Fig. 3). No hyperventilation-apnea reaction was observed in the other five patients, indicating permanent occlusion of the bypass (Fig. 4). Angiography was performed in ten patients of the flow increase-decrease group and confirmed Doppler diagnosis in all cases.

Discussion

Direct Doppler recordings from the EC-IC bypass with the patient at rest to evaluate its patency have been used in other series (3, 5, 14). Since the donor STA changes from an external to an internal carotid type artery, increased diastolic blood flow signals compared to preoperative recordings or to simultaneous recordings from the contralateral STA can be expected (11, 14). Thus, a major increase in diastolic blood flow signals by Doppler generally correlates with significant collateral blood flow through the bypass angiographically. This was also demonstrated angiographically 3-12 months after surgery in 16 of the 33 patients with a major increase in diastolic blood flow signals by Doppler (the other 17 patients had no follow-up angiography). Additional functional testing with hyperventilation-apnea demonstrated a major decrease in diastolic blood flow signals after hyperventilation and an increase after apnea, compared to the registrations with the patient at rest. Thus, bypass patency as well as its functional connection to the brain vasculature can be further confirmed with the hyperventilation-apnea maneuver.

A major increase in diastolic blood flow by Doppler was observed in all 42 patients immediately after the operation. A decrease to preoperative or even lower values occurred in nine patients 2 weeks to 12 months after surgery. Had bypass surgery failed in these patients? Hyperventilation-apnea maneuvers were followed by blood flow alterations in four of these patients, while in the other five blood flow signals remained unchanged during the provocation test. Thus the former patients still had a patent bypass functionally connected to the brain vasculature, while in the latter a functionally insufficient, e.g., occluded bypass had to be assumed. In the former patients collateral blood flow to the brain seemed insignificant, but these patients had at least a potential additional collateral which could be activated if the cerebrovascular territory appropriate to the EC-IC bypass had a need for additional blood, while in the latter patients no such reserve existed (4). The results of noninvasive Doppler recordings from the EC-IC bypass were confirmed with postoperative angiography in six patients of this group (the other three patients had no follow-up angiograms). The reason for blood flow reduction in an EC-IC bypass, or occlusion of the bypass during long-term follow-up remains obscure; speculations on this subject, however, are beyond the scope of this contribution.

Doppler registration from the EC-IC bypass with or without provocation maneuvers such as the hyperventilation-apnea test generally do not allow quantitative assessment of volume blood flow through the bypass to the brain. Doppler registrations represent instantaneous blood flow velocity rather than quantitative blood flow values. Thus, if the lumen of the

EC-IC bypass increases during long-term follow-up, Doppler signals can decrease, while volume blood flow remains equal (10, 12, 13, 14). Since with angiography a likewise qualitative assessment of blood flow through the bypass to the brain can be evaluated, other inexpensive and quickly performable methods are needed. Doppler registrations from the bypass can be used for the quantitative approach if intraoperative recordings are performed and calibrated with additional methods such as electromagnetic flowmeter measurements or the beaker-and-stopwatch method (12, 14). A further approach with Doppler has been made with quantitative recordings of blood flow from the common carotid artery with and without digital compression of the bypass (13). Further information on the efficacy of bypass surgery on intracranial blood flow can be expected from the application of a recently developed transcranial pulsed Doppler system (1).

Conclusions

The evaluation of EC-IC bypass patency by means of continuous-wave Doppler equipment with registrations of blood flow signals directly from the bypass with the patient at rest, after hyperventilation, and after apnea is a valuable and reliable diagnostic tool in the immediate and long-term follow-up of a given patient. The method can be quickly performed in addition to clinical and routine cerebrovascular Doppler examination, and no additional devices, such as 100% O_2 or 5% CO_2 inhalation equipment, are needed. Furthermore, angiography is no longer needed to document bypass patency, even in cases questionable clinically.

References

1. AASLID, R., MARKWALDER, T.M., NORNES, H.: Noninvasive transcranial Doppler ultrasound recordings of flow velocity in the basal cerebral arteries. J. Neurosurg. 57, 796-774 (1982)
2. BÜDINGEN, H.J., von REUTERN, D.M., FREUND, J.J.: Doppler-Sonographie der extrakraniellen Hirnarterien. Stuttgart, New York: Georg Thieme Verlag 1982
3. CAVAILLOLES, F., REDONDO, A., BERTHELOT, J., BOK, B., ABOULKER, J.: Les anastomoses extra-intracraniennes: Controle de leur perméabilité par effect Doppler. Neurochirurgie 24, 361-366 (1978)
4. HALSEY, J.H., MORAWETZ, R.B., BLAUENSTEIN, U.W.: The hemodynamic effect of STA-MCA bypass. Stroke 13, 163-167 (1982)
5. HOPMAN, H., GRATZL, O., SCHMIEDEK, P., SCHNEIDER, I.: Dopplersonographic control of microvascular bypass function. In: SCHMIEDEK, P. GRATZL, O., SPETZLER, R.F. (eds.). Microsurgery for stroke, pp. 230-232. New York, Heidelberg, Berlin: Springer-Verlag 1977
6. HYES, A.C., BAKER, P.-C., REICHMAN, O.H.: Noninvasive evaluation of patients with extracranial to intracranial bypass. Stroke 13, 365-368 (1982)
7. KRIESSMANN, A., BOLLINGER, A., KELLER, H.: Praxis der Doppler-Sonographie. Stuttgart, New York: Georg Thieme Verlag 1982
8. LÜBBERS, D.W.: Physiologie der Gehirndurchblutung. In: GÄNSHIRT, H. (ed.). Der Hirnkreislauf, pp. 214-260. Stuttgart: Georg Thieme Verlag 1972
9. MEYER, J.S., NAKAJIMA, S., OKABE, T., AMANO, T. CENTENO, R., LEE, Y.Y., LEVINE, J., LEVINTHAL, R., ROSE, J.: Redistribution of cerebral blood flow following STA-MCA bypass in patients with hemispheric ischemia. Stroke 13, 774-784 (1982)

10. MORITAKE, K., GRATZL, O.: Morphological and clinical analysis of extra-intracranial bypass I. Clinical and angiographical analysis. Arch Psychiatr Nervenkr 232, 325-340 (1982)

11. MORITAKE, K., HANDA, H., YONEKAWA, Y., NAGATA, I.: Ultrasonic Doppler assessment of hemodynamics in superficial temporal-middle cerebral artery anastomosis. Surg Neurol 13, 249-257 (1980)

12. MÜLLER, H.R.: Evaluation of cranial blood flow by means of ultrasonic Doppler techniques. In: BARNETT, J., PAOLETTI, P., FLAMM, E., BRAMBILLA, G. (eds.). Cerebrovascular diseases: New trends in surgical and medical aspects, pp. 77-90. Amsterdam, New York, Oxford: Elsevier/North Holland Biomedical Press 1981

13. MÜLLER, H.R., GRATZL, O.: Quantitative Funktionsprüfung des ATS/ACM-Bypasses mittels eines neuartigen Ultraschall-Flowmeters. Ultraschall in der Medizin 1, 217-222 (1980)

14. MÜLLER, H.R., SAIA, A., PISTOLLATO, G., GRATZL, O.: Dopplersonographische Verlaufskontrollen nach ATS/ACM-Bypassoperationen. In: HINSELMANN, M., ANLIKER, M., MEUDT, R. (eds.). Ultraschalldiagnostik in der Medizin, pp. 300-301. Stuttgart, New York: Georg Thieme Verlag 1980

15. TANAKA, K., NUKADA, T., YONEDA, S., MAIZUMI, M., IWATA, Y.: Ultrasonic Doppler studies after superficial temporal-middle cerebral artery anastomosis. Angiology 32, 128-136 (1981)

16. ZUMSTEIN, B., KELLER, H.M., LUETOLF, U.: Noninvasive management of stroke patients by Doppler sonography and dynamic brain scanning. In: PEERLESS, S.J., McCORMICK, C.W. (eds.). Microsurgery for cerebral ischemia, pp. 89-94. New York, Heidelberg, Berlin: Springer-Verlag (1980)

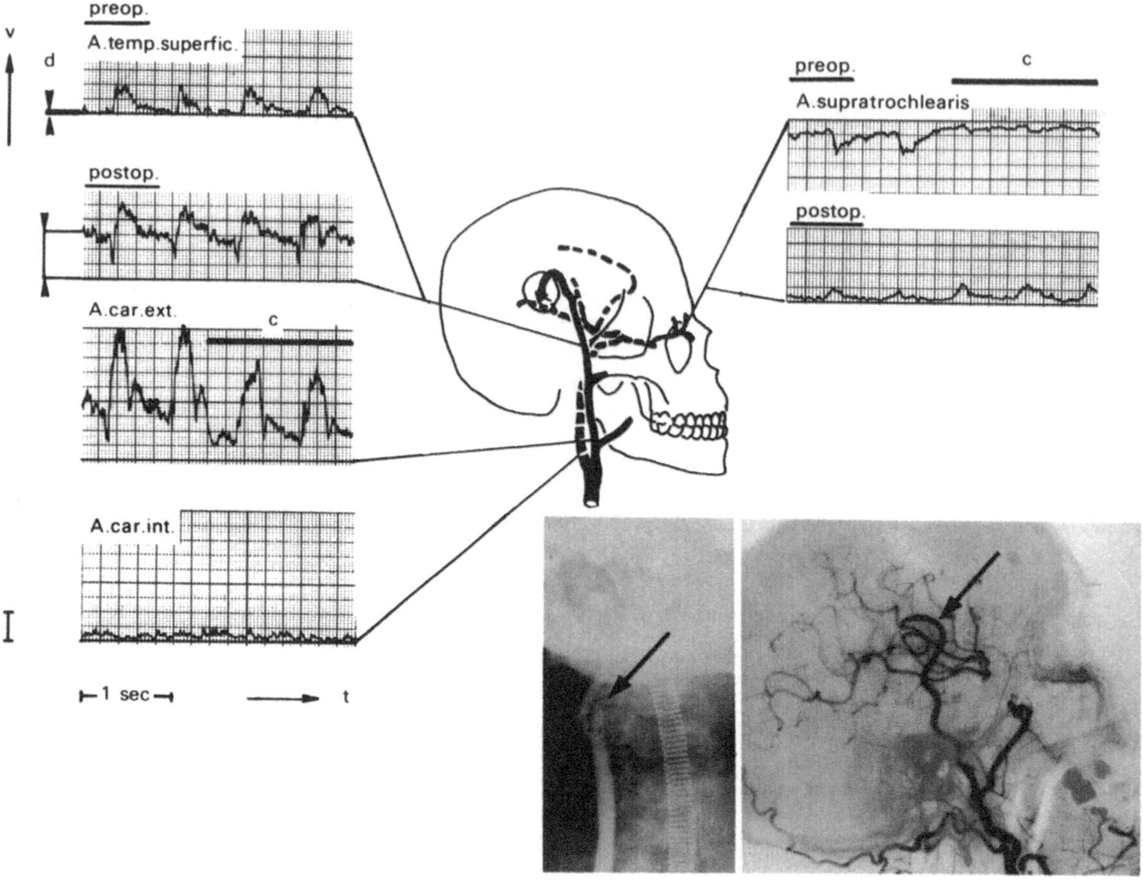

Fig. 1. Doppler blood flow recordings in a 61-year-old patient with symptomatic occlusion of the right internal carotid artery (marked with an *arrow* on the left angiogram). Low diastolic blood flow signals from the right STA before the operation changed to permanently and markedly increase values after the operation (top two registrations on the left side). Blood flow signals recorded from the right external carotid artery decreased if the bypass was compressed digitally (compression phase *c*, third registration from top). No blood flow signals were obtained by Doppler from the right internal carotid artery (bottom registration). Furthermore, a "long-distance" effect of blood flow through the bypass could be observed: Blood flow in the right supratrochlear artery was reverse before the operation with major filling from the right facial artery, proved by the flow decrease if this artery was compressed digitally (compression phase c, top registration on the right side of the figure). After surgery, blood flow direction was reinverted (second registration on the right side). Angiography was performed 9 months after the operation and demonstrated major filling of cerebral arteries through the bypass (angiogram on the right side). *v*, velocity (blood flow); *d*, diastolic value; *c*, compression phase; *t*, time

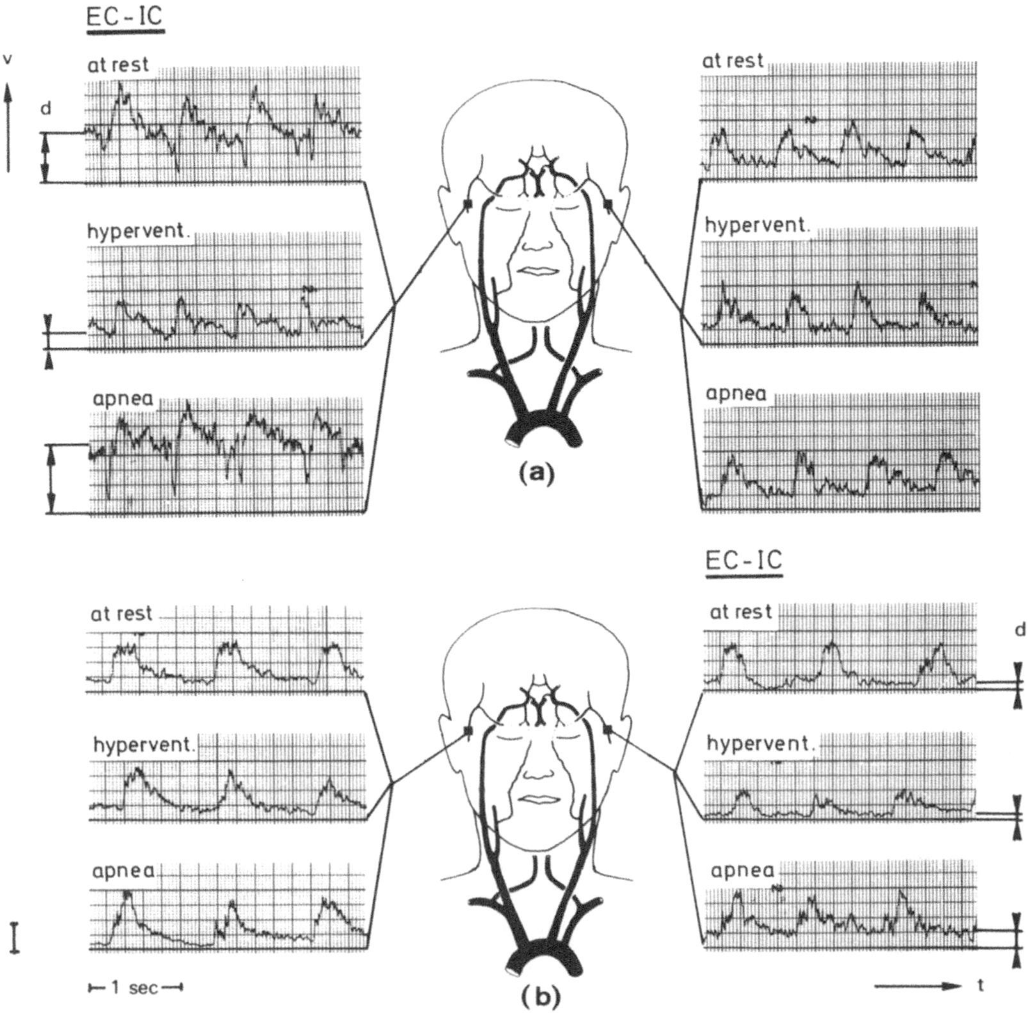

Fig. 2a, b. Effect of the hyperventilation-apnea test on Doppler blood flow recordings from a patent EC-IC bypass. a A permanent increase in diastolic blood flow signals was present in a 54-year-old patient with occlusion of the right internal carotid artery after bypass surgery. A major decrease in diastolic blood flow signals could be recorded after hyperventilation, while after apnea an increase occurred compared to the recordings with the patient at rest. No or only minor alterations of blood flow signals were observed in the contralateral STA. b A transient increase in diastolic blood flow signals was observed in a 60-year-old patient with occlusion of the left internal carotid artery. One year after surgery, however, blood flow in the bypass was decreased, and no difference in the Doppler recordings from the bypass and the contralateral STA was present. The hyperventilation-apnea test, however, was normal on the side of the bypass, i.e., a flow decrease occurred after hyperventilation and an increase in diastolic blood flow recordings after apnea, indicating a functional connection between the bypass and the brain vasculature. No such alterations could be observed on the right side

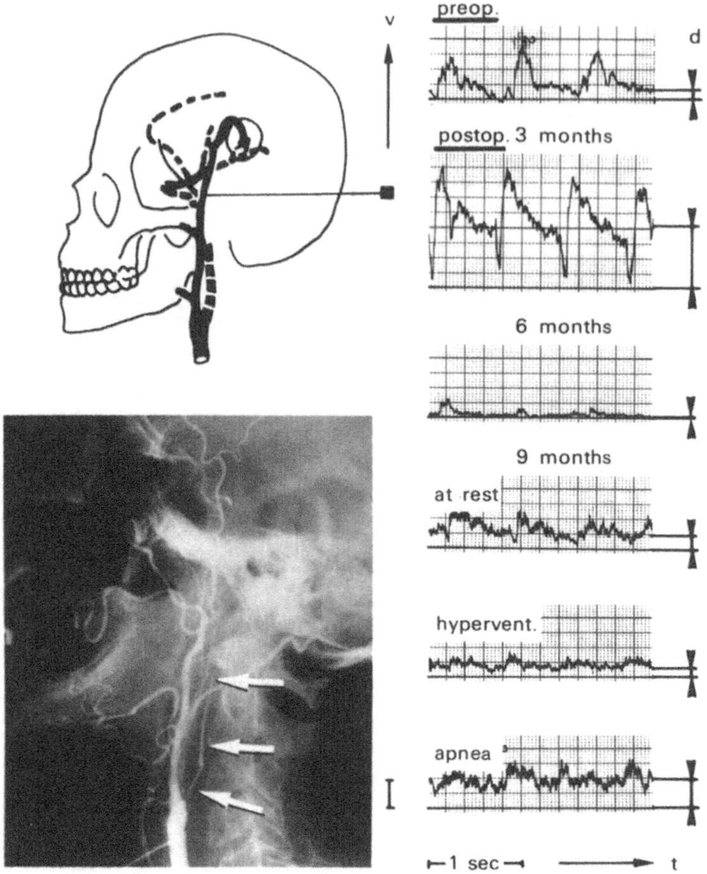

Fig. 3. Results of Doppler EC-IC bypass testing in a 58-year-old patient with symptomatic obstructions in the left internal carotid artery (preoperative angiogram demonstrates high-grade stenosis at the bifurcation marked with three *arrows*, and occlusion near the base of the skull). Diastolic blood flow signals of the bypass were significantly increased during the first 3 months after surgery (top two registrations). A major decrease was observed 3 months later, but the hyperventilation-apnea test was normal (third registration from top with the patient at rest). Another 3 months later blood flow recordings with Doppler indicated increased blood flow, which was still weaker than during the first 3 months after operation. The hyperventilation-apnea test was normal (bottom three registrations). Thus the EC-IC bypass obviously was "redimensioned" between the 4th and 9th months postoperatively.

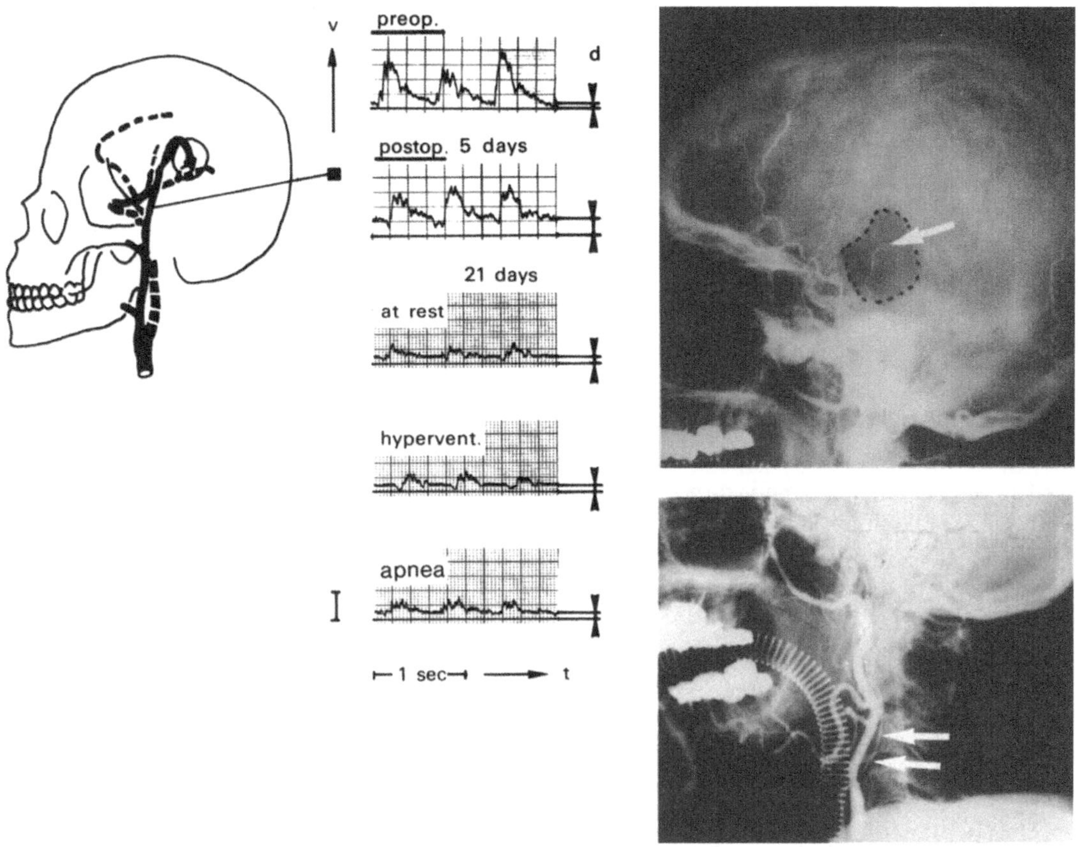

Fig. 4. Results of Doppler EC-IC bypass testing in a 52-year-old female patient with high-grade stenosis of the left internal carotid artery between the bifurcation and the clinoidal portion and occlusion in the supraclinoidal region. The bypass was patent until the patient was discharged from the hospital (increased diastolic blood flow signals after the operation compared to preoperative recordings, top two registrations, normal hyperventilation-apnea reaction). One day after discharge, the patient suffered a TIA with aphasia and paresis of the right leg lasting 1 min. Bypass blood flow signals were markedly reduced, and hyperventilation-apnea maneuvers did not influence blood flow recordings from the bypass (bottom three registrations). During further follow-up examination blood flow signals from the bypass remained pathological, indicating occlusion of the vessel. Angiography performed 3 months later demonstrated occlusion of the bypass within the region of the craniotomy (marked with an *arrow* in the upper angiogram)

Transcranial Doppler Findings in Extracranial-Intracranial Bypass Surgery

A. Harders, J. Gilsbach, and W. Haßler
Neurochirurgische Universitätsklinik, Klinikum der Albert-Ludwigs-Universität, Hugstetter Straße 55, D-7800 Freiburg

Introduction

Intracranial hemodynamics that change after the cervical or intracranial occlusion of the carotid artery until now have been investigated by angiography or by cerebral blood flow measurements (xenon). Using transcranial Doppler sonography, we are now preoperatively able to determine flow velocities and flow directions of the larger vessels of the circle of Willis. Postoperatively, the hemodynamic effect of the bypass on cerebral vessel circulation can be investigated by compressing the donor artery. Our experiences after using this method of investigation for one year are described on the basis of 20 patients with occlusion of the carotid artery.

Materials and Methods

Using a 2 MHz Doppler system with pulsed ultrasound emission developed by AASLID (1-3), it is possible for the first time to measure the flow velocity in the cerebral vessels. Measurements are made through "cranial windows" of thin bony areas, either temporally, frontally, or through the orbit. The depth of measurement can be varied by means of range-gating. The Doppler frequency spectrum is demonstrated by a real time frequency analyzer. A flow adapter identifies the direction of flow. The following vessels are investigated through the temporal and frontal bone openings: the middle cerebral artery at a depth of 3-5 cm, the horizontal part of the anterior cerebral artery and the posterior cerebral artery at a depth of 6-7 cm, and the terminal internal carotid artery at 5.5-6.0 cm. The flow in the carotid siphon is recorded transorbitally at a depth of 7 cm using the ophthalmic artery as a guide.

Figure 1 shows the frequency spectra of cerebral vessels with normal flow velocities and pulse waveforms. The time averaged maximum velocity is 1.6 ± 0.3 kHz in the middle artery, 1.3 ± 0.3 kHz in the proximal anterior cerebral artery, and 1.1 ± 0.3 kHz in the posterior cerebral artery. Furthermore, compression tests can be carried out to identify the arteries. While the velocities in the middle cerebral artery are being measured and compression of the homolateral cervical carotid artery is being done, the flow velocity will decrease. During measurement of the proximal part of the posterior cerebral artery, there will be an increase in flow due to an increased flow from the basilar artery. It is difficult to register a signal from the proximal part of the anterior cerebral artery, since there are anatomical variations in the anterior part of the circle of Willis. However, if there is a marked increase in flow during compression of the contralateral cervi-

Advances in Neurosurgery, Vol. 13
Edited by H. Dietz, M. Brock, and M. Klinger

cal carotid artery and if the flow goes away from the probe, we then know that there is good cross-flow through the proximal part of the anterior cerebral artery. On the other hand, the direction of flow is towards the probe following compression of the ipsilateral cervical carotid artery.

Among patients with symptomatic occlusion of the internal carotid artery, preoperatively the flow pattern of the vessels on the affected side show damped waveforms and reduced velocities. On the other hand, we find high velocities in the vessels that take part in the collateral circulation (Fig. 2). A reversed flow in the proximal part of the anterior cerebral artery is a reliable sign of low resistance in the internal carotid artery system. High velocities with increased diastolic flow can also be measured in the posterior cerebral artery.

Using the 20 MHz microvascular Doppler (4), we can determine - intraoperatively and postoperatively - whether the bypass joins the brain circulation. With the 2 MHz transcranial Doppler we find postoperatively at a depth of 2 cm an "internal type" waveform with a high diastolic flow in the superficial temporal artery if the bypass is working properly (Fig. 3). By compressing the STA and measuring the velocities in the middle cerebral artery, we found the following reaction types: (1) flow reduction, (2) no flow, and (3) reversed flow (Fig. 4).

Discussion

The transcranial 2 MHz Doppler with pulsed ultrasound emission is a new and important tool for the diagnostics and follow-up of cerebral vascular disease. The noninvasive method can be repeated as often as necessary. Besides being able to determine whether the donor artery contributes to the brain circulation, one can establish the hemodynamic changes in some of the cerebral vessels. In patients with symptomatic occlusion of the internal carotid artery, the bypass causes an increase in velocity in the middle cerebral artery while the physiological collateral flow in the proximal part of the anterior cerebral artery can remain constant.

Postoperative control angiography is no longer necessary for patency control.

References

1. Aaslid, R., Markwalder, T.-M., Nornes, H.: Noninvasive transcranial Doppler ultrasound recording of flow velocity in basal cerebral arteries. J. Neurosurg. 57, 769-774 (1982)
2. Aaslid, R., Huber, P., Nornes, H.: Evaluation of cerebrovascular spasm with transcranial Doppler ultrasound. J. Neurosurg. 60, 37-41 (1984)
3. Aaslid, R., Nornes, H.: Musical murmurs in human cerebral arteries after subarachnoid hemorrhage. J. Neurosurg. 60, 32-36 (1984)
4. Gilsbach, J.M.: Intraoperative Doppler sonography in neurosurgery. Springer, Wien New York 1983

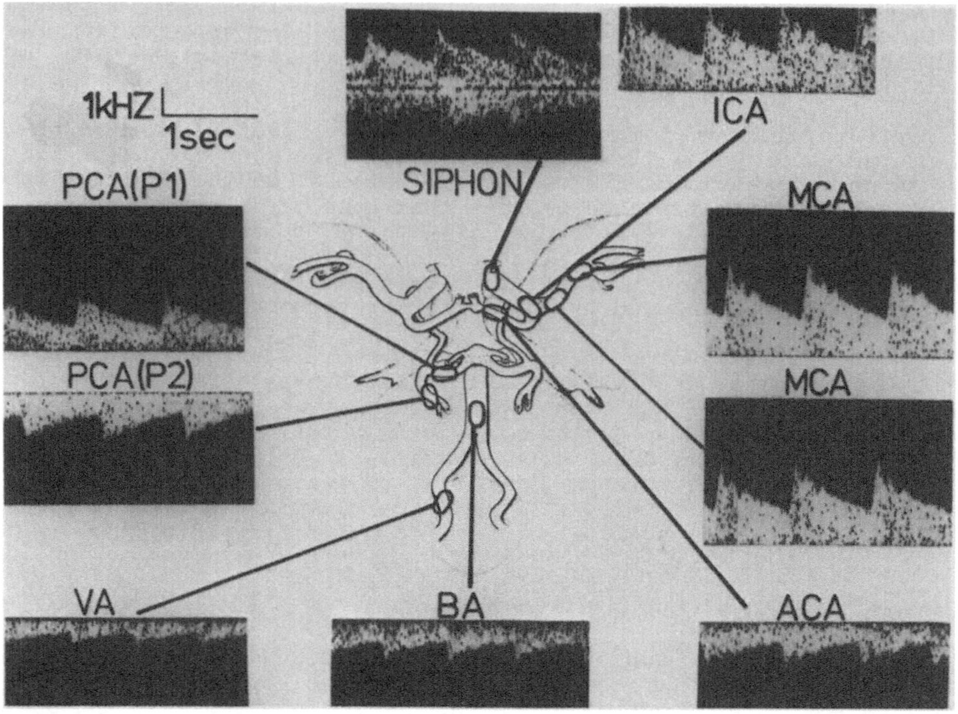

Fig. 1. Flow patterns of intracranial vessels with normal flow velocities

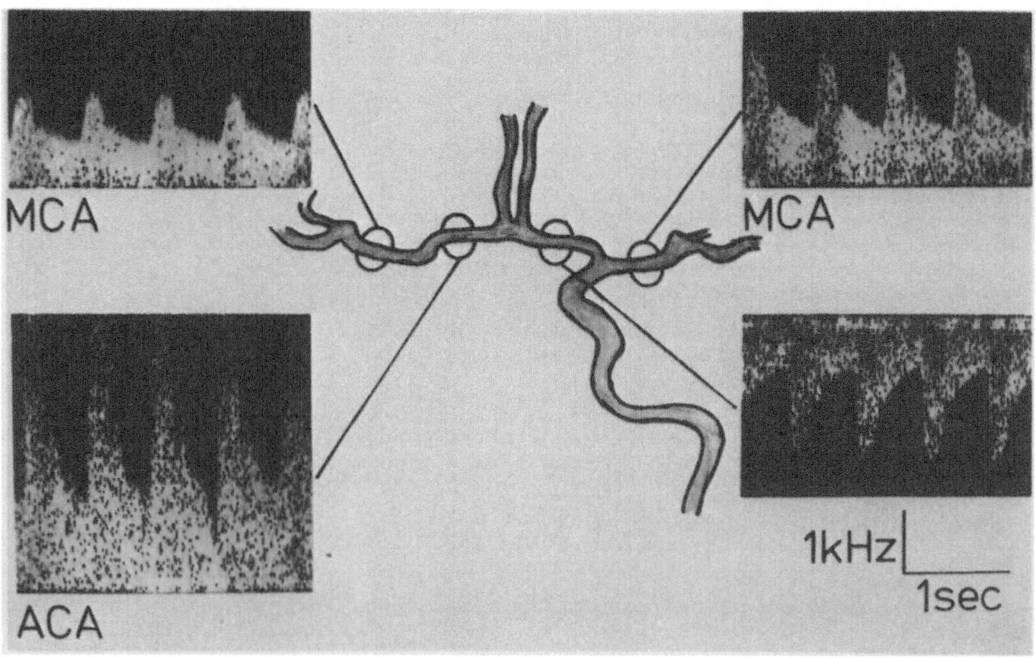

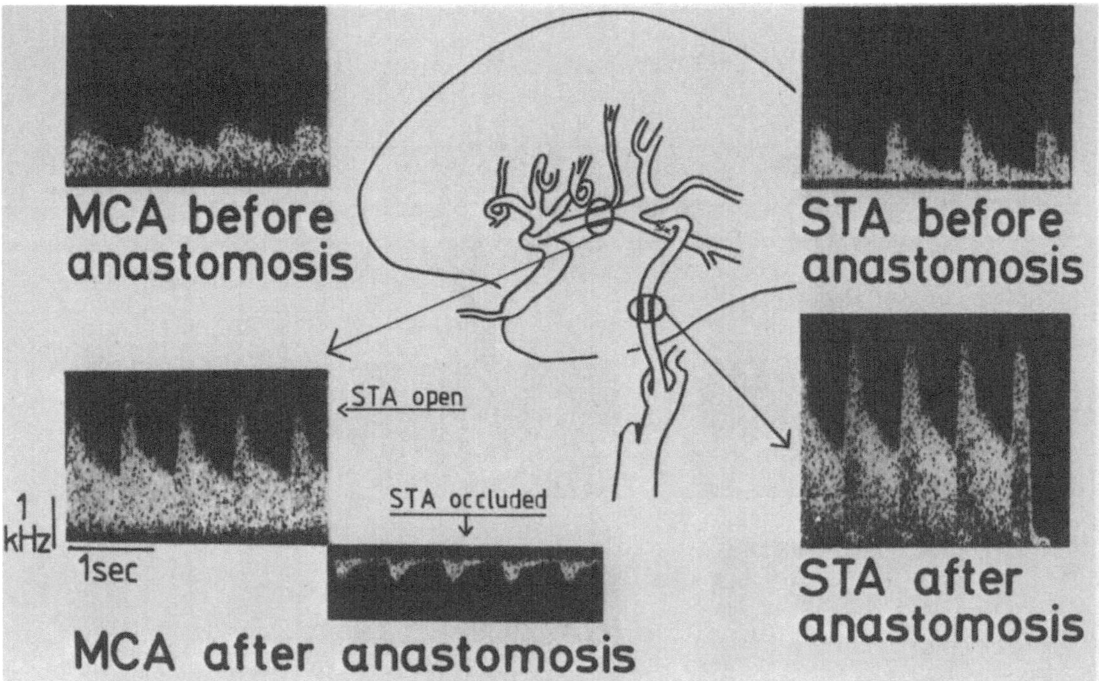

Fig. 3. Hemodynamic changes following a superficial temporal-middle cerebral artery bypass operation. The flow pattern of the donor artery changed from an "external type" with high resistance to an "internal type" with low resistance. This indicates that the bypass is connected to the brain circulation. In the MCA the flow velocity increases. After compression of the STA the high bypass-induced flow in the MCA stops and the original slow flow can be measured

---

Fig. 2. Flow patterns of a 63-year-old patient with occlusion of the cervical internal carotid artery on the right side. The velocities in the MCA are reduced and the pulse waveforms are damped. In the left proximal ACA the velocity is increased and the direction of the blood flow is retrograde due to the high collateral flow

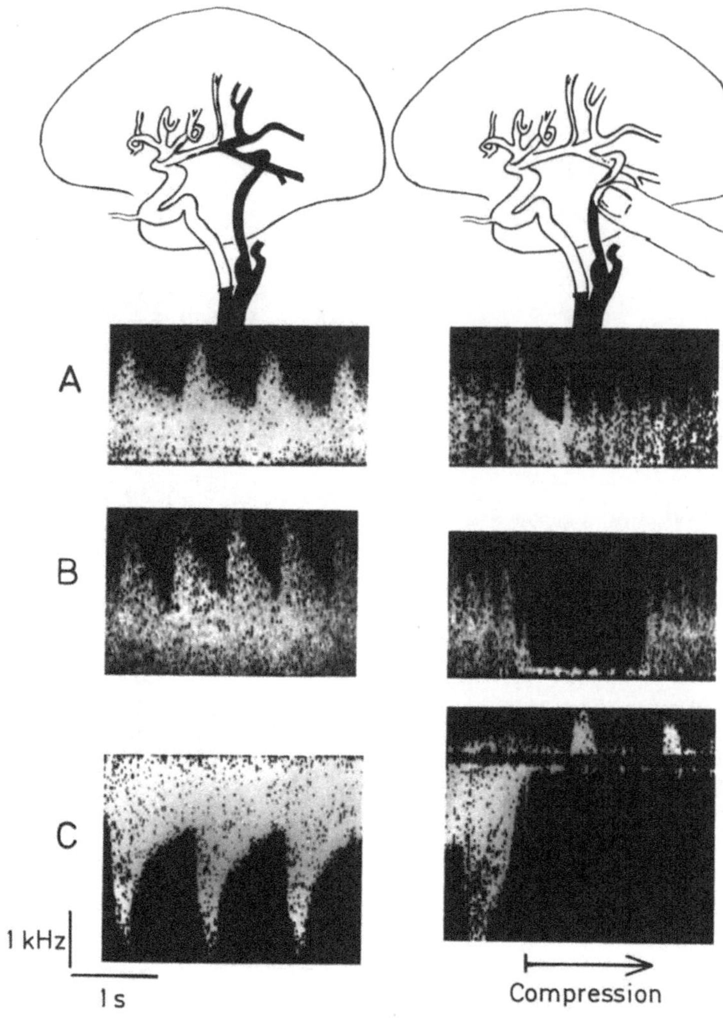

Fig. 4A-C. Three types of hemodynamic changes after bypass surgery and compression test of STA. A Flow reduction; B no flow (clinically followed by TIA); C reversed flow

Is an Intra-Extracranial Reversal of Flow Possible Following EIAB Operation?

J. Jansen
Abteilung Neurochirurgie im Zentrum Neurologische Medizin der Universität Göttingen, Robert-Koch-Straße 40, D-3400 Göttingen

Introduction

Doppler sonographic findings for patients with an extra-intracranial arterial bypass have led to discussion of the possibility of an intra-extracranial reversal of flow in the anastomosis. These Doppler sonographic observations were the starting point for an investigation as to whether and under which extra-intracerebral pressure conditions an intra-extracranial steal would be possible. Blood pressures were measured intraarterially in the radial artery (RA), the superficial temporal artery (STA), and the cortical branch of middle cerebral artery (cMCA). These data provide information about the pressure drop from extra- to intracranial circulation.

Methods

The intraoperative measurements were taken in patients who had been given a fentanyl anesthesia. During the preparation of the parietal branch of the STA, a relatively large branch – about 1.5 cm in length – is left on the artery. A short silicon tube is slipped over this branch up to the STA. After the STA and the cMCA have been anastomosed, the intraarterial pressure is measured over this silicon tube and a tube extension with the aid of a pressure converter. The pressure converter is placed at heart level. The intraarterial pressures – which are averaged electronically – are measured simultaneously (a) in the radial artery (RA) and the STA, (b) in the RA and the cMCA, and (c) in the RA and the proximal section of the cortical middle cerebral artery (cMCAp). The pressure curves appear continuously on a monitor. When pressure is constant, the pressure pairs are read simultaneously from the digital recording. Measurement of pressure in the STA is carried out by pinching it off on the distal portion of the catheterized branch. Pressure in the cortical artery is measured after the STA has been pinched off on the proximal portion of the branch. The pressure in the proximal portion of the cMCA is measured by an additional pinching off of the distal part of the cMCA. During individual measurements, there were fluctuations in the system pressure which is registered by means of the radial artery. Thus, in order to calculate the relative pressure drop from the STA to the cMCA and from the STA to the cMCAp, the STA pressures were computed from the system pressure at the time of the cMCA and cMCAp measurements with the aid of the measured relative pressure drop from the RA to the STA. The mathematical determination of the STA pressure is permitted because the arterial relative drop is as good as constant. This has been shown in other investigations carried out by the author (2-4).

Advances in Neurosurgery, Vol. 13
Edited by H. Dietz, M. Brock, and M. Klinger

Table 1. Summary of intraoperative intraarterial pressures of 29 patients measured in the radial artery (RA), the superficial temporal artery (STA), and the cortical branch of the middle cerebral artery (cMCA); the pressure drop (PD) from corrected STA (STA') to cMCA was calculated

No.	Pat.	Age	Mean pressures (mmHg)					PD(%)	Site of vascular disease
			RA	STA	RA	cMCA	STA'	cMCA/ STA'	
1	G.W.♀	45	86	92	87	71	93	23.7	Infraclinoidal aneurysm
2	G.W.♂	46	77	54	76	29	53.3	45.6	ICA stenosis r
3	E.F.♀	68	83	83	82	43	82	47.6	ICA stenosis r
4	M.E.♀	68	100	104	95	87	98.8	11.9	ICA stenosis l
5	W.B.♂	49	93	73	92	46	72.2	36.3	ICA stenosis l
6	G.R.♂	29	77	73	70	48	66.4	27.7	ICA stenosis l
7	H.H.♀	47	77	78	75	65	76	18.4	ICA stenosis l
8	R.Z.♂	55	77	71	80	63	73.8	14.6	MCA stenosis r
9	D.G.♂	47	91	79	88	27	76.4	64.6	ICA occlusion l
10	K.R.♂	50	87	82	84	26	79	67	ICA occlusion l
11	H.M.♂	63	84	72	84	24	72	66.7	ICA occlusion r
12	H.F.♂	57	100	100	100	57	100	43	ICA occlusion l
13	M.B.♂	66	96	92	96	54	92	41.3	ICA occlusion l
14	W.S.♂	63	110	110	90	67	90	25.6	ICA occlusion l
15	P.K.♂	57	72	73	74	62	75	17.3	ICA occlusion r
16	W.H.♂	40	90	70	90	16	70	77.1	ICA occlusion l
17	K.H.♂	67	102	94	102	52	94	44.7	ICA occlusion l
18	H.O.♂	66	103	80	112	25	87	71.3	ICA occlusion r
19	M.G.♂	52	100	106	107	37	113	67.3	ICA occlusion l
20	H.M.♂	59	92	104	91	67	102.9	34.9	ICA occlusion r
21	K.G.♂	52	93	83	82	41	73.2	44	ICA occlusion r
22	H.K.♂	59	81	82	85	28	86	67.4	ICA occlusion l
23	T.S.♂	50	100	73	105	55	76.7	28.3	ICA occlusion r
24	A.M.♀	65	96	96	85	30	85	64.7	ICA occlusion r and contralateral stenosis l
25	U.S.♂	58	84	88	76	39	79.6	51	
26	B.S.♂	68	88	88	88	54	88	38.6	
27	H.W.♀	46	112	104	110	35	102	65.7	
28	H.S.♂	56	79	76	85	55	81.8	32.8	
29	R.K.♂	66	75	71	75	39	71	45.1	

Table 2. Summary of intraoperative intraarterial pressures of 29 patients measured in the radial artery (RA), the superficial temporal artery (STA), and the proximal part of the cMCA (cMCAp); pressure drop (PD) from corrected STA (STA") to cMCAp was calculated

No.	Pat.	Age	Mean pressures (mmHg)					PD(%) cMCAp/ STA"	Site of vascular disease
			RA	STA	RA	cMCAp	STA"		
1	G.W.♀	45	86	92	87	79	93.1	15.1	Infraclinoidal aneurysm
2	G.W.♂	46	77	54	78	36	54.7	34.2	ICA stenosis r
3	E.F.♀	68	83	83	81	63	81	22.2	ICA stenosis r
4	M.E.♀	68	100	104	94	92	97.8	6	ICA stenosis l
5	W.B.♂	49	93	73	92	52	72.2	28	ICA stenosis l
6	G.R.♂	29	77	73	70	50	66.4	24.7	ICA stenosis l
7	H.H.♀	47	77	78	75	62	76	18.4	ICA stenosis l
8	R.Z.♂	55	77	71	79	68	72.8	6.6	MCA stenosis r
9	D.G.♂	47	91	79	91	39	76.4	48.9	ICA occlusion l
10	K.R.♂	50	87	82	87	30	82	63.4	ICA occlusion l
11	H.M.♂	63	84	72	86	28	73.7	62	ICA occlusion r
12	H.F.♂	57	100	100	100	68	100	32	ICA occlusion l
13	M.B.♂	66	96	92	94	55	90.1	39	ICA occlusion l
14	W.S.♂	63	110	110	90	69	90	23.3	ICA occlusion l
15	P.K.♂	57	72	73	74	66	75	12	ICA occlusion r
16	W.H.♂	40	90	70	90	20	70	71.4	ICA occlusion l
17	K.H.♂	67	102	94	103	60	94.9	36.8	ICA occlusion l
18	H.O.♂	66	103	80	108	27	83.9	67.8	ICA occlusion r
19	M.G.♂	52	100	106	100	40	106	62.3	ICA occlusion l
20	H.M.♂	59	92	104	91	78	102.9	24.2	ICA occlusion r
21	K.G.♂	52	93	83	85	48	75.9	36.8	ICA occlusion r
22	H.K.♂	59	81	82	90	33	91	63.7	ICA occlusion l
23	T.S.♂	50	100	73	104	61	75.9	19.6	ICA occlusion r
24	A.M.♀	65	96	96	90	30	90	66.7	ICA occlusion r and contralateral stenosis l
25	U.S.♂	58	84	88	76	40	79.6	49.6	
26	B.S.♂	68	88	88	90	62	90	31	
27	H.W.♀	46	112	104	107	39	99.4	60.8	
28	H.S.♂	56	79	76	79	55	76	27.6	
29	R.K.♂	66	75	71	75	40	71	43.7	

Table 3. Mean arterial pressure drop (PD) from the superficial temporal artery (STA) to the cortical branch of the middle cerebral artery (cMCA) and from the STA to the proximal part of the cMCA (cMCAp) in percent

Site of arterial disease	Mean arterial pressure drop (%)	
	STA → cMCA	STA → cMCAp
ICA aneurysm (infraclinoidal)	23.7% (n=1)	15.1% (n=1)
ICA stenosis (unilateral)	28.9% (n=7)	20.0% (n=7)
ICA occlusion (unilateral)	50.7% (n=15)	44.2% (n=15)
ICA occlusion with contralateral ICA stenosis	49.7% (n=6)	46.6% (n=6)

Results

Tables 1, 2, and 3 show the measured and calculated pressures along with the pressure drop from the calculated STA pressure (STA') to the cMCA and from the STA pressure (STA") to the cMCAp. The distribution is in accordance with the degree of arterial disease. Patients with unilateral intracranial stenosis of the internal carotid artery (ICA) (n = 7) show a mean relative pressure drop of 29% (28.87%) from the STA to the cMCA and of 20% to the cMCAp. For patients with a unilateral internal carotid occlusion, a mean pressure drop of about 51% (50.7%) from the STA to the cMCA and a mean drop of about 44% (44.2%) from the STA to the cMCAp were calculated. The mean pressure drop from the STA to the cMCA was also about 50% (49.7%) and from the STA' to the cMCAp about 47% (46.6%) in patients with ICA occlusion and contralateral ICA stenosis. One aneurysm patient showed pressure drops of about 24% to the cMCA and about 15% to the cMCAp.

Discussion

A drop in arterial pressure from the aorta to the cortical branches of the middle cerebral artery is unknown in healthy brains. BAKAY and SWEET (1) measured a 17% pressure drop from the internal carotid artery to the cortical branches of the MCA in tumor patients. This relative pressure drop is certainly somewhat too low, especially in view of the fact that, as a result of an increase in volume, an intracranial increase in pressure is to be expected and consequently an increase in the intracranial intraarterial resistance. In experiments with dogs, SYMON (5) found a mean pressure drop of 10% from the aorta to the cortical branch of the MCA (250-400 µm in diameter), and in experiments with monkeys, he found a mean drop of 13%. My own experimental investigations on cats (2-4) revealed a 25% pressure drop from the aorta to the cortical branch of the MCA (250-300 µm in diameter) (chloralose-urethan anesthesia).

A pressure drop of about 24% (23.7%) from the STA to the cMCA was calculated for the aneurysm patient - where an almost normal pressure drop can be expected. For patients with unilateral internal carotid stenosis, there is a mean relative pressure drop from STA to cMCA of about 29%. Patients with unilateral occlusion of the internal carotid artery or also with additional contralateral internal carotid stenosis exhibit a mean relative pressure drop of about 50% from the STA to the cMCA. In view of this registered pressure drop, an intra-extracranial reverse of flow is not possible. Only a reduction of the relative pressure drop of more than 24% (aneurysm), of more than 29% (ICA stenosis), or of more than 51% (ICA occlusion) can lead to a reversal of flow. Such a reduction of the relative pressure drop can occur either when the intraarterial pressure in the cortical artery increases or when the temporal pressure drops. The increase in pressure in the cortical branch of the MCA and thus the reduction of the relative pressure drop from the STA to the cMCA is only possible when the ICA is recanalized, collateral circulation is improved, or the peripheral portion of the cMCA is occluded. Occlusion is coupled with an increase in pressure in the proximal portion of the cortical branch of the MCA. Assuming a nearly normal pressure drop between 17% (5) and 24% (aneurysm), found in human investigations, or between 10% (5) and 25% (2-4), found in animal investigations, an ICA recanalization would not result in a reversal of flow. During occlusion of peripheral cMCA, the decrease in pressure to be expected – from about 29% to 20% for ICA stenosis or from about 51% to about 44% for ICA occlusion or from about 50% to about 47% for ICA occlusion and contralateral stenosis – would likewise not result in a reversal of flow.

Arterial stenoses in the arteries (common carotid artery, external carotid artery) before the anastomosis lead to an increase in the intraarterial flow resistance. Assuming that the blood supply is constant, pressure is directly proportional to the arterial resistance (Ohm's law). Then – with an increase in arterial resistance of about 29% (ICA stenosis) or 50% (ICA occlusion) – a pressure drop can be expected. This drop would lead to a termination of flow and, if the increase in the arterial resistance exceeds 29% or 50%, respectively, to a reversal of flow in the anastomosis. The Hagen-Poiseuille law

$$R = \frac{8 \cdot \eta \cdot l}{\pi \cdot r^4}$$

shows that even a very minor reduction in the radius of the artery leads to a considerable increase in arterial resistance. It does demonstrate how important it is, both before and after an EIAB operation, to recognize arterial stenoses early and to eliminate them.

Conclusion

An intra-extracranial reversal of flow is not possible after EIAB operations without an increase in the resistance in the arteries before the anastomosis. If, however, a constriction in the diameter of the artery does occur in this arterial area and there is an increase in the resistance of 29% or more in the case of ICA stenosis or of 51% or more in the case of ICA occlusion with or without contralateral stenosis, then there is a danger of a termination of flow (which would lead to a thrombosis in the anastomosis) or of an intra-extracerebral steal phenomenon.

References

1. Bakay, L., Sweet, W.H.: Cervical and intracranial intra-arterial pressure with and without vascular occlusion. Surg. Gynec. Obstet 95, 67-75 (1952)
2. Jansen, J., Berndt, U., Kanzow, E.: Anpassungsmechanismen der Widerstandsverteilung im Hirnkreislauf. Folia Angiologica 21, 353-355 (1973)
3. Jansen, J., Kanzow, E.: Pressure drop and vascular resistance in cerebral circulation. In: Klug, W., Brock, M., Klinger, M., Spoerri, O. (eds.) Advances in neurosurgery, Vol. 2, pp. 314-315. Springer, Berlin Heidelberg New York 1975
4. Kanzow, E., Jansen, J., Dieckhoff, D.: Druckabfall und Strömungswiderstand in den Arterien des Gehirn- und Extremitätenkreislaufs. In: Betz, E. (ed.) Vascular smooth muscle, pp. 80-83. Springer, Berlin Heidelberg New York 1972
5. Symon, L.: A comparative study of middle cerebral pressure in dogs and macaques. J. Physiol. 191, 449-465 (1967)

Regional Cerebral Blood Flow Measurement as a Supportive Indication for Vascular Surgical Procedures*

J. Bockhorn, A. Brawanski, and W. Ullrich
Neurochirurgische Klinik und Poliklinik der Universität Würzburg, Josef-Schneider-Straße 11, D-8700 Würzburg

The indication for surgical procedures to improve the cerebral perfusion is usually given by the clinical findings and course as well as by the results of the angiographic examination. This is true for extra-intracranial arterial bypass operations as well as for vascular surgical treatments at the internal carotid. In those cases lowered perfusion values in the regional cerebral blood flow (rCBF) measurement will be found (1), corresponding with the clinical and the angiographic findings. A change in the indication given by the clinical and angiographic findings as a result of the rCBF measurement is unusual. The clinical findings and course, the angiographic results, and the values of the rCBF measurement fit together, each supporting the indication.

The measurement of rCBF is performed with a cerebrograph with 32 detectors. Up until the beginning of 1984 the detectors were arranged in parallel (2), the flow data being calculated according to the OBRIST (4) and RISBERG (6) method. Since March 1984 we have used a helmet system with 32 detectors. With the change in the detector arrangement, the calculation modus was also changed. The values are now calculated according to OBRIST et al. (4) and using the dual artifact program of PROHOVNIK et al. (5). The graphic presentation of the values was changed with the change in the detector system.

Different to the above-mentioned situation is the indication in cases where one or more of the three parameters – clinical findings, angiographic findings, and rCBF measurement – will not match. In most cases this occurs in patients in whom screening methods, e.g., ultrasound Doppler sonography, have revealed changes in the region of the cervical carotid bifurcation during check-up for general vascular disease prior to surgical treatment of vascular changes in the extremities. In such patients more or less extensive changes in the course of the carotid arteries with regular clinical findings or only minimal clinical disturbances may be found. Often the indication for a vascular surgical procedure at the brain supplying arteries is not given, if the rCBF measurement shows normal values in the total hemispheric as well as in the regional calculations (Fig. 1). The decision against an operative procedure is based on the fact that with a sufficient perfusion of the brain, an improvement in perfusion cannot be established either by endarterectomy of a low-grade stenosis of the internal carotid artery or by an extra-intracranial arterial bypass.

A similar situation pertains in respect of patients in whom no or only minimal vascular alterations are diagnosed by ultrasound Doppler sonography, without clinical findings. In the case of a diffuse decrease

* Supported by grants of the Deutsche Forschungsgemeinschaft (Br 843/2-1)

of the cerebral perfusion in the rCBF measurement, it can be assumed that the reason for this is arteriolosclerotic changes of the small cerebral vessels (Fig. 2). An improvement of this sitation by vascular surgical procedures or by microneurosurgical revascularization measures is hardly to be anticipated. Those procedures take place at the medium-sized and large brain supplying vessels; the precapillary vessels in the area of the arterioles, however, are not reached. Therefore also in this group of patients operative measures are not indicated.

An improvement of the clinical situation certainly cannot be expected – and therefore rCBF measurement can provide a contraindication to surgical procedures – in patients in whom a generalized or localized severe decrease of the perfusion in certain brain areas is found (Fig. 3). With corresponding clinical findings it can be assumed that ischemia caused by a CVA has led to destruction of brain tissue with absence of a functional metabolism and even absence of the structural metabolism, and that only a flow through the necrotic brain areas without any participation in a useful metabolism takes place. If the perfusion values lie below the "stroke threshold", i.e., at or below values of 25 ml/100 g brain/min (3), operative measures with reconstruction of brain-supplying vessels will not improve the clinical findings.

Problematic is the indication for procedures which improve the brain perfusion in patients with regular angiographic findings and more or less severe clinical disturbances, and in whom the rCBF measurements show a decrease in perfusion localized under several detectors, in the sense of a "focal ischemia" (Fig. 4). An indication for a surgical procedure is not given on the basis of angiographic findings. In accordance with the findings of the cerebral blood flow measurements, the indication for a procedure to improve the brain perfusion has to be considered and cannot be rejected without discussion. The only procedure that can be discussed is extra-intracranial arterial bypass, for there is no reason for an endarterectomy in a normal brain-supplying vessel. However, one has to bear in mind that an extra-intracranial arterial bypass may not function owing to an insufficient pressure gradient from extra- to intracranial or that there may even be a retrograde flow from intra- to extracranial, with a steal effect.

References

1. Bockhorn, J., Brawanski, A., Gaab, M.R.: Regional cerebral blood flow and extra-intracranial bypass surgery. In: Driesen, W., Brock, M., Klinger, M. (eds.) Advances in neurosurgery, Vol. 10, pp. 333-339. Springer, Berlin Heidelberg New York 1982
2. Brawanski, A., Gaab, M.R., Bockhorn, J.: Nichtinvasive Messung der regionalen cerebralen Durchblutung. Acta Medicotechn. 30, 7-9 (1982)
3. Deshmukh, V.D., Meyer, J.S.: Noninvasive measurement of regional cerebral blood flow in man. Spectrum, New York London 1978
4. Obrist, W.D., Thompson, H.K., Wang, H.S., Wilkinson, W.E.: Regional cerebral blood flow estimated by 133-xenon inhalation. Stroke 6, 245-256 (1975)
5. Prohovnik, I., Knudsen, E., Risberg, J.: Accuracy of models and algorithms for determination of fast-compartment flow by noninvasive 133-xenon clearance. In: Magistretti, P.L. (ed.) Functional radionuclide imaging of the brain, pp. 87-115. Raven Press, New York 1983
6. Risberg, J.: Regional cerebral blood flow measurements by 133-xenon inhalation: Methodology and applications in neuropsychology and psychiatry. Brain and Language 9, 9-34 (1980)

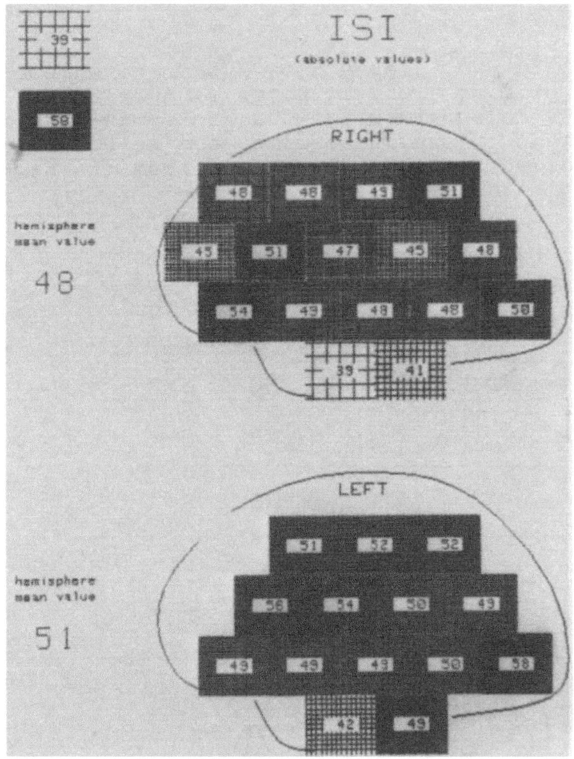

Fig. 1. Normal rCBF values in a patient with internal carotid occlusion on the left, without clinical disturbances. Found during check-up for femoral artery disease. No indication for vascular surgical procedures (EIAB)

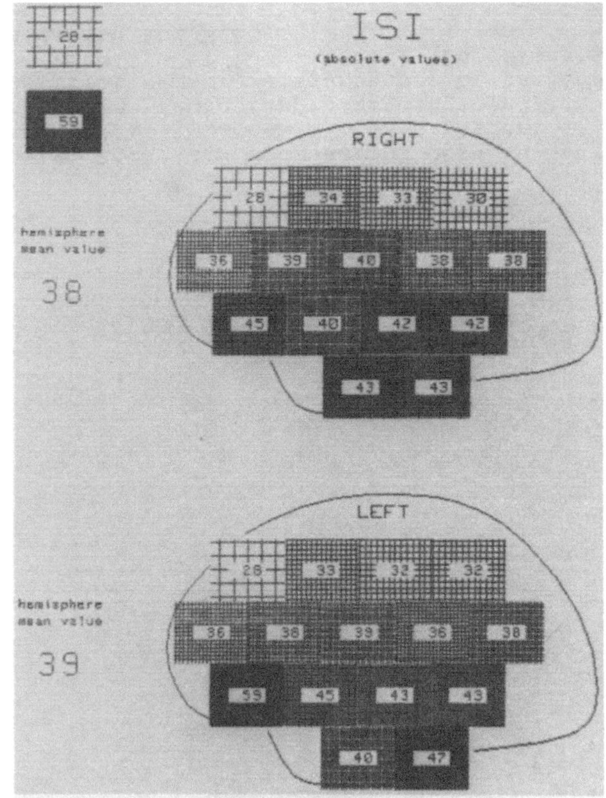

Fig. 2. Diffuse decrease of rCBF values (mean hemispheric flows 38 and 39 ml/100 g brain/min) as a sign of generalized vascular disorders in the distribution of precapillary vessels (arteriolosclerosis)

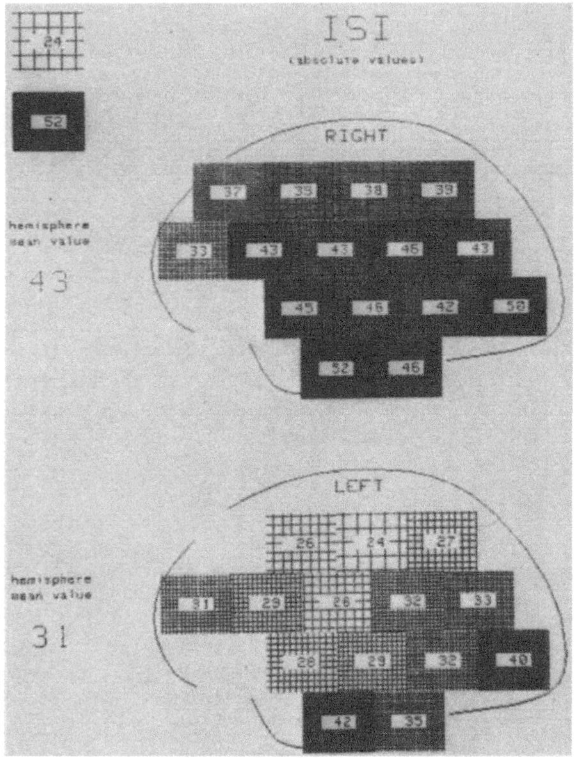

Fig. 3. Decrease of the cerebral perfusion below the "stroke threshold" over large areas of the left hemisphere. Angiography revealed internal carotid occlusion on the left side

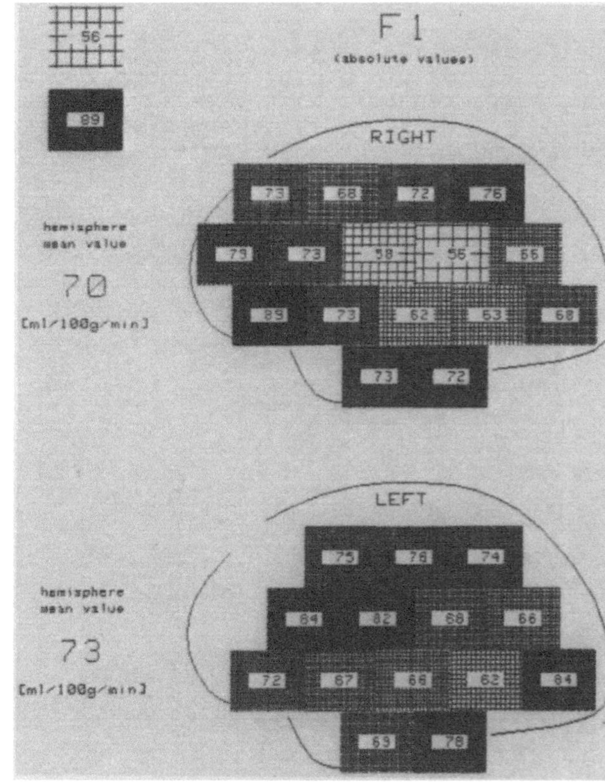

Fig. 4. Localized decrease of cerebral perfusion ("focal ischemia") in a patient with normal angiographic findings and intermittent sensory disturbances of the left arm (tingling of the fingers). Questionable indication for EIAB

Long-Term Control of Completed Stroke: rCBF Measurements and Psychological Assessment Before and After Extra-Intracranial Bypass Surgery

W. H. Heienbrok and M. Krupp

Neurochirurgische Klinik, Alfried-Krupp-Krankenhaus, Alfried-Krupp-Straße 21, D-4300 Essen

The indication for extra-intracranial bypass operation in transient ischemic attacks (TIA) is undisputed. By contrast, since the chance of the operation being successful in completed stroke is reduced owing to severe morphological changes, the question of whether to operate remains a subject of discussion (2, 4, 6). However, we have observed that despite severe neurological disorders, the mental activity of patients with cerebral infarction improved considerably following surgery. In a prospective study we aimed to verify this observation. To this end patients were submitted to pre- and postoperative radiological and neurological examination as well as series of regional cerebral blood flow (rCBF) measurements and psychological tests.

In the selected patients, stroke had, on average, occurred a year previously, and with two exceptions their condition had not improved following conservative treatment for at least three months prior to operation.

To date, 35 patients have been selected for study (Table 1), of whom 29 have been male (83%), with an average age of 55 years (ranging from 34 to 74 years), and six female, with an average age of 63 years (within a narrower age range). In 29 cases the cause of stroke had been either uni- or bilateral internal carotid occlusion; this was associated with contralateral carotid stenoses in 15 cases, with less than 50% narrowing of the vascular lumen in seven and more than 50% narrowing in eight (Table 2).

Computerized axial tomographic scanning (CAT scan) revealed severely depleted brain tissue in 31 patients, particularly in the region supplied by the middle cerebral artery; this was left-sided in almost two-thirds of the cases, as illustrated in Table 3. In the neurological control examinations, emphasis was placed particularly on patients' use of the extremities and speech ability. These results, as well as the medical evaluation of overall handicap, were categorized in several subgroupings (Table 4). Hence, the worst result would be 15 points and the best result 1 point. Changes during the observation period were determined by means of the average points evaluation. Reports on the condition of patients immediately following the attack were largely taken from external case histories. The average point evaluation at onset of stroke was 9.9. A year prior to operation this value was remarkably reduced, to 7.9, as shown in Fig. 1. Noticeable postoperative improvement had occurred by the time of discharge, and this continued significantly during the first few postoperative months. Statistics on further improvements over the next year have not been considered relevant.

Advances in Neurosurgery, Vol. 13
Edited by H. Dietz, M. Brock, and M. Klinger

Table 1. Age range of patients examined

Average age:	56.7 ± 8.7 years (34-74 years)
Average age of 29 males:	55.4 ± 8.9 years
Average age of 6 females:	62.7 ± 5.4 years

Table 2. Preoperative findings of angiography

Carotid occlusion - unilateral		12
bilateral		2
Carotid occlusion and contralateral carotid stenosis	(<50%)	7
Carotid occlusion and contralateral carotid stenosis	(>50%)	8
Intracranial stenoses	(>50%)	2
Occlusion of middle meningeal artery		3
Occlusion of the carotid and middle meningeal arteries (contralateral)		1
		35

Table 3. Preoperative CAT scan findings

Severe	31
Mild	2
General cerebral atrophy	1
Inconspicuous	1
	35
Left-sided	21
Right-sided	13
Bilateral	1
	35

As illustrated in Table 5, follow-up angiography generally showed good intracranial vessel filling through the bypass. In four cases, only regional vessel demonstration was apparent, while one case showed no anastomotic function. Accordingly, in these five cases the improvement was less than the average of the others, whereby two cases showed isolated improvement of speech impairment. Our overall appraisal was that in relation to the other disorders, speech impairment improved remarkably.

rCBF measurement was performed prior to surgery in all 35 patients, and was repeated in 26 patients approximately a year following operation. Due to a change in methods during the installation of our own facilities, only trend analysis without differential statistical evaluation was possible.

Table 4. Neurological findings

Upper extremity	Lower extremity
0 No loss of function	1 Well able to walk
1 Slightly handicapped	2 Ability to walk impeded
2 Heavy work impeded	3 Ability to walk severely impeded
3 Movements against gravity impeded	4 Unable to walk
4 Suggestion of movement, plegia	
Speech	*Overall handicap*
0 Unimpeded	0 Not handicapped
1 Mild dysphasia	1 Slightly handicapped
2 Simple sentences	2 Moderately handicapped
3 Words, fragmentary sentences	3 Severely handicapped
4 Stammering, aphasia	
Overall assessment	
Best possible no. of points: 1	Worst possible no. of points: 15

Table 5. Results of follow-up angiography

Good retrograde filling of the middle cerebral artery	23	2.5 points
Additional filling of anterior cerebral vessels	3	
Only regional vessel demonstration	4	1.3 points
No anastomotic function	1	
Doppler control only	4	
	35	

As shown in Table 6, the reduction in blood circulation is graded in four groups, from normal to extremely reduced. None of the patients was in the normal range in the area of the lesioned vessel at the preoperative stage. The main contingency showed clear circulatory impairment, at between 20%-40%. A year after surgery the situation had improved remarkably, only seven cases having clearly extreme reduction whereas six had normalized. With regard to the initial slope index (5, 7), we found a postoperative mean value of $x_{26} = 38.6 \pm 5.2$ for the lesioned side and 43.1 ± 5.6 for the contralateral side. Altogether, 17 patients improved, seven remained unchanged, and two worsened compared to the preoperative starting values without worsening of the clinical condition.

Unless the patient considers the results of surgery beneficial, even the best operation is of no avail. A year following operation 22 pa-

Table 6. Trend analysis of the pre- and postoperative rCBF measurements. The postoperative values are based on the initial slope index

rCBF	Normal	↓Mild	↓Significant	↓High-grade
Preop. $n = 35$	0	5	22	8
Postop. (1 year) $n = 26$	6	13	6	1

Postop. (1 year) $n = 26$	Affected side	Contralateral side
$\bar{X}$ ISI	38.6 ± 5.2	43.1 ± 5.6

Table 7. Assessment of the operative results

	Very good	Good	Slight improvement	No change	Deterioration
Subjective assessment	4	18	8	4	1
Medical assessment	2	11	17	4	1

tients assessed the achieved results as ranging from good to very good. Objective results proved this to be true in only 13 cases. Eight patients noticed a slight improvement, four felt unchanged, and one had worsened. Subjectively, 86% of the patients felt that some benefit had accrued from the operation (Table 7). The explanation for the positive assessment must lie in the psychometric results.

Series of psychological tests were performed preoperatively and about 7.5 months after the operation. Concentration was examined with BRICKENKAMP's D2-test (1) and memory with a test based on HAWIE numbers (8); in addition, tests were carried out on special intelligence factors (3). All tests were selected to avoid as far as possible a reduction in validity due to aphasic and paretic disabilities.

As can be seen in Fig. 2, our results in 30 patients show that there was a statistical improvement in ability to concentrate, although no significant changes occurred in respect of memory capacity.

Of the intelligence factors, there were significant improvements in verbal communication and spatial conception (Fig. 3). Moreover, the improvement in logical thinking was only narrowly short of being statistically significant. There was no change in the flexibility of imagination, i.e., the ability to abstract substantial elements from an entire concept. However, preoperatively this factor did not deviate from findings in the normal population. Therefore, in the essential areas of the spectrum of psychological factors tested, there was a distinct improvement.

The conclusion is that despite severe neurological disorders, bypass surgery is justified. Apart from the neurological and circulatory improvement demonstrated by angiography and rCBF measurement, we determined, particularly from the psychological tests, that brain organic function had improved. The patients became more able to cope with their situations.

References

1. Brickenkamp, R.: Test d2, Aufmerksamkeits-Belastungs-Test, 6. Aufl., Göttingen Toronto Zürich 1978
2. Gratzl, O., Schmiedeck, P., Spetzler, P., Steinhoff, H., Marguth, F.: Clinical experience with extra-intracranial arterial anastomosis in 65 cases. J. Neurosurg. 44, 313 (1976)
3. Horn, W.: Leistungsprüfsystem (L-P-S). Göttingen 1962
4. Kletter, G.: The extra-intracranial bypass operation for prevention and treatment of stroke. Springer-Verlag, Wien New York 1979
5. Obrist, W.D., Wilkinson, W.E.: The non-invasive Xe-133 method: Evaluation of CBF indices. Proceedings of the International Congress on Cerebral Circulation. Exerpta Medica, Amsterdam Oxford Princeton 1979
6. Peerless, S.J., McCormick, C.W.: Microsurgery for cerebral ischemia. Springer-Verlag, New York Heidelberg Berlin 1980
7. Risberg, J.H., Ali, Z., Wilson, E.M., Wills, E.L., Halsey, J.H.: Regional cerebral blood flow by ^{133}Xenon inhalation. Stroke 6, 142 (1975)
8. Wechsler, D.: Hamburg-Wechsler-Intelligenztest für Erwachsene (HAWIE). Deutsche Bearbeitung von Hardesty, A., Lauber, H. 3. Aufl. Bern Stuttgart 1964

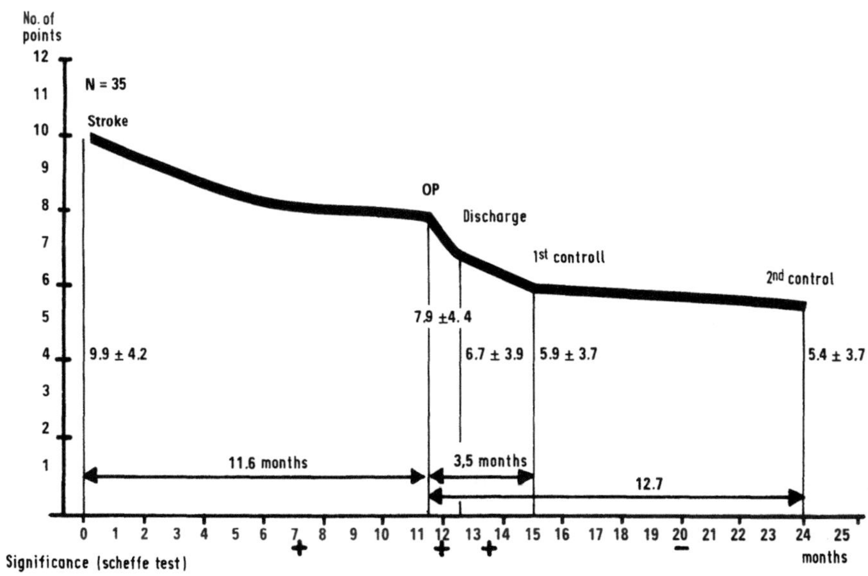

Fig. 1. Legend see p. 146

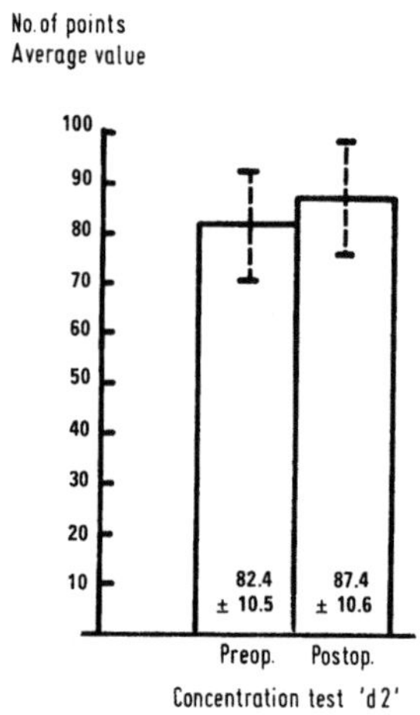

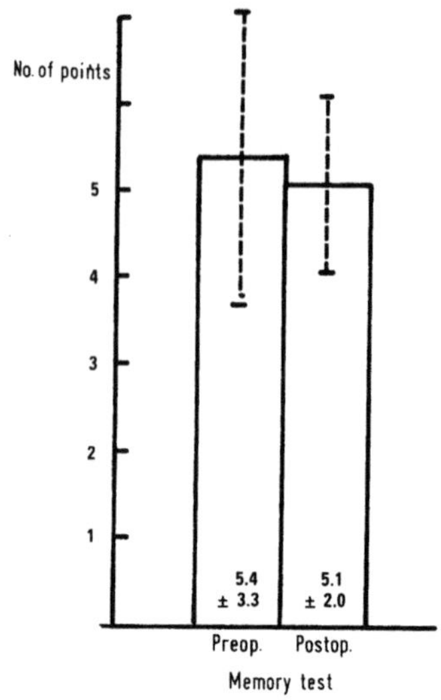

Fig. 2. Results of pre- und postoperative tests on concentration, using Brickenkamp's test, and memory, based on HAWIE numbers ($n = 30$)

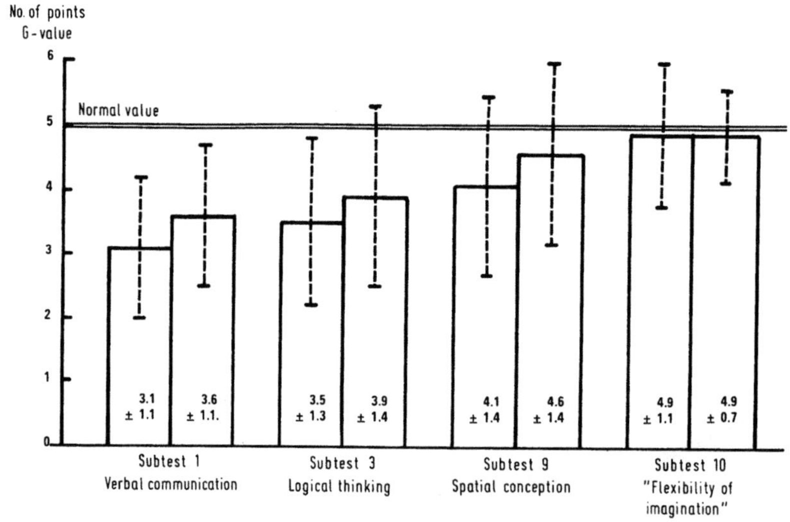

Fig. 3. Results of four pre- and postoperative mental ability tests, performed on 30 patients

---

Fig. 1. Changes in neurological findings within the observation period compared to the average number of points (± standard deviation). Significant improvements occurred between onset of stroke and operation, between operation and time of discharge (2-4 weeks postoperatively), and between discharge and the first control examination (3.5 months postop.). There were no significant changes between the first and second control examinations (approx. one year postoperatively)

Psychometric Follow-Up Studies in Patients with Transient Ischemic Attacks and Completed Stroke Treated by Extra-Intracranial Arterial Bypass

W. I. Steudel[1] and P. Jacobi[2]

[1] Abteilung für Allgemeine Neurochirurgie der Johann Wolfgang Goethe-Universität Schleusenweg 2–16, D-6000 Frankfurt 71

[2] Abteilung für Medizinische und Klinische Psychologie der Universität des Saarlandes, D-6500 Homburg/Saar

Introduction

The indication for bypass operation after a completed stroke is appraised very dissimilarly by different surgeons. The indication extends from mild to moderate deficits up to complete neurological syndrome. There are differences with regard to the extent of the neurological symptoms, the time of operation after occurrence of the stroke, as well as the size and localization of the infarction. The brain infarction leads to a large number of neurological and psychopathological effects which can be classified in different groups such as cognitive and perceptive disorders, alteration of mood and behavior, reduced ability to master the tasks of daily life, and somatic symptoms (5, 7, 23).

The value of a carotid endarterectomy (8, 9, 11-17, 19, 20, 22, 24) or extra-intracranial arterial bypass surgery (3, 4, 10, 21) for restoration of neuropsychological disorders is controversial (1). Whereas some investigations indicate an improved intellectual and cognitive performance (4, 8, 12, 15, 22) even in patients with dementia (16, 21), other authors (3, 24) do not see any or only minimal positive effects which can be objectively documented.

In the quantification of psychopathological findings, measurement of psychometric functions has proved suitable, especially measurement of the reaction times in patients with cerebrovascular processes (18). To demonstrate the long-term effect of extra-intracranial bypass on cerebral function using psychometric tests, we investigated prospectively 15 patients with a completed stroke and for comparison 14 patients with transitory ischemic attacks (TIA).

Patients and Methods

Since 1982, 55 patients (25 with TIA, five with PRIND, and 25 with a completed stroke) have been investigated prospectively. Besides the cliniconeurological status, Doppler sonography, angiography, computer tomography, perfusion scintigraphy, and EEG, the investigations comprised neuropsychological tests. The investigations were carried out preoperatively and repeated in the second postoperative week and after six months. Twenty-nine patients – 14 with TIA (age range 41-69, mean age 57 years) and 15 patients with previous stroke (age range 41-69, mean age 54.5 years) – have so far been investigated completely.

In the patients with completed stroke, there was a mild or moderate neurological deficit with a small subcortical infarction in the com-

Advances in Neurosurgery, Vol. 13
Edited by H. Dietz, M. Brock, and M. Klinger

puter tomogram in 12 cases, and severe neurological deficits with a large infarction in three cases. The bypass operation was carried out within three months after the stroke in ten cases, after six months in two cases, and after two years in three cases.

The psychological examination comprises measurement of simple acoustic and optical reaction times as well as the complex reaction time under standardized conditions (18). The reaction time is that which the patient requires in order to press a button when a lamp lights up or when he hears a signal. In the complex reaction time, 48 light stimuli are presented in accordance with a random pattern via a configuration of 12 lamps. The performance of the test subjects consists in an adaptation of the motor reaction to the objective of as short a time as possible, with presence of a feedback in that the corresponding light is extinguished by a correct reaction.

In addition, the State Trait Anxiety Inventory (STAI), which detects fear, anxiety, and threats to the patient, was tried out (6).

The results were analyzed by univariate analyses of variance. The analysis of variance had two factors: time (pretest or posttest) and type of cerebrovascular disorder (TIA or stroke).

Results

Measurement of the simple optical and acoustic and the complex optical reaction time reveals different values for the group of TIA and the stroke group. Stroke patients have poorer preoperative performance values than TIA patients (Fig. 1). Six months after bypass surgery, the values of the stroke patients correspond almost completely to those of the TIA patients. This means that the postoperative improvement is relatively greater in patients with infarction ($P < 0.1$). In the TIA patients, there was no statistically significant improvement of the reaction times.

The complex reaction time for the two investigation groups and the different times of investigation did not show any appreciable alteration.

The performance values in the second postoperative week deteriorated markedly for all patients.

In addition, all patients were presented with the STAI. The two groups are the same with regard to their anxiety before the impending operation. The postoperative anxiety development in the two groups is also the same. This is one of the major effects of a subjective alleviation after the operation (Table 1).

With regard to the time of operation, two groups are distinguished among the stroke patients: group I comprises patients with a bypass operation within six months after the infarction and group II those with a bypass operation more than six months after the infarction. The two groups differ to a statistically significant extent only after six months ($P < 0.025$). Group I patients showed faster reaction times throughout and are evidently stabilized emotionally immediately and for a long period after the operation. Group II patients can clearly no longer be influenced favorably with regard to emotionality (Table 1, Fig. 2).

Table 1. Review of results on the State Trait Anxiety Inventory[a]

Time of examination		TIA	Stroke		
			n	Group I	Group II
t_1 preoperative	$\bar{x}$	44	43	44	40
	n	14	14	9	5
t_2 2nd week postoperative	$\bar{x}$	37	36	34	40
	n	14	14	9	5
t_3 6th month postoperative	$\bar{x}$	37	39	33	44
	n	13	12	8	4

[a]Sum value from 20 scaled single questions. Higher value = more pronounced anxiety and fears

Table 2. Review of results on optical and acoustic reaction times in stroke patients before and six months after the operation

Stroke patients[a]	Optical reaction time	Acoustic reaction time
Group I	$\bar{x}$ = 3.6	$\bar{x}$ = 3.1
	(s) = 0.3	(s) = 0.4
	n = 8	*n* = 8
Group II	$\bar{x}$ = 4.9	$\bar{x}$ = 3.8
	(s) = 0.5	(s) = 0.2
	n = 3	*n* = 3
Kolmogorov-Smirnov test	$P < 0.025$	$P < 0.025$

[a]Group I: patients with bypass operation within six months after the infarction. Group II: operation six months after the infarction

Discussion

Because of the often pronounced psychological disorders in stroke patients, the improvement of the clinical picture is difficult to quantify. A particular possibility in cerebrovascular processes is afforded by psychometric tests such as measurement of the reaction time (18). The optical and acoustic reaction times show marked differences. The complex reaction time is not suitable for this investigation group.

Our investigation shows that in infarct patients, an improvement of the reaction times is present postoperatively. Such an improvement cannot be detected in TIA patients. Since an unoperated group for comparison is lacking, it is not possible to describe the spontaneous course of the clinical psychopathological disorders after a mild or severe stroke (1, 3). Pathophysiologically, it appears likely that the ischemic threshold for neuronal electrical failure and the threshold for neuronal death are distinctly different (2, 16). This concerns in particular patients with bilateral carotid occlusion or with a carotid occlusion and contralateral stenosis (16).

Since it is assumed that in patients with infarction almost without exception a further recovery cannot be expected after 6-9 months (23), our results indicate a useful effect of the bypass operation even in those patients. The detection of small infarctions in TIA or PRIND is known. In agreement with OWENS et al. (1980) – with reference to patients with endarterectomy – our results show that there was a postoperative improvement in the stroke group with regard to their psychometric performance.

The STAI test serves to exclude possible effects arising from the psychological stress of the operation. A clinical improvement may be at least partially due to a psychological alleviation after the operation (1, 24). A reduction of performance due to the preoperative psychological stress could be excluded by the comparison with the TIA group.

Conclusion

Our investigations show that compared to patients with TIAs, patients with a completed stroke reveal a psychometric improvement after an extra-intracranial bypass operation. The comparison between early and late operative stroke patients shows that patients operated on early benefit more from a bypass operation than those operated on late.

References

1. Asken, M.J., Hobson, R.W.: Intellectual change and carotid endarterectomy, subjective speculation or objective reality: A review. J. Surg. Res. 23, 367-375 (1977)
2. Astrup, J., Siesjo, B.K., Symon, L.: Thresholds in cerebral ischemia – The ischemic penumbra. Stroke 12, 723-725 (1981)
3. Binder, L.M., Tanabe, C.T., Waller, F.T., Wooster, N.E.: Behavioral effects of superficial temporal artery to middle cerebral artery bypass surgery. Neurology 32, 422-424 (1982)
4. Bollbach, R., Wassmann, H., Holbach, K.-H., Payk, T.: Psychometric follow-up studies in patients with occlusive disease of the cerebral arteries treated by extra-intracranial arterial anastomosis. Adv. Neurosurg. 9, 405-409 (1981)
5. Boller, F.: Strokes and behavior: disorders of higher cortical functions following cerebral disease. Disorders of language and related function. Stroke 12, 532-534 (1981)
6. Brickenkamp, R.: Handbuch psychologischer und pädagogischer Tests, erster Ergänzungsband. Verlag für Psychologie, Göttingen 1983
7. Delaney, R., Wallace, J., Egelko, S.: Neuropsychological aspects of transient ischemic attacks. J. Clin. Neuropsychol. 2, 107-114 (1980)
8. Drake, W.E. Jr., Baker, M., Blumenkrantz, J., Dahlgren, H.: The quality and duration of survival in bilateral carotid occlusive disease: A preliminary survey of the effects of thromboendarterectomy. In: Cerebral vascular diseases, Sixth Conference, pp. 242-259. Grune & Stratton, New York 1969
9. Duke, R., Bloor, B., Nugent, G., Majzoub, H.: Changes in performance on WAIS, trailmaking test, and finger tapping test associated with carotid artery surgery. Percept. Mot. Skills 26, 399 (1968)

10. Evans, R.B., Austin, G.: Psychological evaluation of patients undergoing microneurosurgical anastomoses for cerebral ischemia. In: Austin, G.M. (ed.) Microneurosurgical anastomoses for cerebral ischemia, pp. 320-326. Thomas, Springfield (Ill.) 1976

11. Garner, I.T., Tosenstock, J., Field, T.D., Tager, R.M., Jacques, D.B.: Lateralized changes in cognitive function following carotid endarterectomy. Adv. Neurosurg. 7, 9-14 (1979)

12. Goldstein, S., Kleinknecht, R., Gallo, A.: Neuropsychological changes associated with carotid endarterectomy. Cortex 6, 308-321 (1970)

13. Haynes, D., King, G., Dempsey, R.: Improvement of cognitive and personality changes after carotid endarterectomy. Surg. Forum 26, 288 (1975)

14. Haynes, D., King, G., Dempsey, R.: Improvement of cognitive and personality after carotid endarterectomy. Surgery 80, 699-704 (1976)

15. Horne, D., Royle, J.: Cognitive changes after carotid endarterectomy. Med. J. Aust. 1, 316-317 (1974)

16. Jacobs, L.A., Ganji, S., Shirley, J.G., Morrell, R.M., Brinkman, S.D.: Cognitive improvement after extracranial reconstruction for the low flow-endangered brain. Surgery 93, 683-687 (1983)

17. Kelly, M.P., Garron, D.C., Javid, H.: Carotid artery disease, carotid endarterectomy and behavior. Arch. Neurol. 37, 743-748 (1980)

18. Klensch, H.: Die diagnostische Valenz der Reaktionszeitmessung bei verschiedenen cerebralen Erkrankungen. Fortschr. Neurol. Psychiat. 41, 575-581 (1973)

19. Matarazzo, R.G., Matarazzo, J.D., Gallo, A.E., Wiens, A.N.: IQ and neuropsychological changes following carotid endarterectomy. J. Clin. Neuropsychol. 1, 97-116 (1979)

20. Owens, M., Pressman, M., Edwards, A.E., Tourtellotte, W., Rose, J.G., Stern, D., Peters, G., Stabile, B.E., Wilson, S.E.: The effect of small infarcts and carotid endarterectomy on postoperative psychologic test performance. J. Surg. Res. 28, 209-216 (1980)

21. Peerless, S.J., Chater, N.L., Ferguson, F.G.: Multiple vessel occlusions in cerebrovascular disease – a further follow-up of the effects of microvascular bypass on the quality of life and the incidence of stroke. In: Schmiedek, P. (ed.) International symposium on microsurgical anastomoses for cerebral ischemia, 3rd ed., pp. 251-259. Springer-Verlag, New York 1977

22. Perry, P., Drinkwater, J., Taylor, G.: Neuropsychological tests and carotid artery disease. Brit. J. Surg. 61, 922-923 (1974)

23. Toole, J.F.: Cerebrovascular disorders, 3rd ed., pp. 271-279. Raven Press, New York 1984

24. Williams, M., McGee, T.: Psychological study of carotid artery occlusion and endarterectomy. Arch. Neurol. 10, 342 (1964)

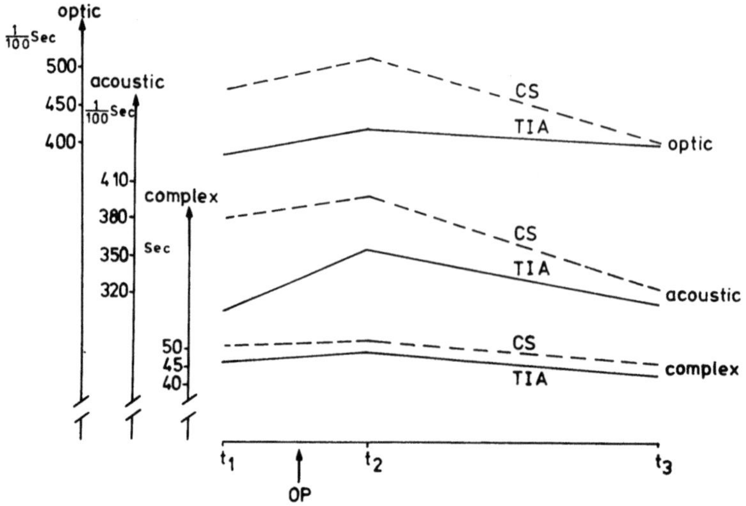

Fig. 1. The performance values (mean values) of the patient groups with transient ischemic attacks *(TIA)* and with a completed stroke *(CS)* at the various times of investigation (t_1 = preoperatively, t_2 = in the second week, and t_3 = six months postoperatively) in the measurement of the optical, acoustic, and complex reaction times. Insult patients have poorer performance values than TIA patients preoperatively. Six months after the operation, the values of the infarct patients approach those of the TIA patients

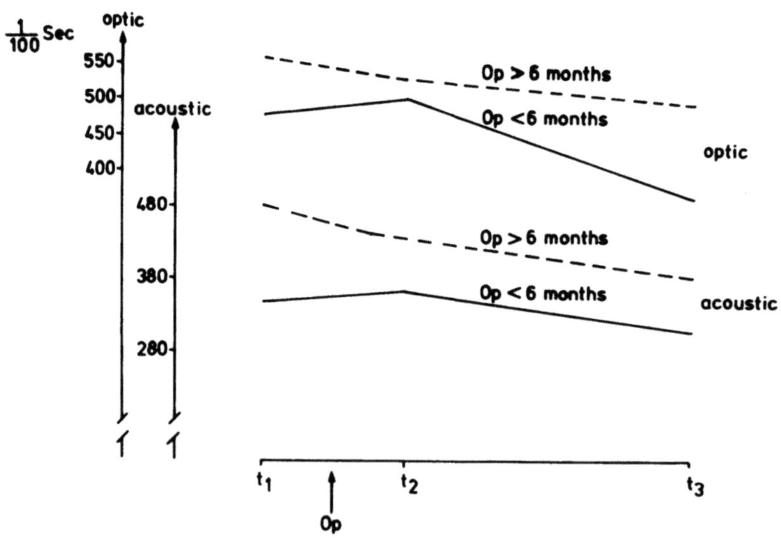

Fig. 2. The performance values (mean values) of the patients with completed stroke. Group I *(Op <6 months)* comprises patients with a bypass operation within 6 months after the infarct and group II *(Op >6 months)* with bypass operation 6 months after the infarct. Group I shows faster reaction times throughout

Application of 3-Fluoro-Deoxyglucose for the Assessment of Cerebral Perfusion and Glucose Transport in Candidates for EC/IC Bypass Surgery

H. M. Mehdorn[1], E. J. Knust[2], H.-J. Machulla[2], and K. Vyska[3]

[1] Abteilung für Neurochirurgie, [2] Institut für Strahlenphysik, Universitätsklinikum der Gesamthochschule Essen, Hufelandstraße 55, D-4300 Essen 1

[3] Medizinisches Institut, Kernforschungsanlage Jülich, D-5170 Jülich

Introduction

Indications for extracranial/intracranial (EC/IC) bypass surgery can be divided into two groups: (1) the prophylactic indication: its value has been accepted but still has to be defined by the ongoing Cooperative Study (8); (2) the therapeutic indication. This indication is based on the observation familiar to everyone performing EC/IC bypass surgery routinely, that there are some patients in whom a neurological deficit is improved immediately after the revascularization and in the following time, more than could have been expected from the natural course of improvement. These are often the most rewarding candidates for EC/IC bypass surgery.

X-ray computed tomography (CT) scanning, regional cerebral blood flow (rCBF) measurements, hyperbaric oxygenation, and EEG analysis and evaluation of evoked potentials in stress situations such as hypotension and hypertension (4-6, 11, 13) have been applied to the noninvasive assessment of EC/IC bypass patients in order to define these optimal candidates. Of late, more information about cerebral three-dimensional perfusion pattern and tissue viability has become available with the introduction of positron emission tomography (PET).

Based on oxygen-15 (O-15) as positron emitter, it has been suggested that patients with a mismatch between CBF and oxygen extraction fraction (OEF) in the sense of a "misery perfusion" (1) would be good candidates for an EC/IC bypass as some of their brain tissue is still viable but in the idling state (3).

Another approach to this problem can be undertaken by using glucose analogues marked with fluorine-18 (F-18). This isotope has the practical advantage over O-15 that its half-life is 110 min. Therefore, it is not necessary to have both the cyclotron and the PET scanner in one center.

In this paper, the experience is reported which has been gained by applying a new glucose analogue, F-18-3-deoxy-3-fluoro-D-glucose (3FDG) (7, 14, 15), to the problem of patient selection for EC/IC bypass surgery. 3FDG is a glucose analogue in which the hydroxyl group at carbon-3 is replaced by F-18. It is transported across the blood-brain barrier (BBB) by the same carrier mechanisms as glucose but is not further metabolized.

Advances in Neurosurgery, Vol. 13
Edited by H. Dietz, M. Brock, and M. Klinger

Methods

Production of 3-Fluoro-Deoxyglucose

F-18 was produced in the compact cyclotron at the University of Essen Medical Center; up to 500 mCi F-18 were obtained in routine production. 3FDG was synthesized as described by KNUST and co-workers (7). In typical routine runs, 30 mCi F-18-3FDG was obtained ready for i.v. injection.

Model

In the present studies, 5 mCi 3FDG was injected into an antecubital vein of the patient, and the transaxial activity distribution in one selected slice of the brain (mostly O.M. +5) was registered with the ECAT II scanner at 30-s intervals for 40 min. Medium resolution shadows and high resolution data collection were used. The measured attenuation correction was applied for image reconstruction.

At different regions of brain scans regions of interest (ROIs) were selected and the activity curves created. Since the blood volume in brain is small (cortex approx. 4%, white matter approx. 2%), the time-activity curves registered over brain were considered as a measure of the brain 3FDG concentration c_2^*.

As an estimate of the capillary blood flow 3FDG concentration, c_B^*, either the arterial or venous 3FDG concentrations can be used. In the present study the activity registered over the superior longitudinal sinus (SLS) was taken as an estimate of the 3FDG venous concentration (14, 15).

According to VYSKA and co-workers (14, 15), in plasma, 3FDG competes with glucose for a common carrier for transport into a primary precursor pool in brain tissue. The rate of 3FDG accumulation in brain tissue is equal to the difference between the rate of 3FDG influx ($K_1^* \cdot c_B^*$) and 3FDG efflux ($k_2^* \cdot c_2^*$):

$$dc_2^*/dt = K_1^* \cdot c_B^* - k_2^* \cdot c_2^*$$

In this equation c_B^* is the concentration of 3FDG in blood, c_2^* is the 3FDG concentration in brain tissue, K_1^* is the observed rate constant for 3FDG influx, and k_2^* is the rate constant for 3FDG efflux.

As demonstrated by SOKOLOFF and co-workers (12), under the conditions of:

- steady state of cerebral glucose utilization during the period of measurement,
- a constant plasma glucose concentration,
- symmetry of glucose transport across BBB, and
- application of 3FDG in tracer amounts,

the rate constants for 3FDG influx and efflux may be considered as true first order constants, which are independent of the plasma 3FDG concentration.

Under these conditions it can be demonstrated that the slope of approach of 3FDG tissue concentration to the steady state is equal to k_2^* and that the local perfusion rate is given by the ratio of the 3FDG concentrations at steady state in blood c_{BSS}^* and in tissue c_{2SS}^* (see Fig. 1.).

The average of brain perfusion rate found with this method was 88±8 ml/100 g/min.

The regions of interest (ROIs) used in the studies were approximated to the major vascular supply territories, that is, the anterior cerebral artery (ACA), middle cerebral artery (MCA), and posterior cerebral artery (PCA) territories.

Patient Selection

Usually, patients were selected for EC/IC bypass surgery on the basis of generally accepted criteria. Six particular patients underwent pre- and postoperative PET evaluation using 3FDG, in addition to pre- and postoperative conventional X-ray CT scan and three vessel angiography.

Results

A patient is presented in detail to show the value of information gained by PET.

This 57-year-old man had suffered two right hemispheric strokes four and two years prior to admission, with residual left hemiparesis, pronounced in the arm. Left eye: amaurosis due to central artery occlusion; right eye: reduced visual capacity due to ischemic retinopathy. Neurologically, he had a left arm spastic paresis.

CT scan (Fig. 2a) showed cortical atrophy, ventricular dilatation, and hypodense lesions high parietally and frontally on the right side. Angiograms (Fig. 2b,c) revealed bilateral ICA occlusion with good filling of intracranial circulation on the left side via ophthalmic collaterals. On the right side there was only late intracranial filling via ophthalmic collaterals. Note the diameter of the superficial temporal artery (STA) on the right side. PET scan (Fig. 2d) showed ventricular dilatation, with perfusion reduced bilaterally; the right side was worse than the left, particularly in the right frontal pole (-20% right, -14% left frontal) and in the watershed area between the MCA and the PCA territory (-12% right occipital lobe). For flow values, see Table 1. After right-sided EC/IC bypass, there was improvement of vision in the right eye, and of left arm paresis and intellectual functions.

Control angiography (Fig. 2e,f) showed excellent filling of the entire right MCA territory through the dilated STA, with only very late opacification of the right ophthalmic artery. On the left side, there was opacification of the MCA territory through the ophthalmic artery; when compared with the right MCA territory, however, there was lesser perfusion.

EC/IC bypass on the left side was not performed upon the patient's request. Follow-up PET scan 10 months postoperatively (Fig. 2g) demonstrated improvement of the perfusion pattern in both hemispheres, particularly in the right MCA (+10%) and ACA (+5%) territory. There was improvement on the left side without reaching normal values: ACA territory, +8%; MCA and PCA territories, no significant changes (see Table 1).

Table 1. Perfusion values (ml/100 g/min) as determined by the 3-FDG method

	Preoperatively		Postoperatively	
	Left	Right	Left	Right
ACA	75.7	69.9	82.4	75.7
MCA	75.2	72.4	73.9	79.6
PCA	77.7	76.9	78.5	77.5

Discussion

By way of an example, a patient with cerebrovascular ischemic disease with hemodynamic consequences has been presented. He was unilaterally symptomatic, with occlusion of both ICAs. The results obtained by PET indicate that the collateralization via the ophthalmic arteries was predominant on the left side; because of the perfusion values it must be assumed that the right hemisphere was the worst perfused area. Postoperatively, there was not only a significant increase in both right-sided ACA and MCA territories but also in the left ACA supply area. This finding suggests that the right EC/IC bypass not only increased the right side perfusion but also eliminated the steal from the left ophthalmic artery.

Under such conditions, if the steal contributing to the right hemispheric perfusion of approx. 7 ml/100 g/min were to be eliminated, the perfusion of the right ACA territory would be only 62 ml/100 g/min, and this might under certain circumstances be beneath the critical threshold values.

The possibility of hemodynamically induced cerebral ischemia is well known under the terms of "terminal supply area infarction" and "watershed infarction" (16). Over recent years, this possibility has often been disregarded, but it has gained increasing attention again lately (2, 9).

It is noteworthy that in this patient, even in the presence of a well functioning bypass, the normal perfusion values were not achieved. However, a high degree of cortical atrophy was observed in the CT scan (see Fig. 2a), and the values observed in this patient correspond well with values obtained in nonstroke patients with a comparable amount of atrophy. This probably means that by EC/IC bypass surgery only those values corresponding to the degree of atrophy can be achieved.

Comparing the pre- and postoperative flow values in the ACA territories, it becomes obvious that an improvement in perfusion of about 12 ml/100 g/min could be achieved. The apparent improvement of the ipsilateral ACA territory perfusion, however, was only 5 ml/100 g/min, whereas another 7 ml/100 g/min must be interpreted as being used to recompensate for the preoperative steal (from the left ophthalmic artery). These 7 ml/100 g/min can be seen in the postoperative improvement of ACA perfusion in the nonoperated contralateral hemipshere. This finding indicates clearly that hemodynamic consequences of EC/IC bypass surgery cannot be considered as effective only for the ipsilateral hemisphere.

The example given here clearly demonstrates the value of PET scan in evaluating the hemodynamic consequences of occlusive processes as well as the therapeutic effects of microsurgical revascularization. By this method it is possible to determine exactly those patients with low perfusion due to major vascular occlusive disease who are candidates for EC/IC bypass surgery. As already mentioned, the method not only provides the possibility of the assessment of local perfusion rate, but also enables the determination of the rate constant of glucose transport across the BBB. Moreover, if the rate constants are determined under normo- and hypoglycemic conditions (14, 15), it is possible to calculate essential enzymatic kinetic parameters such as maximal velocity (v_{max}) and the Michaelis-Menten constant. We started to apply this procedure to EC/IC bypass patients and observed that in ischemic regions v_{max} is significantly lower than in the normal regions. After EC/IC bypass surgery, a tendency for improvement of v_{max} was observed. Further extensive studies are necessary to correlate these data to the development of the clinical picture, to understand their value in predicting the outcome of operated patients, and to better define optimal candidates for bypass surgery.

References

1. Baron, J.C., Bousser, M.G., Rey, A., Guillard, A., et al.: Reversal of focal "misery perfusion syndrome" by extra-intracranial arterial bypass in hemodynamic cerebral ischemia. A case study with 150 positron emission tomography. Stroke 12, 454-459 (1981)
2. Cote, R., Barnett, H.J.M., Taylor, D.W.: Internal carotid occlusion: A prospective study. Stroke 14, 898-902 (1983)
3. Grubb, R.L. Jr., Ratcheson, R.A., Raichle, M.E., et al.: Regional cerebral blood flow and oxygen utilization in superficial temporal-middle cerebral artery anastomosis patients. J. Neurosurg. 50, 733-741 (1979)
4. Heilbrun, M.P., Anderson, R.E.: Preoperative evaluation of STA-MCA anastomosis candidates with rCBF studies. In: Schmiedek, P. (ed.) Microsurgery for stroke, pp. 202-213. Springer, New York Heidelberg Berlin 1977
5. Holbach, K.-H., Wassmann, H., Kutzner, M.: Intracranial vascular reconstructive surgery of the brain – indications. In: Carrea, R. (ed.) Neurological surgery, ICS 433, pp. 223-232. Excerpta Medica, Amsterdam Oxford 1977
6. Ito, Z., Susuki, A., Ohta, H.: The induced-hypotension test for TIA or RIND patients with stenotic cerebrovascular lesions. Presented at the 5th Int. Symp. on Microvasc. Anast. for Cerebral Ischemia, Vienna, Sept. 14-17, 1980
7. Knust, E.J., Machulla, H.-J., Dutschka, K.: Radiopharmaceuticals IV: 18F-labelling with water target produced 18F. Synthesis and quality control of 18F-3-deoxy-3-fluoro-D-glucose. Radiochem. Radioanal. Letters 55, 21-28 (1982)
8. Peerless, S.J., Barnett, H.J.M., Sackett, D.L., et al.: Collaborative study of extracranial/intracranial arterial anastomosis – Progress report. In: Barnett, H.J.M., Paoletti, P., Flamm, E.S. (eds.) Cerebrovascular diseases: New trends in surgical and medical aspects, pp. 351-363. Elsevier, Amsterdam New York Oxford 1981
9. Ringelstein, E.B., Zeumer, H., Angelou, D.: The pathogenesis of strokes from internal carotid artery occlusion. Diagnostic and therapeutic implications. Stroke 14, 867-875 (1983)

10. Schmiedek, P., Gratzl, O., Spetzler, R., Steinhoff, H., et al.: Selection of patients for extra-intracranial arterial bypass surgery based on rCBF measurements. J. Neurosurg. 44, 303-312 (1976)

11. Schmiedek, P., Olteanu-Nerbe, V., Gratzl, O., Marguth, F.: Comments on the use of regional cerebral blood flow studies in extra-intracranial arterial bypass surgery. Presented at the 6th Int. Symp. on Microsurg. Anast. for Cerebral Ischemia, Kyoto, Sept. 12-15, 1982

12. Sokoloff, L., Reivich, M., Kennedy, C., et al.: The 14C-deoxyglucose method for the measurement of local cerebral glucose utilization: Theory, procedure, and normal values in the conscious and anesthetized albino rat. J. Neurochem. 28, 897-916 (1977)

13. Spetzler, R.F., Wing, S.D., Norman, D.: Evaluation of patients with cerebral ischemia using computerized tomography. In: Schmiedek, P. (ed.) Microsurgery for stroke, pp. 195-201. Springer, New York Heidelberg Berlin 1977

14. Vyska, K., Profant, M., Schuier, F., et al.: The use of 11C-methyl-D-glucose for assessment of glucose transport in the human brain: theory and application. In: Lambrecht, R.M., Rescigno, A. (eds.) Tracer kinetics and physiologic modeling. Springer, Berlin Heidelberg New York Tokyo 1983

15. Vyska, K., Profant, M., Schuier, F., et al.: In vivo determination of kinetic parameters for glucose influx and efflux by means of 3-O-C 11-methyl-D-glucose, F18-3-deoxy-3-fluoro-D-glucose and dynamic positron emission tomography. Theory, method and normal values. In: Knapp, W., Vyska, K. (eds.) Current topics in tumor cell physiology and diagnostic implications for positron emission tomography, pp. 37-60. Springer, Berlin Heidelberg New York Tokyo 1984

16. Zülch, K.J.: Die Pathogenese von Massenblutung und Erweichung unter besonderer Berücksichtigung klinischer Gesichtspunkte. Acta Neurochir. 7, 51-117 (1961)

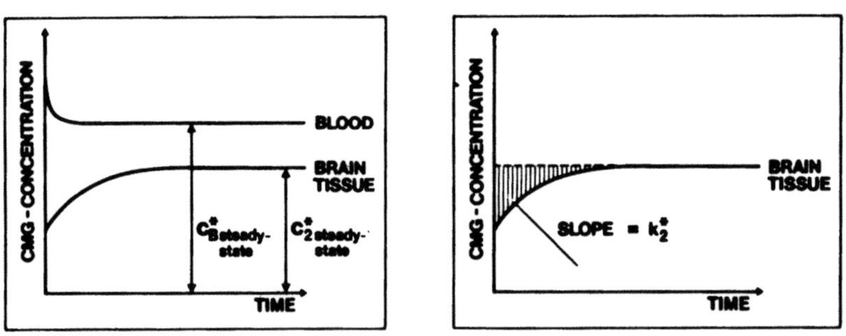

$$\frac{\varkappa_1^*}{k_2^*} = \frac{C^*_{2\,\text{steady-state}}}{C^*_{B\,\text{steady-state}}} \qquad k_2^*$$

$$\varkappa_1^* = \frac{C^*_{2\,\text{steady-state}}}{C^*_{B\,\text{steady-state}}} \cdot k_2^*$$

Fig. 1. Schematic representation of the evaluation of 3FDG data in the theoretical case that the blood 3FDG concentration is constant, that is c = const (14)

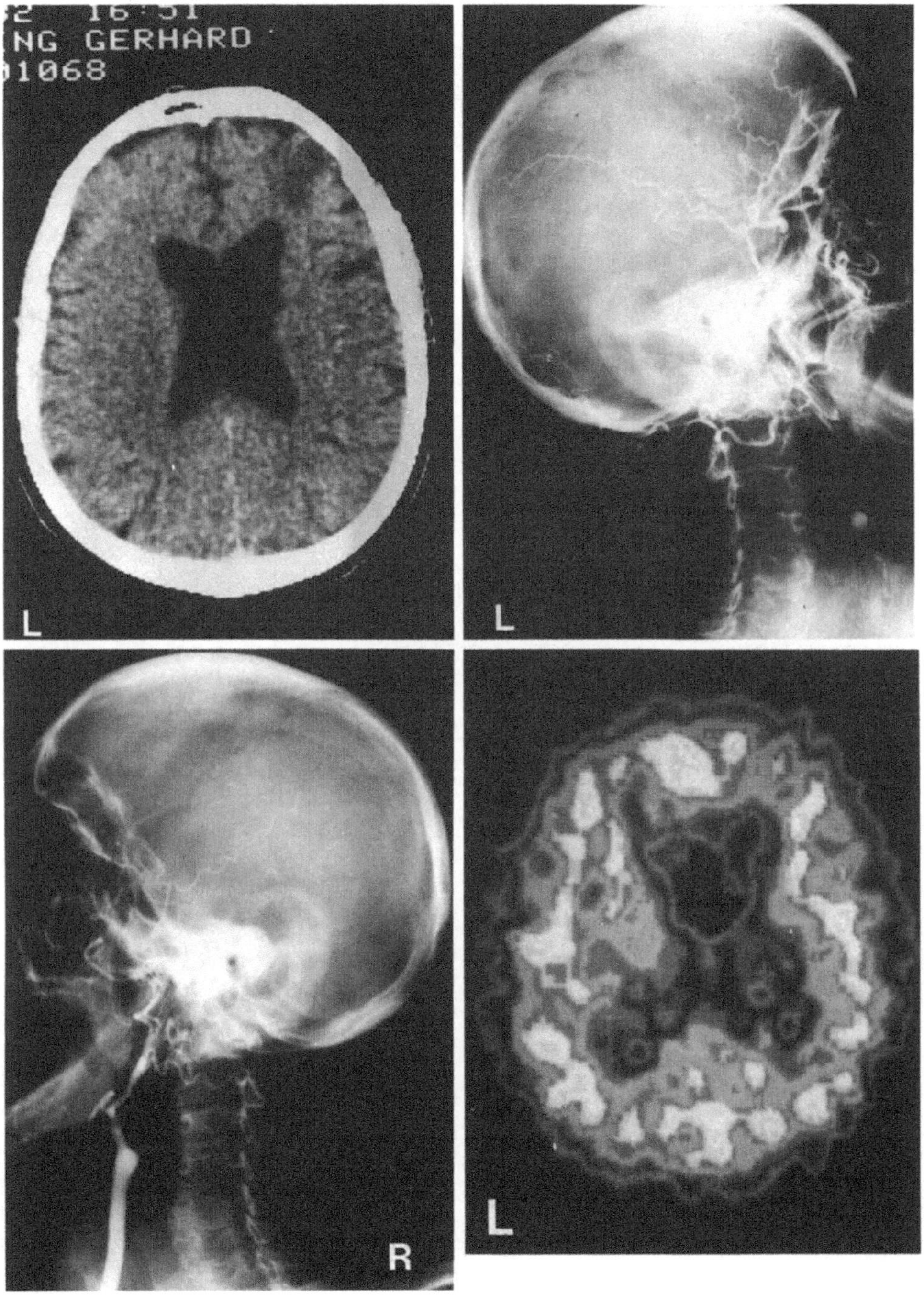

a b c d

Fig. 2a-d. Legend see p. 161

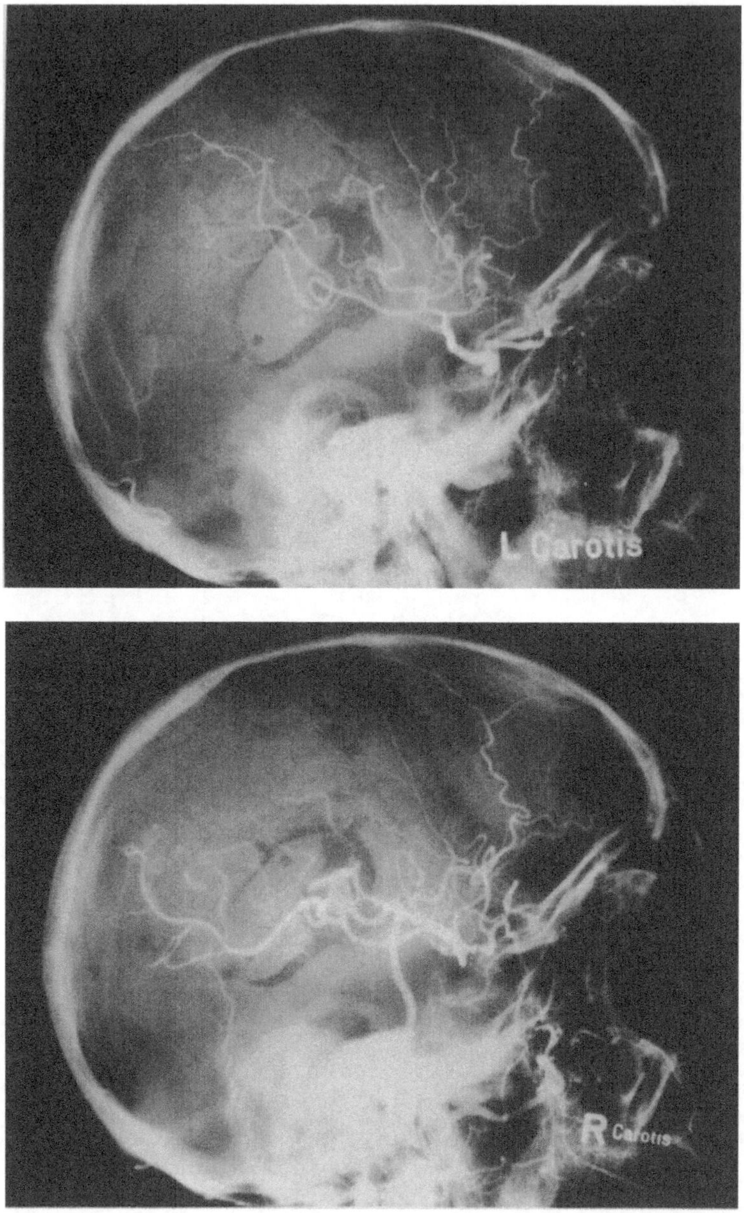

e

f

Fig. 2e,f. Legend see p. 161

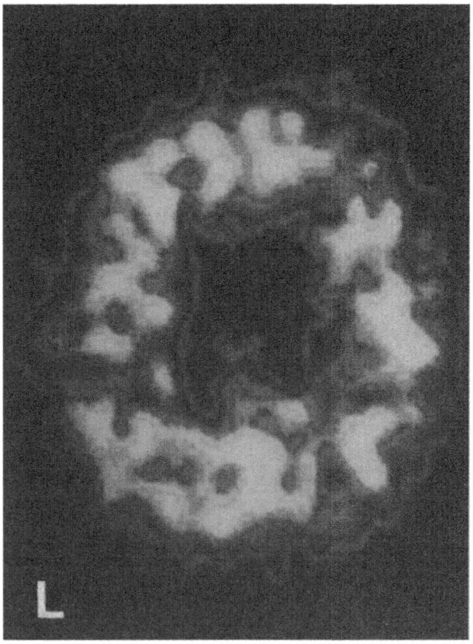

g

Fig. 2a-g. 57-year-old man who had suffered two right hemispheric strokes four and two years prior to admission. a CT scan: cortical atrophy, ventricular dilatation, and hypodense lesions high parietally and frontally on the right side. b,c Preop. angiograms: Bilateral ICA occlusion with good filling of intracranial circulation on the left side via ophthalmic collaterals. On the right side only late filling via ophthalmic collaterals. Note the diameter of superficial temporal artery (STA) on the right side. d PET scan preop.: Ventricular dilatation, perfusion reduced bilaterally, right side worse than left, particularly in the right frontal pole (-20% right, -14% left frontal), and in the watershed area between the MCA and the PCA territory (-12% right occipital lobe. For flow values, see Table 1. e,f Control angiography: Excellent filling of the entire right MCA territory through the dilated STA. On the left side, opacification of the MCA territory through the ophthalmic artery; when compared to right MCA territory, however, lesser perfusion. g Follow-up PET scan, 10 months postop.: Improvement of perfusion pattern in both hemispheres, particularly in the right MCA (+10%) and ACA (+5%) territory. Left side improvement without reaching normal values: ACA territory (+8%); MCA and PCA territories without significant changes (see Table 1)

Dynamic Single Photon Emission Computerized Tomography in Extra-Intracranial Bypass Patients with Internal Carotid Artery Occlusion

P. Schmiedek, T. Kreisig, E. A. Moser, C. M. Kirsch, G. Leinsinger, V. Olteanu-Nerbe, K. Einhäupl, and U. Buell

Abteilung für Neurochirurgie und Abteilung für Nuklearmedizin, Klinikum Großhadern, Universität München, Marchioninistraße 15, D-8000 München 70

Measurement of cerebral blood flow (CBF) has been used previously by various investigators to study the effect of extra-intracranial arterial bypass surgery on brain blood flow. The results, however, are inconclusive. While postoperative CBF was found to be only slightly increased by some (2, 3, 6, 8), others were unable to document any significant change in CBF or even found a decrease in brain blood flow during later postoperative studies (7, 11). Since different techniques for the measurement of CBF were used in these studies, it remains difficult to assess to what extent these findings may have been affected by inherent limitations of the individual method. Measurements obtained by intracarotid xenon-133 are of limited use because of their invasiveness and also because blood flow can usually be studied in only one hemisphere of the brain. Noninvasive techniques using inhaled or intravenously administered 133 Xe and stationary external detectors provide imformation on bilateral brain blood flow; however, they were found to be less accurate in the presence of cerebral infarcts because of the so-called look-through phenomenon (5). With the more recent introduction of the dynamic single photon emission computerized tomography (d-SPECT) technique, it is now possible to measure three-dimensional regional CBF, which allows the detection and localization of even small subcortical ischemic brain areas (4, 9). In the present report, the d-SPECT technique was used to investigate CBF before and after bypass surgery in a selected group of patients with symptomatic unilateral internal carotid artery occlusion.

Clinical Material

The series comprised two groups with a total of 29 male patients. In the first group there were 21 patients ranging in age from 32 to 72 years (mean age 55.5 years). All patients had a history of cerebral ischemia due to angiographically verified unilateral internal artery occlusion. Based on clinical findings, eight patients had no clinical deficits but had a history of previous transient cerebral attacks (TIA). Prolonged reversible ischemic neurologic deficits (PRIND) were found in eight patients and five patients had minor completed strokes (CS). Following routine preoperative work-up, bypass surgery was performed on the symptomatic side. There was no operative mortality or serious morbidity in this series. Bypass patency was confirmed in all patients by postoperative angiography which was done either at the end of the first postoperative week or several weeks later during follow-up studies. In all of these patients pre- and postoperative CBF measurements were done at resting state conditions. In another group of eight cases cerebral hemodynamics were studied following intravenous injection of 1 g acetazolamide (Diamox), which results in a significant increase of

Advances in Neurosurgery, Vol. 13
Edited by H. Dietz, M. Brock, and M. Klinger

CBF under normal conditions (10). Five of these cases were patients with internal carotid artery occlusion who underwent bypass surgery, and the Diamox response was studied pre- and postoperatively in addition to CBF measurements at rest. Finally, in three male volunteers with no evidence of cerebral ischemia CBF was measured before and at various intervals following intravenous injection of Diamox with a total of three studies in each case.

Measurement of CBF

The CBF was measured by the xenon-133 inhalation method and single photon emission tomography, which has been described in detail elsewhere (4, 9). The tomograph (TOMOMATIC 64, Medimatic Inc., Copenhagen, Denmark) has a rotating array of 64 Na-I-crystals which are arranged in four banks of 16 individual detectors. Three tomographic slices of the brain are obtained simultaneously with each slice 2 cm in thickness. The slices are positioned 1 cm, 5 cm, and 9 cm above the orbitomeatal plane. Following 1 min inhalation of 133 Xe with a maximum concentration of 10 mCi/l, the uptake and subsequent wash-out of the isotope is monitored over a 3-min period. A single detector is positioned over the right lung and the recorded activity is used to estimate the arterial input. By a conventional filtered back projection algorithm, flow values are calculated for each pixel in a 32 x 32 matrix and the resulting CBF maps are displayed on a colour-coded screen. At the end of each study an arterial blood sample is taken for measurement of the arterial pCO_2. For further analysis of data, a semiautomatic computer program was developed by which each tomographic slice is subdivided into 2 x 6 axially symmetric areas. This not only allows estimation of CBF in small region of interest but in addition provides interhemispheric flow ratios by comparing mean CBF of corresponding areas of the right and the left hemisphere (1). Since the second tomographic slice includes most of the middle cerebral artery territory which also would be primarily influenced by a revascularization procedure, only flow data of four areas - two on each side - of slice 2 were evaluated in this study. For internal standardization of the method, d-SPECT studies were performed in 35 normal volunteers.

Results

Group A (Fig. 1). Mean preoperative CBF (slice 2, areas 3 and 4 or 9 and 10) in 21 patients was found to be 63.1 ± 8.2 ml/100 g/min over the occluded side and 70.7 ± 13.2 ml/100 g/min over the contralateral side as opposed to a value of 72.5 ml/100 g/min which was obtained from 35 normal volunteers for the same area. At the end of the first postoperative week, the study was repeated in 17 patients and the respective values were now 61.6 ± 7.7 ml/100 g/min over the operated side and 65.6 ± 11.1 ml/100 g/min over the contralateral side. In 12 patients follow-up studies were done 2-6 months postoperatively, revealing mean CBF values of 62.9 ± 11.3 (operated side) and 67.3 ± 10.9 ml/100 g/min (contralateral side).

Group B. In all three normal volunteers a significant increase in CBF - 38%, 31%, and 22% above resting flow - was noted as early as 5 min following an intravenous injection of 1 g Diamox. Repeat measurements at 30, 60, and 120 min showed a gradual decrease in CBF but even after 120 min CBF was still 14% above the resting value in one case. No change in the arterial pCO_2 was noted following administration of Diamox. In five patients in whom the Diamox response was tested before bypass surgery, a significant increase in CBF was again seen over the contralateral side whereas almost no effect was found over the occluded site.

Postoperative results are as yet inconclusive, but there were two cases where the Diamox test suggested a markedly improved reserve capacity of CBF over both hemispheres.

Case Report (Figs. 2, 3). This 55-year-old patient had a history of intermittent right-sided deficits and was now presenting with mild aphasia and weakness of his right arm. Angiography disclosed a left internal carotid artery occlusion. Preoperative CBF showed ischemic flow values over the left side with almost no response to Diamox, which resulted in a significant increase in CBF over the contralateral side. One week after surgery, the study was repeated and a slight improvement in the Diamox response was noted over both hemispheres. Two months later another follow-up study was done and at this time a marked improvement in the Diamox response was noted over the operated side. Control angiography showed a well functioning bypass.

Discussion

Our understanding of the hemodynamic effect of extra-intracranial bypass surgery on brain ischemia is still incomplete and is primarily based on postoperative angiographic findings and additional evidence derived from previous two-dimensional CBF studies. Considering the advantage of the tomographic CBF technique which was used in this study, it can be assumed that the herein reported results will more precisely reflect the hemodynamic situation before and after surgery. Two observations are of particular interest. First, in the present study we were unable to find any significant change in CBF following bypass surgery despite angiographic proof of bypass patency in all patients and excellent intracranial filling of middle cerebral artery vessels in many of them. The number of the study population seems to be sufficient to make this more than just a preliminary finding. Whether, however, this conclusion, namely that bypass surgery has no effect on the resting blood flow, is generally correct needs to be further evaluated because in this study we have only included patients with internal carotid artery occlusions and the situation may be different in patients with, for example, occlusion of the middle cerebral artery. The other observation concerns the results that were obtained with the Diamox activation test. These studies were performed in order to evaluate the hypothesis that bypass surgery, even if it has no effect on resting CBF, might increase the reserve capacity of brain blood flow. While the mechanism by which Diamox acts on brain blood flow is as yet speculative, it was found to have a potent effect, resulting in an immediate and long-lasting increase in CBF. The results obtained with Diamox before and after surgery are too few to allow any definite conclusion. Preliminary evidence, however, suggests that the Diamox-induced flow increase is more pronounced in both hemispheres postoperatively. This would be in support of the concept that the hemodynamic effect of bypass surgery is primarily to improve the demand potential of the ischemic cerebral circulation.

References

1. BUELL, U., MOSER, E.A., KIRSCH, C.M., SCHMIEDEK, P.: 133 Xe-DSPECT (Dynamische Single Photon Emission CT). Fortschr. Röntgenstr. 139, 351-358 (1983)
2. HALSEY, H.J., MORAWETZ, R.B., BLAUENSTEIN, U.W.: The hemodynamic effect of STA-MCA bypass. Stroke 13, 163-167 (1982)

3. HEILBRUN, M.P., REICHMAN, O.H., ANDERSON, R.E., ROBERTS, T.S.: Regional cerebral blood flow studies following superficial temporal-middle cerebral artery anastomosis. J. Neurosurg. 43, 706-716 (1975)

4. LASSEN, N.A., HENRIKSEN, L., PAULSON, O.: Regional cerebral blood flow in stroke by 133-xenon inhalation and emission tomography. Stroke 12, 284-288 (1981)

5. LASSEN, N.A.: Editorial. Regional cerebral blood flow measurements in stroke: the necessity of a tomographic approach. J. Cereb. Blood Flow Metabol. 1, 141-142 (1981)

6. LITTLE, J.R., YAMAMOTO, Y.L., FEINDEL, W., MEYER, E., HODGE, C.P.: Superficial temporal artery to middle cerebral artery anastomosis. J. Neurosurg. 50, 560-569 (1979)

7. MEINIG, G., ULRICH, P., KÖSTER, E., SCHÜRMANN, K.: Ergebnisse der atraumatischen Hirndurchblutungsmessung mittels Xenon-Inhalation nach EC/IC-Anastomose. Akt. Neurol. 10, 208-211 (1983)

8. SCHMIEDEK, P., GRATZL, O. STEINHOFF, H., OLTEANU-NERBE, V.: Blood flow and cerebral revascularization. Clin. Neurosurg. 23, 270-286 (1976)

9. STOKELEY, E.M., SVEINSDOTTIR, E., LASSEN, N.A., ROMMER, P.: A single photon dynamic computer assisted tomography (DCAT) for imaging brain function in multiple cross sections. J. Comput. Assist. Tomogr. 4, 230-240 (1980)

10. VORSTRUP, S., ENGELL, H.C., LINDEWALD, H., LASSEN, N.A.: Hemodynamically significant stenosis of the internal carotid artery treated with endarterectomy. Case report. J. Neurosurg. 60, 1070-1075 (1984)

11. YONEKURA, M., AUSTIN, G., HAYWARD, W.: Longterm evaluation of cerebral blood flow, transient ischemic attacks and stroke after STA-MCA anastomosis. Surg. Neurol. 18, 123-130 (1982)

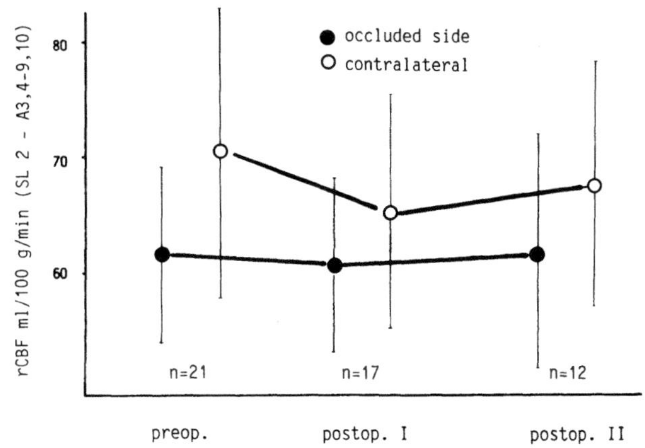

Fig. 1. Mean values of serial CBF measurements in 21 patients with internal carotid artery occlusion before and after extra-intracranial bypass surgery

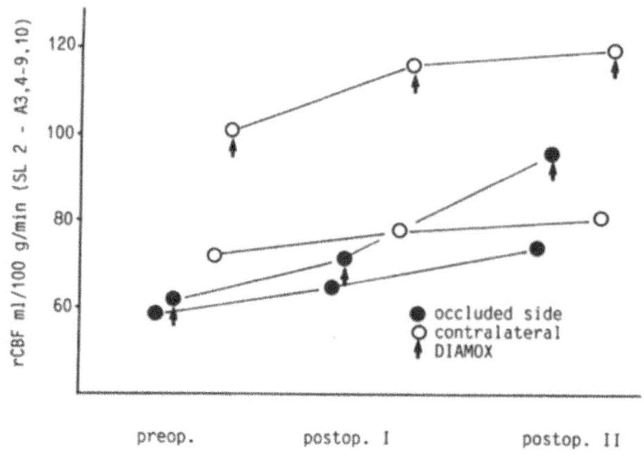

Fig. 2. CBF at rest and following injection of 1 g Diamox before and after bypass surgery. For details, see Case Report

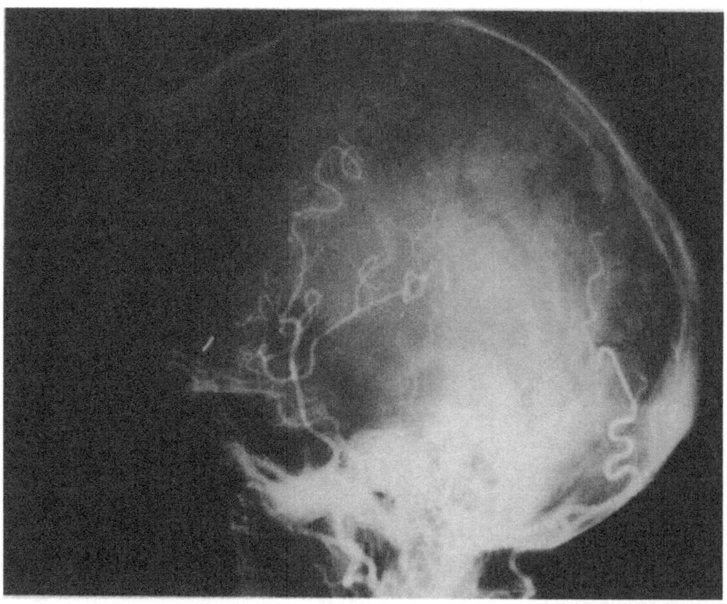

Fig. 3. Postoperative angiogram with patent bypass

Magnetic Resonance Imaging of Cerebral Infarcts Before and After Extra-Intracranial Anastomoses

H. Becker[1], R. Schwarzrock[2], and H. Friedrich[3]

[1] Abteilung Neuroradiologie, [2] Abteilung Nuklearmedizin, [3] Neurochirurgische Klinik, Medizinische Hochschule Hannover, Konstanty-Gutschow-Straße 8, D-3000 Hannover 61

Magnetic resonance imaging (MRI) is a new noninvasive imaging technique which can directly reveal cerebral infarcts (2-4, 6). One advantage of MRI over CT is that encephalomalacious foci can be visualized 3-6 h after vessel occlusion whereas CT needs approximately 24 h. Cerebral infarcts cannot be visualized in native CT scans during the "fogging effect" (isodensity of the infarct and missing signs of expansion) in the second or third week after the insult (1). However, MRI clearly identifies the infarct.

It is also possible to distinguish between fresh and old cerebral infarcts by using different modes. While the encephalomalacious foci can be detected during the stage of necrosis and resorption by T2 accentuated spin echo sequences, it can be demonstrated with proton density and T1 accentuated spin echo sequences during the stage of cyst and glial scarring. An additional advantage of MRI is the identification of infarcts in areas problematic for CT owing to superimposing artifacts, especially basal and posterior cranial fossa areas. The purpose of this study was to investigate cerebral infarcts before and after extra-intracranial arterial bypass grafting (EIAB), to establish whether there is a change of signal intensity in the infarcted areas after successful anastomoses. For comparison, parallel CT studies were performed.

Material and Methods

Ten patients with occlusions of the internal carotid artery and one with an occlusion of the middle cerebral artery, all clearly identified by angiography, were examined with MRI and CT before EIAB.

A postoperative angiography was performed to ensure the function of the bypass. If functioning, another MRI and another CT scan were done two months after surgery. This was possible for eight patients. The Siemens MRI Scanner had a magnetic resistance of 0.2 Tesla and a high frequency system with 8.25 mHz. The slice thickness was 10 mm. The spin echo mode and inversion recovery mode were employed in axial, coronal, and sagittal planes. The computer tomographic scans were performed on a General Electric 9800 CT scanner. To get comparable axial slices, the same slice thickness of 10 mm was chosen.

Results

The encephalomalacious foci were detected in the stage of cyst and glial scarring in 10 of 11 patients. The areas of infarction were shown more impressively by MRI because of the greater contrast of the adjacent brain tissue than the contrast of the hypodense zones in CT

Advances in Neurosurgery, Vol. 13
Edited by H. Dietz, M. Brock, and M. Klinger

scans. With increasing delay, this difference in contrast in MRI scans could be further intensified. No differences between MRI and CT regarding the number and size of the infarctions were found. Comparing the pre- and postoperative results that existed for eight patients, we found no change in five cases. Three patients showed additional encephalomalacious foci, which appeared in two cases in the area of surgery (Figs. 1, 2). None had additional neurological deficits.

Discussion

The invention of CT was a major breakthrough in the detection of cerebral vascular disease. In every case where cerebral ischemia leads to morphological changes of the cerebral parenchyma, CT can be the instrument of decision in determining the possibility of EIAB (5). MRI has the same ability. Although the infarction area can be seen even more clearly with MRI, it does not offer advantages over CT while the cerebral infarction is in the stage of cyst and glial scarring. MRI especially does not provide clues that EIAB leads to proton shifts to the margin of the infarction area as a sign of revitalization. Information concerning improvement in regional blood flow after EIAB cannot be obtained with MRI, which remains reserved for functional methods of nuclear medicine (rCBF, PET, SPECT, etc.). As a noninvasive method, MRI has the ability to identify progression of infarctions and postoperative complications, but similar results can be obtained with CT.

Conclusion

After extra-intracranial arterial bypass grafting, MRI does not show a change in signal intensity in cerebral infarctions which are in the stage of cyst and glial scarring. Due to greater contrast differences in the adjacent tissues, infarctions can be visualized more clearly than with CT. No differences regarding the number and size of the infarctions were demonstrated between MRI and CT.

Pre- and postoperative CT and MRI show progressing infarctions and secondary surgical complications with equal diagnostic accuracy.

References

1. Becker, H., Desch, H., Hacker, H., Pencz, A.: CT fogging effect with ischemic cerebral infarcts. Neuroradiology 18, 185-192 (1979)
2. Bryan, R.N., Willcott, M.R., Schneiders, N.J., Rose, J.E.: NMR evaluation of occlusive stroke in the rat. AJNR 4, 242-244 (1983)
3. Bryan, R.N., Willcott, M.R., Schneiders, N.J., Ford, J.J., Derman, H.S.: Nuclear magnetic resonance evaluation of stroke. Radiology 149, 189-192 (1983)
4. Levy, R.M., Mano, J., Brito, A., Hosobuchi, Y.: NMR imaging of acute experimental cerebral ischemia: time course and pharmacologic manipulations. AJNR 4, 238-241 (1983)
5. Schmiedek, P., Lanksch, W., Olteanu-Nerbe, V., Kazner, E., Gratzl, O., Marguth, F.: Combined use of regional cerebral blood flow measurement and computerized tomography for the diagnosis of cerebral ischemia. In: Schmiedek, P. (ed.) Microsurgery for stroke. Springer, New York Heidelberg Berlin 1977
6. Sipponen, J.T., Kaste, M., Ketonen, L., Sepponen, R.E., Katevuo, K., Sivula, A.: Serial nuclear magnetic resonance (NMR) imaging in patients with cerebral infarction. J. Comput. Assist. Tomogr. 7, 585-589 (1983)

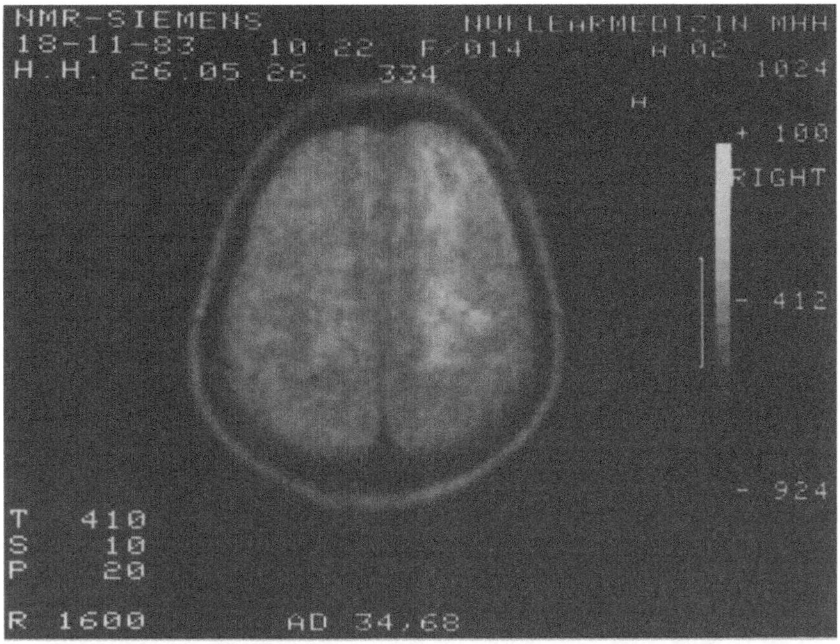

a

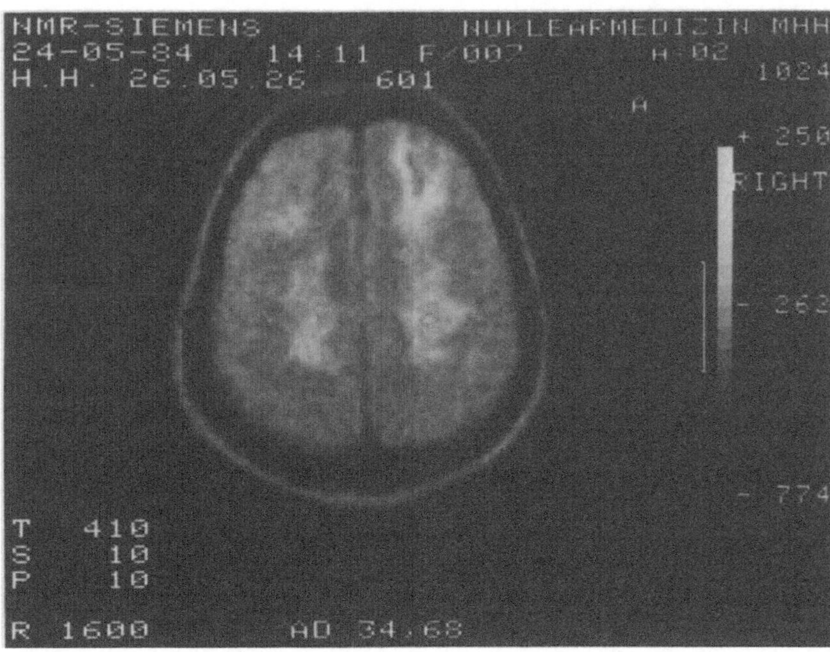

b

Fig. 1. a 58-year-old man with occlusion of the right internal carotid artery. MRI scan before EIAB; right and left parietal infarctions. b Postoperative control after right EIAB, in the meantime additional cerebral infarctions had occurred

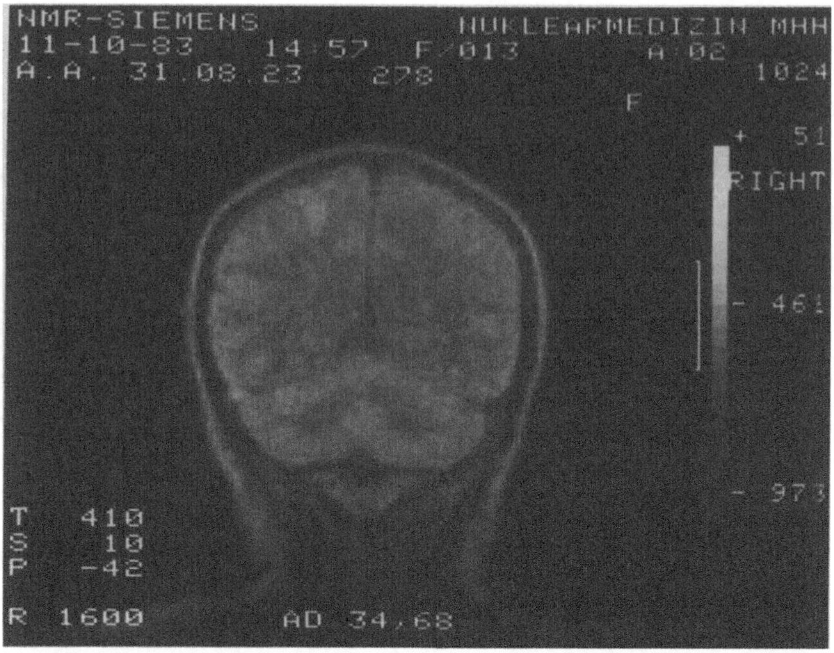

a

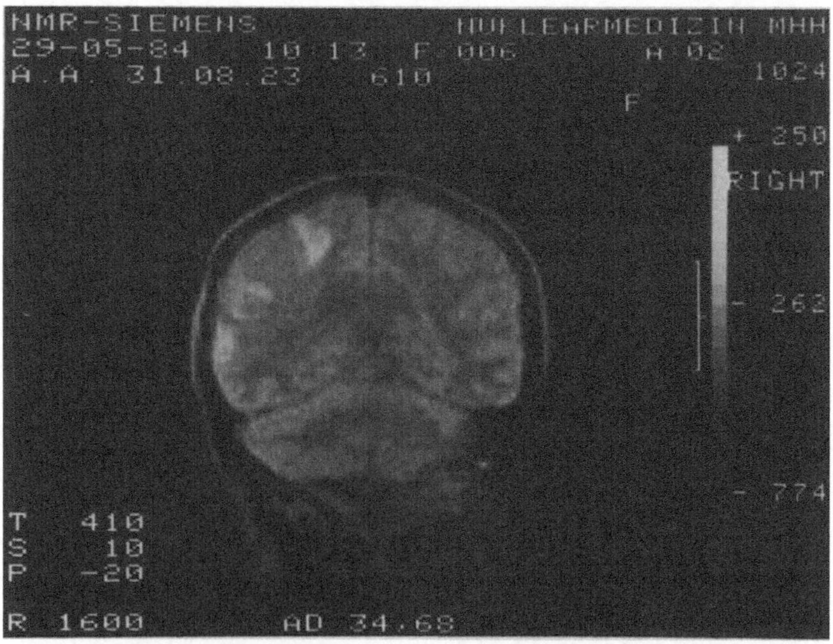

b

Fig. 2. a 60-year-old man with left internal carotid occlusion. MRI scan before EIAB; left parietal cerebral infarction. b Postoperative control after left EIAB. Demonstration of additional cerebral infarctions in the surgical area secondary to prolonged temporary clipping at the time of saphenous vein interposition

Microsurgery at the Edge of the Tentorium

Anatomy of the Tentorial Margin

J. Lang
Anatomisches Institut der Universität, Koellikerstraße 6, D-8700 Würzburg

Tentorial Margin (Fig. 1)

The tentorium cerebelli and its medial margin are composed of collagen fibers. This rigid construction is fixed anteriorly on the clinoid processes by two folds. The upper and posterior part of the tentorial notch rises more steeply than the lower part and finally merges into an arch running rostrally. In this part the tentorium cerebelli rises relatively steeply to a central ridge, which is bounded on both sides of the median plane by a strand of fibers known as the plica limitans fastigii.

The *anterior petroclinoid fold* is mainly composed of fibers from the tentorial notch. It is usually sharp edged but may sometimes be rounded where it is in relation to the side wall of the sinus. In the vicinity of the anterior clinoid process, which is embraced by this group of fibers, the medial fibers radiate above the optic nerve and unite with the transverse fibers of the dura mater on the planum sphenoidale (3). The lateral fibers run along the posterior margin of the lesser wing of the sphenoid and contribute to the relatively thick dural layer at this site. The fibers in the basin region of the transverse plate of the cavernous sinus are likewise largely derived from the anterior radiation of the tentorium. The entry portal for the oculomotor nerve is formed by a concave border, sharp rostrally and rounded dorsally. That part of the basin situated behind the oculomotor nerve consists of fibers which originate from the ramification zone of both petroclinoid folds and form dense bundles dorsally. Anteriorly, these fibers diverge into a relatively thin roof layer for the cavernous sinus.

The *posterior petroclinoid fold* is fixed on the posterior clinoid process and represents the basal medial extension of the tentorial notch. The angle enclosed between the two petroclinoid folds averages 37.92° ($25-50^{\circ}$) on the right and 36.86° ($20-55^{\circ}$) on the left. Most values for the angle were between 30° and 50° on right and left alike. Surprisingly enough, large cranial widths seem to be associated with narrow angles between the clinoid folds. There is no correlation between the width of the cavernous sinuses, measured at the level of the posterior clinoid process, and the size of the angle.

The anterior petroclinoid fold lies against part of the parahippocampal gyrus. The fold produces the so-called uncal notch in the latter, but when the fold is rounded this notch may not be apparent. The oculomotor nerve may be pressed against and involved by the posterior petroclinoid fold in displacement of the brain.

Advances in Neurosurgery, Vol. 13
Edited by H. Dietz, M. Brock, and M. Klinger

Cisterna Ambiens

The cisterna ambiens acts as a liquor cushion against the tentorial margin and communicates basally with the interpeduncular cisterna, surrounds the lateral sides of the cerebral peduncles, and continues dorsally into the cisterna of the lamina tecti and the cisterna of the great cerebral vein. Dorsally it overlaps both surfaces of the free border of the tentorium cerebelli and the notch. Posteriorly and below it communicates with the lateral pontine cisterna and the subarachnoid spaces of the cerebellum, while above the tentorium it communicates with the subarachnoid spaces of the occipital lobe. Within the cisterna are situated segments of the posterior cerebral artery, the tectal artery, and the posterior choroidal ramus. The lateral mesencephalic vein is the largest supra-infratentorial vessel. The superior cerebellar artery and basal vein run dorsally, while the trochlear nerve runs basally. The peripeduncular cisterna is demarcated by its appositional surfaces on the mesencephalon. Above the cisterna of the lamina tecti, there is a wide connection between the two halves of the peripeduncular cisterna; they also communicate behind and above the pineal body and via a narrow connecting channel (1-1.5 mm wide) immediately dorsal to the epithalamic (posterior) commissure and below the pineal body. Apart from these connections, this segment communicates with the retrosplenial part of the unpaired pericallosal cisterna. Cerebrospinal fluid from the cisterna ambiens also runs rostrally into the cisterna of the transverse fissure.

Mesencephalon (Fig. 2)

The mesencephalon connects those parts of the brain in the hypophyseal region (diencephalon) with those in the posterior cranial fossa (rhombencephalon).

Cerebral Peduncles

The interpeduncular fossa is bounded laterally by the cerebral crura. Situated in the depths of the fossa is the tegmentum of the mesencephalon, with the crura lying basal and lateral to it.

Tegmentum of the Mesencephalon

The tegmentum of the midbrain contains the substantia nigra, the red nucleus, the nuclei of the oculomotor and trochlear nerves, and parts of the nuclei of the trigeminal nerve. Other structures within the tegmentum include the central matter of the midbrain, the decussation of the superior cerebellar peduncles, the lemnisci, and parts of the reticular formation. The lamina tecti forms the dorsal part of the mesencephalon. The principal structures which it contains are the superior and inferior quadrigeminal bodies (cranial and caudal colliculi) and the brachia of the midbrain (brachia colliculorum).

Crus Cerebri

At the point where it joins the pons, the lateral aspect of the crus cerebri measures between 14 mm and 16 mm, and in its upper part the corresponding dimension averages 18.54 mm. On the basal surface it has an average length of 13.03 mm. When the optic tract is dissected off, a further segment of the crus cerebri, averaging 4.01 mm in length, comes into view. The crus cerebri contains long and short projection pathways arranged in a somatotopic pattern. Laterally and above run the fibers from the temporal lobe to the nuclei of the pons: the temporopontine fibers (Türck). Some of the latter also run into the substantia nigra. In the middle zone is the corticospinal tract; the dorsolateral fibers in this tract run to the lower limb; next come the fibers for the trunk and basally the fibers for the upper limb and cranial nerve nuclei (corticonuclear tract). Situated mediobasally, and extending as far as the medial sulcus of the crus, are the fibers running from the frontal lobe to the pontine nuclei (the frontopontine fibers of Arnold) together with other fibers destined for the substantia nigra.

Interpeduncular Fossa

The average length of the interpeduncular fossa in adults is 11.72 mm (7-20 mm). In its posterior part it deepens to form the caudal recess of the interpeduncular fossa. In this area the average depth (measured from the basal surface of the crura cerebri) is 6.94 mm (5-13 mm). In the anterior part there is a smaller rostral recess, which is situated an average of 2 mm posterior to the dorsal surfaces of the mamillary bodies. When the subject is standing upright, it forms the highest point of the interpeduncular fossa, and in our material the fossa had an average depth of 5.80 mm (4-12 mm) in this region. A shallow median longitudinal furrow divides the interpeduncular fossa indistinctly into two halves. The lateral boundary is formed by the medial crurotegmental sulcus, in the neighborhood of which the substantia nigra is often visible and the oculomotor nerve leaves the midbrain.

The term "caudal perforated fossa", sometimes applied to the interpeduncular fossa, is based on the existence of numerous holes in the basal surface of the tegmentum. Arteries to the midbrain, diencephalon, and pons enter through these holes and veins emerge. The majority of the arteries which plunge into the interpeduncular fossa (interpeduncular arteries) supply the nuclei and white matter of the midbrain and, more importantly, parts of the diencephalon. In view of this fact, we have designated them as the posterior inferior diencephalic branches. For the nuclei and pathways of the mesencephalon, see Fig. 2.

Blood Supply to the Mesencephalon (Fig. 3)

Anterior Choroid Artery

In our material (1) the anterior choroid artery is derived from the internal carotid artery in 96% of bodies. In 2% it arises from the posterior communicating artery, and in a further 2% the artery is double, one vessel coming from the internal carotid artery and the other from the posterior communicating artery. Its origin is situated an average of 2.9 mm (0.5-5.0 mm) proximal to the division of the carotid. The artery has an average diameter of 0.77 mm (0.4-1.25 mm) and runs at first towards the optic tract. It crosses the tract medially and upwards and gives off fine twigs to the diencephalon: the posterior lateral inferior diencephalic branches. It consistently supplies fine twigs to the surface of the optic tract, and in 53% there are arteries 0.25-0.5 mm in thickness running through the tract. Twigs (0.38 mm) also run into the diencephalon, passing lateral to the optic tract in 35% and medial to it in 39%. Fine twigs run to the lateral geniculate body and to the mesencephalon.

Blood Supply to the Lateral Geniculate Body

The anterior parts of the lateral geniculate body are mostly supplied by twigs from the anterior choroid artery, and the posterior parts by twigs from the lateral posterior choroid branch and directly by twigs from the posterior cerebral artery (thalamogeniculate branches).

Posterior Cerebral Artery

Some fine twigs of the PCA reach the lateral surface of the midbrain (see Fig. 3).

Artery of the Lamina Tecti (A. quadrigemina)

In approximately 58% of cases the artery of the lamina tecti arises from the precommunicating part of the posterior cerebral artery proximal to the posterior communicating artery. The artery has an average diameter of 0.37 mm (0.2-0.4 mm) and divides 16.2 mm (1-43 mm) distal to its origin into two branches, first giving off interpeduncular branches to the interpeduncular fossa and then passing around the crus cerebri. In this segment it gives off an average of 3.6 (1-6) twigs to the cerebral peduncle and in 22.8% of cases also sends twigs to the trigonum lemnisci. Having divided into two branches, the artery of the lamina tecti reaches the territory of the quadrigeminal bodies and gives off twigs, chiefly to the superior quadrigeminal body. These twigs frequently form fine anastomoses with one another. In only 4% were there twigs to the inferior quadrigeminal body and medial geniculate body and in only 1.6% twigs to the thalamus. In 36% the artery anastomoses with the medial posterior choroid branch, and in 1.6% with the posterior cerebral artery (5).

Medial Posterior Choroid Branch

In 95% of our material (5) the medial posterior choroid branch arose from the posterior cerebral artery distal to its junction with the posterior communicating artery. In 75.2% the twig was situated proximal to the division of the posterior cerebral artery, in 3.2% in the area of its division, and in 21.6% distal to its bifurcation. When its origin was distally situated, 19.1% arose from the medial occipital artery and 2.5% from the lateral occipital artery.

In 69% there was one artery which followed this course, in 23.9% there were two, in 6.2% three, and in 0.9% four.

The medial posterior choroid branch has an average diameter of 0.5 mm (0.1-1.0 mm). It usually runs in a more or less straight line around the peduncle and below the posterior cerebral artery, passing backwards and upwards within the cisterna ambiens. During this part of its course, it gives off an average of 1.9 (0-5) peduncular branches to the lateral and upper surface of the cerebral peduncle. In 22% we found twigs to the trigonum lemnisci and in 2.8% twigs to the pedunculogeniculate sulcus. The diameter of these twigs averaged 0.12 mm (0.1-2.0 mm).

During its peripeduncular course, an average of 1.2 (0-4) branches to the medial geniculate body arise from the artery. They supply the medial geniculate body, the relay and transmission station of the central auditory pathway. These twigs have an average diameter of 0.16 mm

(0.1-0.3 mm). Fine twigs from this vessel to the lateral geniculate body were demonstrable in only 1.6% of cases and twigs to the trigonum lemnisci in only 0.8%.

Thalamic branches arising from the medial posterior choroid branch were present in roughly 50% of our material. In 36.0% they pierced the posterior surface of the pulvinar and in 28% its upper surface. In 18.6% they ran into the pedunculopulvinar sulcus, and in 17.4% they passed lateral to the pulvinar into the diencephalon. The posterior thalamic branches have an average diameter of 0.16 mm (0.1-0.3 mm). After its peripeduncular segment, the artery runs medially and upwards in the direction of the pineal body and then turns rostrally within the cisterna of the transverse fissure. In 97.3% dissection revealed a branch to the pineal body and in 2.7% there were two such twigs. The average diameter of this vessel was 0.16 mm (0.1-0.3 mm). As a rule, the medial posterior choroid branch forms loops in the vicinity of the pineal body. In 36.3% the medial posterior choroid branch anastomoses with the plexus of the superior quadrigeminal body via twigs which are given off at the level of the brachium of the inferior quadrigeminal body. In 20.5% there are anastomoses with the artery of the lamina tecti and in 2.7% with the posterior cerebral artery.

Where the medial posterior choroid branch runs into the cisterna of the transverse fissure, it is still single in 91.3% of cases, but in 9.7% it has divided into two branches. In this segment the average diameters are 0.31 mm (0.1-0.5 mm). Within the cisterna of the transverse fissure, it gives off twigs to the surface of the thalamus and the choroid plexus of the third ventricle. In 22.4% these twigs enter the posterior quarter of the plexus, in 45.9% the second quarter, in 28.2% the third quarter, and in 3.5% the anterior quarter (5).

Superior Cerebellar Artery

In 99% of our cases (1) there were twigs from the superior cerebellar artery to the lamina tecti. These arose from the medial branch of the superior cerebellar artery or from its twigs (superior artery of the vermis). They run to the vicinity of the inferior quadrigeminal body and anastomose with the twigs from the artery of the lamina tecti supplying the superior quadrigeminal body. The anastomoses with the latter vessel average 0.2 mm in diameter. The twigs from the superior cerebellar artery to the lamina tecti average 6.1 (1-14) in number and have the same diameter. The superior cerebellar peduncle is also supplied by an average of 5.1 (1-11) twigs from the superior cerebellar artery with average diameters of 0.13 mm (0.1-0.4 mm).

Pontomesencephalic Artery

In 60% of bodies LANG and BRUNNER (4) demonstrated a pontomesencephalic artery which arises a few millimeters after the origin of the superior cerebellar artery and, concealed by the latter, runs around the midbrain. The pontomesencephalic artery encroaches upon the lateral portion of the pons and gives off twigs to its anterior and lateral surfaces. Its terminal ramifications, coming from above and behind, reach as far as the sensory and motor roots of the trigeminal nerve and sometimes the superior cerebellar peduncle as well. The vessel has an average diameter of 0.5 mm (0.4-0.75 mm).

Veins of the Midbrain Region (Fig. 4)

Termination of the Basal Vein

In our material the basal vein most frequently drained into the internal cerebral vein, and less frequently into the union between the two internal cerebral veins or into the great cerebral vein. In the average case the junction is situated just rostral to the union between the internal cerebral veins. Several veins drain into the terminal segment of the basal vein: they include the posterior mesencephalic vein, the dorsal vein of the corpus callosum, the internal occipital veins, and the posterior choroid veins. In addition, the precentral cerebellar vein (present in roughly equal percentages on one or both sides), together with other cerebellar veins, regularly drains into the posterior aspect of the terminal segment of the basal vein, into the great cerebral vein (the commonest termination), or directly into the straight sinus. The vein of the superior vermis, the preculminal vein, the culminal vein, and the medial anterior cerebellar vein also discharge into this region, independently of the precentral vein.

Relations between the Basal Vein and Medial Posterior Choroid Branch

In 39.5% of cases the medial posterior choroid branch runs into the cisterna of the transverse fissure at a point lateral to the basal vein, with or without forming a loop directed dorsally. In 46.5% the medial posterior choroid branch runs medial to the basal vein, often forming a lateral loop directed dorsally. In 14% the medial posterior choroid branch bifurcated, one twig running medial and the other lateral to the basal vein on their way to the cisterna of the transverse fissure.

Lateral Affluents

The veins draining into the basal vein from the lateral side are the inferior ventricular vein, the vein of the temporal horn, and frequently also a vein from the apex of the temporal horn and a vein from the floor of the temporal horn.

In the vicinity of the peripeduncular segment and within the cisterna ambiens, there are numerous supra-infratentorial anastomoses. Connections between the interpeduncular veins and the rete venosum of the pons are known as basal anastomoses, while connections on the lateral surface of the cerebral peduncle are termed basolateral anastomoses, and connections between the basal vein and the petrosal vein are termed lateral anastomoses or v. mesencephalica lateralis. The petrosal vein drains into the superior petrosal sinus in the vicinity of the portal for the trigeminal nerve. According to DUVERNOY (2), the vessel is present in 75% and of very large caliber in 10%. In 15% it is absent.

Great Cerebral Vein (of Galen)

The great cerebral vein is formed by the confluence of the two internal cerebral veins. In 28% the confluence is situated on the surface of the pineal body, in 21% on its posterior border, and in 51% occipital to the pineal body. The vein is 1 cm (0.5-1.5 cm) in length and relatively wide. It runs around the posterior margin of the splenium of the corpus callosum to reach the straight sinus, which it usually enters at a right angle.

Clinical Significance of the Tentorial Notch and Midbrain (Fig. 5)

Between the midbrain and the tentorial margin is a narrow space about 1.5 mm in width. Space-occupying lesions in the middle and anterior cranial fossae or in the diencephalon may force parts of the hypothalamus and the medial segments of the temporal lobe through the tentorial notch into the posterior cranial fossa. The posterior cerebral artery may be involved in such cases: the result is contralateral homonymous hemianopia with sparing of the macula. Also the third nerve becomes stretched and according to SUNDERLAND (6) may come in contact with the posterior clinoid process.

During these events it is the anterior and upper surface of the ipsilateral oculomotor nerve which is the first to be damaged. The pupilloconstrictor fibers are believed to run in this part. Accordingly, the first abnormality is narrowing of the pupil (as a result of irritation); this is later followed by dilatation of the pupil and loss of the pupillary reflexes. The next change to be observed is weakening of the other ocular muscles supplied by the oculomotor nerve.

The basal vein may also be compressed by brain shifts. Although it possesses collaterals, this usually results in brain swelling. Infratentorial tumors may cause herniation of the contents of the posterior cranial fossa forwards and upwards through the tentorial notch.

The great cerebral vein (of Galen) may be squeezed against the splenium of the corpus callosum and in these circumstances the variable amounts of cerebellar tissue in the tentorial notch may exert further pressure on the vein. The superior cerebellar arteries may also be compressed against the free border of the tentorium.

References

1. Brunner, F.X.: Über die Arterien des Hirnstammes, Vorkommen, Zahl, Durchmesser und Variationen. M.D. Thesis, University of Würzburg 1979
2. Duvernoy, H.M.: The superficial veins of the human brain. Springer, Berlin Heidelberg New York 1975
3. Lang, J.: Eintritt und Verlauf der Hirnnerven (III, IV, VI) "im" Sinus cavernosus. Z. Anat. Entwickl.-Gesch. 145, 87-99 (1974)
4. Lang, J., Brunner, F.X.: Über die arterielle Versorgung der Medulla oblongata und des Pons. Verh. Anat. Ges. 73, 101-105 (1979)
5. Lang, J., Käpplinger, E.: A. laminae tecti (quadrigemina) und Rami thalamogeniculati. Anat. Anz. 147, 1-11 (1980)
6. Sunderland, S.: The tentorial notch and complications produced by herniation of the brain through that aperture. Br. J. Sur. 45, 422-438 (1957/58)

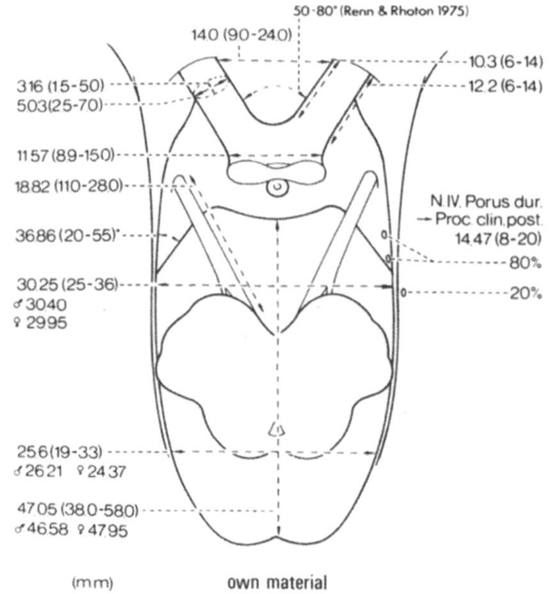

Fig. 1. Tentorial notch and brain structures, measurements. Given are the distance between the optic nerves and its angle (RENN and RHOTON 1975), the heights and the medial and lateral length of the optic nerve, and the width of the chiasm. Also indicated is the length of the oculomotor nerve, the angle between the petroclinoidal folds, the entrance zone of the IVth nerve in the dura mater, and the lower and upper width and length of the tentorial notch

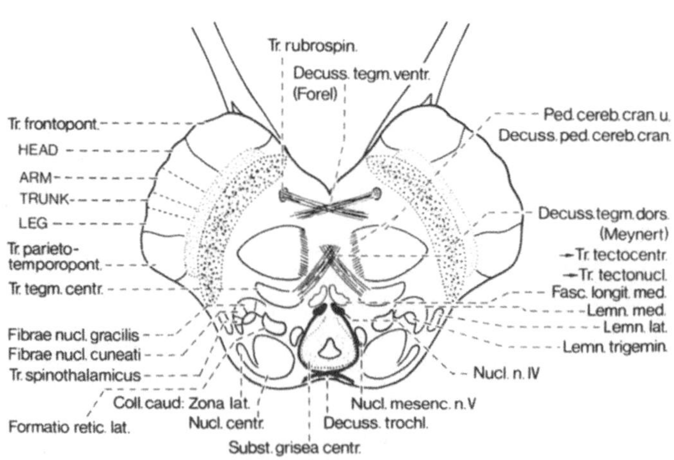

Fig. 2. Mesencephalon, fiber tracts, and nuclei at the level of the caudal colliculus

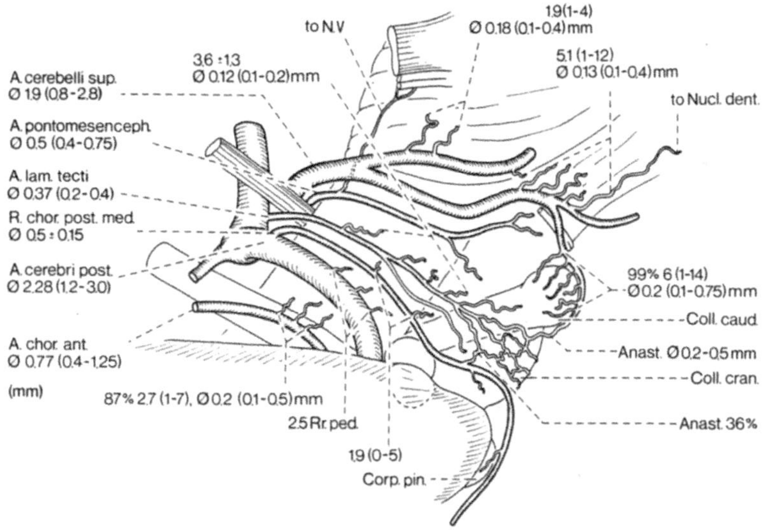

Fig. 3. Arterial mesencephalic branches from different arteries (diameters and numbers)

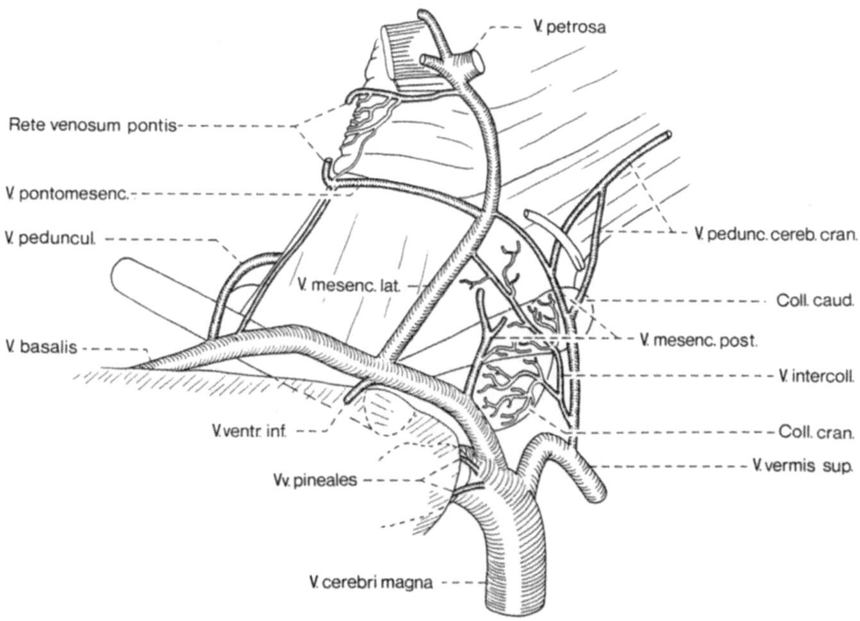

Fig. 4. Superficial mesencephalic veins and their drainage

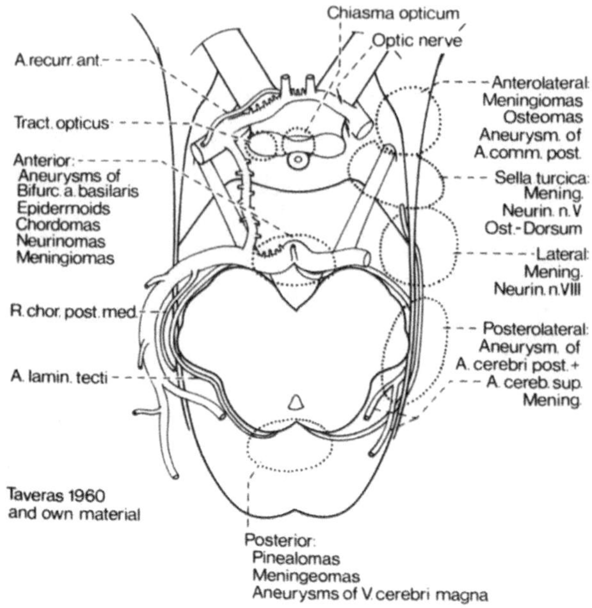

<u>Fig. 5.</u> Tentorial notch and space-occupying lesions

Meningiomas at the Tentorial Edge

H. Arnold and H.-D. Herrmann
Neurochirurgische Abteilung des Universitätskrankenhauses, Martinistraße 52, D-2000 Hamburg 20

Owing to their close relationship to cranial nerves, brain-stem, and brain-stem supporting vasculature, meningiomas at the tentorial edge continue to challenge neurosurgeons, although neurosurgical techniques as well as peri- and postoperative intensive care have improved considerably. The risk to the patient, however, could be reduced, since refined diagnostic tools have provided the facilities for precise planning of surgical access and procedure. Here we outline our experience during the period 1951 through 1983.

Eighty-three patients were admitted because of meningiomas located at the tentorial edge, 79 of whom were operated on. In the remaining four cases, a cerebrospinal fluid drainage system only was installed, or operation was refused. Two periods of treatment are compared, the first lasting from 1951 until 1978, the second from 1979 until 1983. In the first period the mean age of the patients operated was 49 years, with a range of 27-74 years, while in the second period the mean age was 54 years, with a range of 30-72 years. Cranial nerve palsy, symptoms of the increased intracranial pressure, ataxia, and pyramidal deficits were the most common findings. Tumor sites and their frequency are schematically demonstrated in Fig. 1. The current neurosurgical approaches are drawn in. Instead of the combined subtemporal and retromastoidal approach, a parapyramidal route of access can be used by cutting the transverse sinus and severing the tentorium near the pyramid.

Twenty-seven tumors situated in the cerebellopontine angle originated from the tentorium and the pyramid ridge. Partially, they extended into the supratentorial space. Eighteen tumors originated from the tentorial edge at the region of Meckel's cavum, the pyramid tip, and the posterior clinoidal process. Another 17 tumors were located at the tentorial edge, pyramid ridge and tip, and upper clivus, most of them being restricted to the infratentorial space. Eight tumors occupied the region of anterior straight sinus, vein of Galen, and paracollicular space. Thirteen tumors had grown at the dorsolateral tentorial edge, expanding into the supra- and infratentorial spaces.

Operative mortality (Table 1) and postoperative morbidity were mainly linked to tumors located at the clivus and the medial pyramid region. Severe lasting postoperative neurological deficit was present in five patients. In another case, serious neurological disturbances, which had presented preoperatively, failed to improve following microsurgical tumor removal.

From Fig. 1 it is obvious that precise planning of the neurosurgical approach and avoidance of intraoperative complications was difficult

Advances in Neurosurgery, Vol. 13
Edited by H. Dietz, M. Brock, and M. Klinger

Table 1. Operative mortality and morbidity among 79 patients operated on for tentorial edge meningiomas: Relation of results to tumor site

Tumor site	1951-1978		1979-1983	
	n	Died	n	Died
Tentorium/petrous ridge	16 (+2[a])	3	9	0
Tentorial edge Pyramid tip	11	3	5 (+2[a])	0
Tentorium/clivus Pyramid apex	13	6	4	1
Straight sinus Tentorial edge	1	0	7	1
Dorsolateral tentorial edge	9	2	4	0
Total	50	14/50	29	2/29

[a]Patients treated by CSF drainage only, or who refused operation

before cranial computerized tomography had been introduced. For the most part, the high operative mortality of former years resulted from incomplete preoperative knowledge about tumor topography and from inadequate access. As is shown in Table 2, the results have improved impressively during the last five years. This is at least in part due to careful choice of surgical approach and refined microsurgical technique.

During the first period reported, cranial nerve laceration represented a major cause of postoperative fatalities and disability. In total, there were 13 cases among 79 patients with one to seven cranial nerves being surrounded and compressed by the tumor. In 29 additional patients, cranial nerves were only displaced and stretched. Cranial nerve transection during tumor removal was performed five times in the first period, and twice in the period from 1979 through 1983. Persistent cranial nerve damage due to operation presented in ten cases operated on before 1979, and in another three cases operated on between 1979 and

Table 2. Operative mortality and morbidity among 79 patients operated on for tentorial edge meningiomas: Comparison of results between two periods of treatment

	1951-1978	1979-1983
n	52	31
Operated	50	29
Mortality	14	2
Severely disabled[a]	4	2
Slightly disabled	6	3

[a]Need help for common activities

1983. Today, the crucial point for the neurosurgeon is the preservation of tumor-related veins of the pons and midbrain more than that of cranial nerves.

Tumor recurrence developed in seven out of 50 cases of the first period and in two out of 29 cases of the second period. Generally, recurrence became evident within three years following the first operation.

During recent years, by using selected operative approaches and skilful microsurgical techniques, operations on tentorial edge meningiomas have been made safer, though operative procedures have become more extensive.

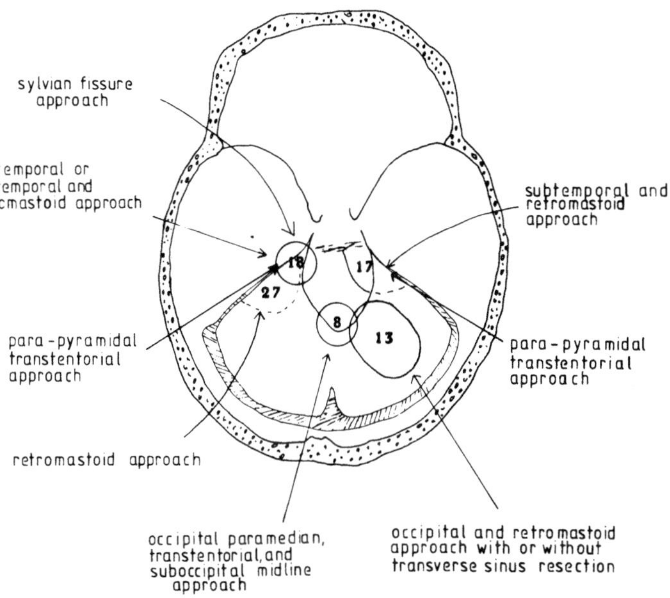

Fig. 1. Site and frequency of 83 meningiomas at the tentorial edge treated between 1951 and 1983, as well as operative approaches

Approaches to the Tentorial Edge, Demonstrated by Reference to 30 Cases of Tentorial Edge Meningioma

A. Perneczky and A. Horaczek
Neurochirurgische Abteilung, Universität Wien, Alser Straße 4, A-1090 Wien

Introduction

The tentorial edge and its relationship to the mesencephalon and the adjacent structures on the one hand and its role as a border between the supra- and infratentorial region on the other hand play a special part in surgical and anatomical publications. Surgical exposure of the tentorial edge can be performed by various approaches, each possibility having topographic and anatomical limits. The appropriate approach is chosen according to the relationship of the process to the tentorial edge. The present paper discusses the various approaches to this region by reference to 30 cases of tentorial edge meningioma.

Clinical Material

Out of 30 patients suffering from tentorial edge meningioma, 21 were female and nine male. The average age was 58 years at the time of surgery. In 27 cases the tumor was radically removed, and in six of them surgery was performed in two stages due to tumor size and age of the patient. In three cases we refrained from radical removal given the advanced age of the patient (more than 70 years), and the portion of tumor attached to the mesencephalon was left. Two patients died following surgery (6.7%) and two further patients had a postoperative peduncular hemiparesis (6.7%). Nine patients suffered from ipsilateral oculomotor paresis following surgery (30%). In five of these patients paresis receded within a few months.

Operative Approaches (Table 1)

1. The *transsylvian-pterional approach* was chosen in six cases. In all of these cases 90% of the meningioma mass was above the tentorial plane. The origin of the meningiomas was adjacent to the oculomotor nerve.
2. The *anterior subtemporal approach* was used in three patients who had a similarly located tumor as previously described for the transsylvian approach.
3. The *posterior subtemporal approach* was chosen in four patients. The tumor was mainly located posteriorly in the falx-tentorium angle. In two cases the tentorium was partially resected and thus the infratentorial part of the tumor was extirpated.
4. The *transtemporal approach* through the angular gyrus was used in four cases, three times on the right and once on the left side. In these cases the origin of the tumor was in the falx-tentorium angle, expanding more superiorly. It was located directly beneath the

 Advances in Neurosurgery, Vol. 13
Edited by H. Dietz, M. Brock, and M. Klinger

Table 1. Surgical approaches to the tentorium edge

	No. of cases
1. Transsylvian	6
2. Anterior subtemporal	3
3. Posterior subtemporal	4
4. Transtemporal	4
5. Paramedian parieto-occipital	1
6. Occipital-transtentorial	1
7. Infratentorial-supracerebellar	3
8. Retromastoid	5
9. Combined supra-infratentorial	3

collateral trigone of the lateral ventricle. In none of these cases was neurological deficit confirmed following surgery.

5. The *paramedian parieto-occipital approach* was employed in one patient. Here the tumor originated from the tentorium-falx angle and grew up along the falx to the superior sagittal sinus.
6. The *occipital-transtentorial approach* was chosen in one patient with a large median located meningioma of the falx and tentorium with supra- and infratentorial extension.
7. The *infratentorial-supracerebellar approach* was chosen in three cases. Here the tumor was located in the pineal region.
8. The *lateral suboccipital* or *retromastoid approach* was predominantly located infratentorially, originating more from the anterolateral portion of the tentorial edge.
9. The *combined supra- and infratentorial approach* was used in three patients who had large tumors growing more laterally as well as supra- and infratentorially. The approach is a combination of the subtemporal and the retromastoid approach.

Discussion

In choosing the most suitable approach for a process of the tentorial edge, we have to take the following topographic criteria into account:

1. Which portion of the tumor is located supratentorially and which portion infratentorially?
2. Is the tumor rather located in the anterior portion of the tentorial notch or in its posterior part?

The combination of the answers to these two questions provides an indication of the most appropriate surgical approach (Table 2, Figs. 1, 2).

If the main part of the tumor is located supratentorially and in the anterior half of the tentorial notch *(Group A)*, the transsylvian-pterional and the subtemporal approach seem to be most suitable. Both approaches allow excellent visualization of the region and, if necessary, they can easily be combined with other approaches. In some cases a transtemporal approach (through the median temporal gyrus) seems indicated, especially if the process reaches far into the medial portion of the temporal lobe.

If the process is located in the anterior half of the tentorial notch, but its main portion is situated infratentorially *(Group B)*, it can be exposed through the cerebellopontine angle from retromastoid. The subtemporal transtentorial approach is especially appropriate for pro-

Table 2. Surgical approach to processes of the tentorial edge in relation to the tumor location

Tumor location	Anterior half of the tentorial edge	Posterior half of the tentorial edge
>50% supratentorial	A 1. Transsylvian 2. Subtemporal 3. (Transtemporal)	C 1. Transtemporal (transangular) 2. Subtemporal 3. Occipital-parasagittal
>50% infratentorial	B 1. Retromastoid 2. Subtemporal-transtentorial 3. Transsylvian-transtentorial Ev. combined supra-infratentorial Ev. two-stage procedure	D 1. Infratentorial-supracerebellar 2. Occipital-transtentorial

cesses part of which has grown supratentorially. For the latter the transsylvian-transtentorial exposure is an alternative approach.

Processes in the posterior region of the tentorial edge with a predominantly supratentorial localization *(Group C)* can be reached through the posterior subtemporal approach. In tumors that have grown along the falx far into its superior portion, the transtemporal exposure (through the angular gyrus) is a safe approach. This approach may even be applied on the dominant side without postoperative neurologic deficit. Another approach is the occipito-parasagittal route, which, however, is known to cause frequent visual field defects postoperatively.

If the tumor is in the posterior region of the tentorial edge with its main part located infratentorially *(Group D)*, two approaches may be chosen. The infratentorial-supracerebellar approach is an elegant and safe microsurgical approach to this region. Alternatively, an occipital-transtentorial exposure may be performed, this mainly being recommended in processes that have grown both supra- and infratentorially.

Especially large tumors which expand both supra- and infratentorially and possibly involve the entire tentorial edge, require a combination of two approaches. Most frequently, the posterior subtemporal approach is combined with retromastoid exposure of the cerebellopontine angle and resection of the tentorium. In patients with large tumors and a critical general condition, the previously described combination can be performed in two stages.

In choosing the appropriate surgical exposure it is important that the surgeon remains flexible and thus chooses the most suitable approach for the individual patient. Of course, the choice of approach does not only depend on the above-mentioned topographic criteria, but also on the type of process, vascularization, the localization of the bridging veins, the general condition of the patient, and a number of other factors.

Summary

Different surgical approaches to the tentorial edge are discussed by reference to 30 cases of tentorial edge meningioma. The advantages and disadvantages of each approach are presented. The clinical and intraoperative findings are supported by anatomical studies. The following approaches are analyzed:

- -Transsylvian
- -Anterior subtemporal
- -Posterior subtemporal
- -Transtemporal
- -Paramedian parieto-occipital
- -Occipital-transtentorial
- -Infratentorial-supracerebellar
- -Retromastoid
- -Combined supra-infratentorial

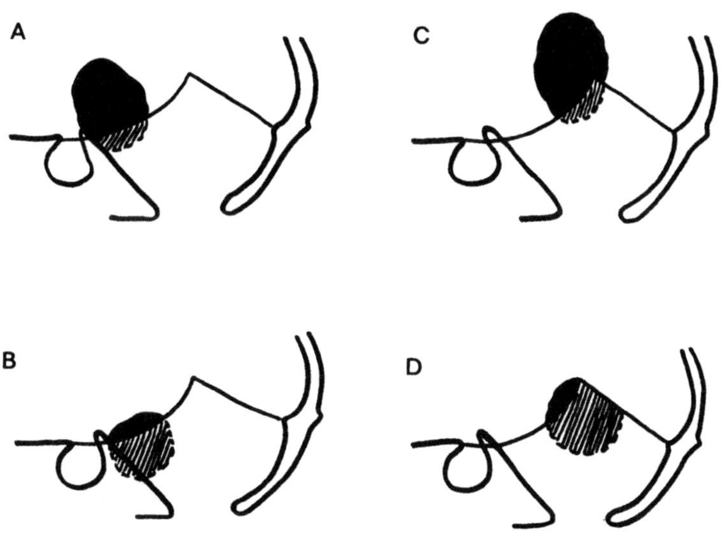

Fig. 1. Scheme of the tumor location as described in Table 2

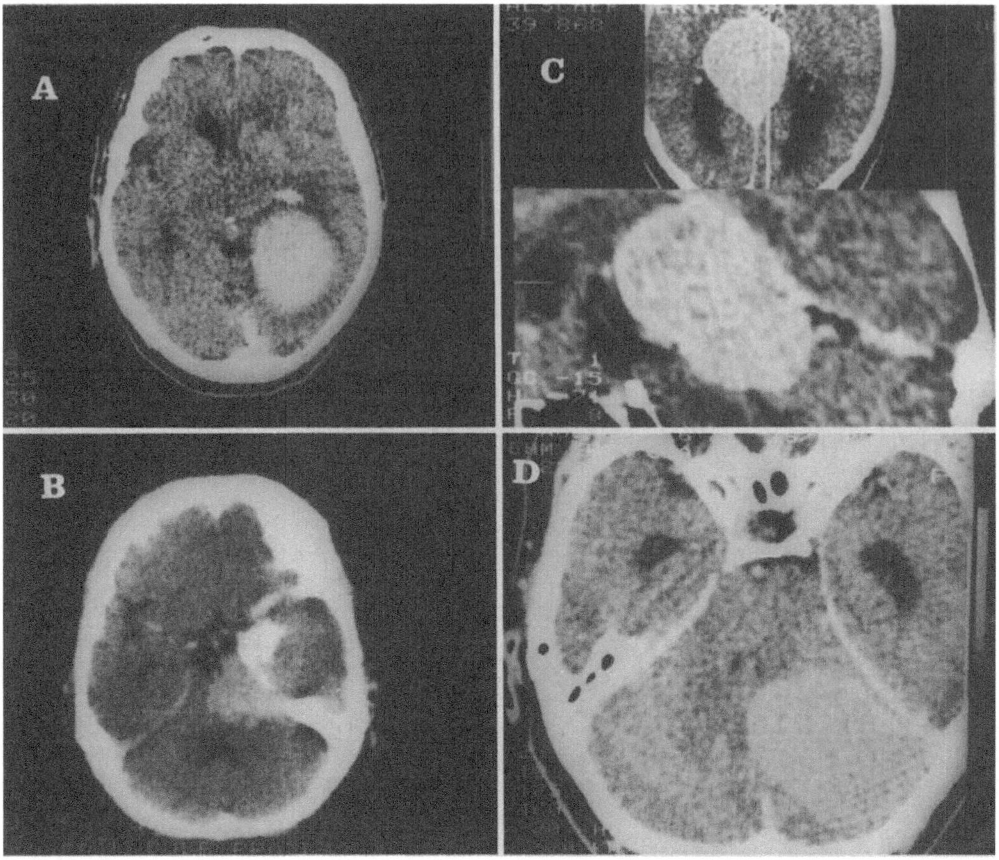

Fig. 2. Examples of the four different location groups according to Table 1 and Fig. 1

Surgical Management of Dysontogenetic Tumors and Cysts in the Region of the Tentorial Incisura and the Ambient Cistern

E. Kazner and H. Collmann
Neurochirurgische Abteilung, Klinikum Charlottenburg, Freie Universität Berlin, Spandauer Damm 130, D-1000 Berlin 19

The ambient cistern and the adjoining CSF spaces are typical locations of epidermoid cysts, lipomas, and arachnoid cysts (2, 3, 4, 7, 8). Since 1975 at the neurosurgical departments of Munich (1975-1979) and Berlin-Charlottenburg (1980-1984), 17 patients with epidermoid cysts, arachnoid cysts, and lipomas of this region have been observed. Surgical treatment has been performed in 14 of them. This group contained 10 epidermoid cysts, two arachnoid cysts, one lipoma, and one so-called simple cyst (6). In the remaining three patients the lesion was found incidentally and did not produce signs and symptoms. The probable diagnoses in these cases are: lipoma (two patients) and arachnoid cyst (one patient). The mean age of the operative group was 34.2 years, the youngest being three years old (arachnoid cyst), the oldest 49 (epidermoid). Both sexes were affected equally.

Table 1 and Fig. 1 a and b give a synopsis of the clinical data and the CT findings confirmed at operation. Five patients showed a considerable infratentorial portion of the lesion, in most cases extending into the cerebellopontine cistern. The predominant clinical findings were episodic headache, cerebellar signs, and cranial nerve dysfunctions. Hemiparesis due to brain-stem compression occurred in some cases of extended epidermoid cysts. An obstruction of CSF pathways resulting in hydrocephalus was observed only twice.

In our personal experience the occipital paramedian transtentorial approach to these lesions at the edge of the tentorium has proved to be most suitable, especially with lesions on the side of the dominant hemisphere. Eleven patients out of 14 were operated on by this approach, seven of them on the left side. Complete removal of epidermoid cysts in this region was possible only when the tentorium was split and a wedge-shaped incision of the tentorium close to the sinus rectus was performed. In case 8 a left subtemporal transtentorial approach was chosen, and in two cases (12, 13) operated upon using the suboccipital petrosal approach; some difficulties arose in removing the most cranial portions of the tumor near the oculomotor nerve. Besides this, major technical problems were not encountered since most of these lesions are avascular. However, complete removal of the cyst wall in an epidermoid cyst may cause considerable difficulties as the wall is often adherent to the underlying structures (1, 5). Patience and tenacity are mandatory in this situation.

In order to prevent acute postoperative CSF accumulation or aseptic meningitis as well as development of CSF cysts, temporary external CSF drainage for some days proved very useful. The implantation of a permanent shunt was necessary only in one patient.

Advances in Neurosurgery, Vol. 13
Edited by H. Dietz, M. Brock, and M. Klinger

Table 1. Clinical data of 14 patients operated on for dysontogenetic tumors and cysts in the region of the tentorial hiatus

Case No.	Year of operation	Patient	Sex	Age	Length of history	Signs and symptoms	Diagnosis
1	1975	H.L.	F	26	>2 y	Headache, hemispasticity, cranial nerve dysfunction	Epidermoid cyst
2	1976	S.D.	M	30	4 m	Headache, vomiting, papilledema	Epidermoid cyst, hydrocephalus
3	1976	M.O.	M	3	>2 y	Macrocephaly, ataxia, upward gaze palsy	Arachnoid cyst
4	1977	J.H.	M	27	3 m	Giddiness, trigeminal and facial nerve paresis	Epidermoid cyst
5	1977	B.H.	F	36	2 y	Headache, syncopal episodes	Lipoma
6	1977	U.Z.	F	25	8 y	Ataxia	Epidermoid cyst
7	1978	M.F.	F	34	>2 y	Headache, episodic hemiparesis, visual impairment	Epidermoid cyst
8	1978	A.Sch.	M	48	?	Trigeminal nerve paresis	Epidermoid cyst
9	1980	G.O.	F	49	4 y	Psychomotor seizures, trigeminal and facial nerve paresis	Epidermoid cyst
10	1980	A.H.	M	47	6 y	Hemiparesis, hemidysesthesia	Epidermoid cyst, hydrocephalus
11	1980	H.-J.C.	M	40	3 w	Ataxia	So-called simple cyst
12	1983	A.D.	F	25	1 y	Trigeminal nerve paresis, headache	Epidermoid cyst
13	1983	L.D.	M	46	1 y	Ataxia, diplopia	Epidermoid cyst
14	1984	R.Sch.	F	43	10 y	Headache, vomiting, episodic giddiness	Arachnoid cyst

Two of our patients (cases 1, 14) had to be operated on twice because of formation of a new arachnoid cyst with mass effect. There was no operative mortality and neurological deterioration was only a temporary event: Homonymous hemianopia occurred in three patients, upward gaze palsy in two, and deterioriation of other cranial nerve palsies in another. Preoperative complaints and neurological deficits vanished in eight patients and subsided partially in five others. As residual symptoms, slight hemiparesis, upward gaze palsy, and syncopal attacks were encountered. One patient committed suicide for unrelated reasons six months after successful surgery.

In conclusion, the surgical treatment of dysontogenetic tumors and cysts located around the tentorial hiatus promises good to excellent results in the majority of cases. The occipital paramedian transtentorial approach to these lesions bears only a low risk and offers an optimal panoramic view over the midline structures.

References

1. Guidetti, B., Gagliardi, F.M.: Epidermoid and dermoid cysts. Clinical evaluation and late surgical results. J. Neurosurg. 47, 12-18 (1977)
2. Hayashi, T., Kuratomi, A., Kuromoto, S.: Arachnoid cyst of the quadrigeminal cistern. Surg. Neurol. 14, 267-273 (1980)
3. Kazner, E., Stochdorph, O., Wende, S., Grumme, T.: Intercranial lipoma. Diagnostic and therapeutic considerations. J. Neurosurg. 52, 235-245 (1980)
4. Kazner, E., Wende, S., Grumme, T., Lanksch, W., Stochdorph, O. (eds.): Computed tomography in intracranial tumors. Springer, Berlin Heidelberg New York 1982
5. McDonnell, D.E.: Pineal epidermoid cyst: Its surgical therapy. Surg. Neurol. 7, 387-391 (1977)
6. Silverberg, G.D.: Simple cysts of the cerebellum. J. Neurosurg. 35, 320-327 (1971)
7. Vaquero, J., Carrillo, R., Cabezudo, J.M., Nombela, L., Bravo, G.: Arachnoid cysts of the posterior fossa. Surg. Neurol. 16, 117-121 (1981)
8. Zülch, K.J.: Die Hirngeschwülste in biologischer und morphologischer Darstellung. Ambrosius Barth, Leipzig 1956

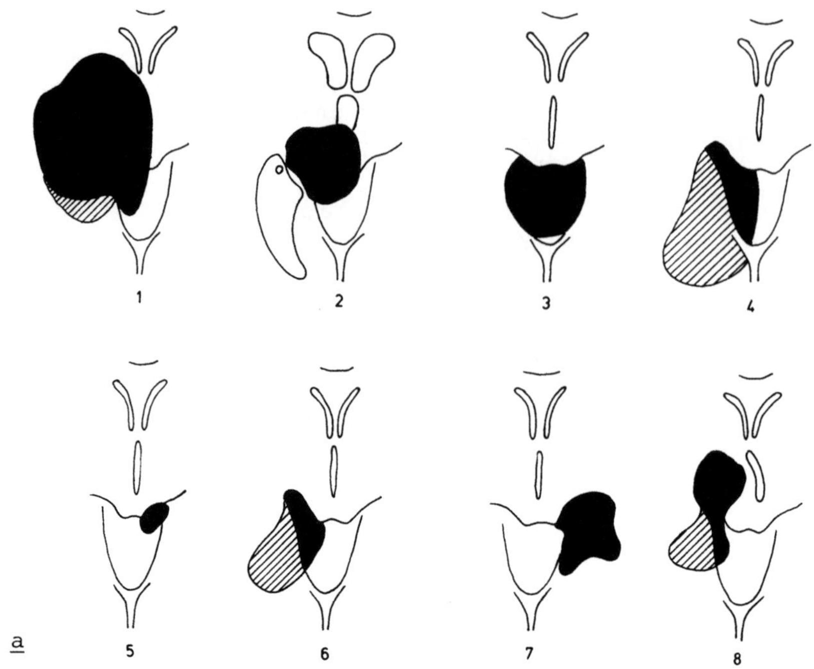

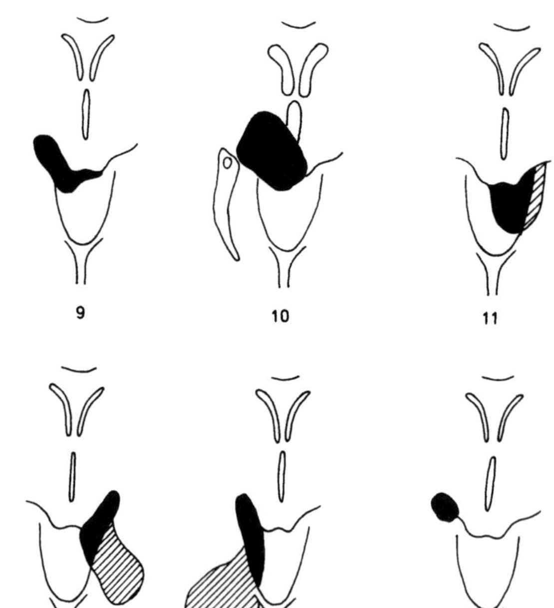

Fig. 1a,b. Synopsis of CT findings of 14 patients operated on for dysontogenetic tumors and cysts in the region of the tentorial hiatus (see also Table 1). Infratentorial tumor portions *hatched*. Patients No. 1-8 were operated on by the senior author at the Neurosurgical Clinic, Klinikum Großhadern, Ludwig-Maximilians-Universität München (director: Prof. Dr. med. Frank Marguth); patients No. 9-14 were treated at the Neurosurgical Department, Klinikum Charlottenburg, Free University of Berlin

Cranial Nerve Lesions Following Operations on Tumors of the Tentorial Edge

H. R. Eggert and J. M. Gilsbach
Neurochirurgische Universitätsklinik, Klinikum der Albert-Ludwigs-Universität, Hugstetter Straße 55, D-7800 Freiburg

Introduction

Since the introduction of computed tomography, we have been able to detect a growing number of meningiomas or other tumorous lesions of the cavernous sinus and the tentorial edge (3). The lesions are normally small or medium sized. They cause protrusions and cranial nerve deficits but often have no space-occupying effect that could be life threatening. The indication for operation is usually the deficit of the cranial nerves. To our knowledge, however, it is still unclear as to whether a surgical procedure on a tumor that usually cannot be totally resected can diminish a nerve lesion or at least prevent further deterioration.

The aim of the retrospective evaluation of our patient material is to establish some criteria for deciding which patients should be operated on, at what time, and by which technique.

Patients

From 1977 to 1982, 21 patients with tumorous lesions mainly involving the tentorial edge were operated upon. The lesions consisted mainly of meningiomas (n = 19). One thrombosed aneurysm of the cavernous section of the internal carotid artery, one chordoma, and one leiomyosarcoma have been included in this series. All patients were operated on by a pterional approach. It seemed advisable to us to discriminate three tumor types according to their growth properties. The term "intracavernous" is confined to tumors growing within the tentorial fold that cause the dura of the middle fossa to bulge and that have no intradural tumor growth (n = 5) (Fig. 1). These tumors are also called tumors of the cavernous sinus or tumors of Meckel's cave. Tumors located within the tentorial edge with bulging of the dura and additional flat intradural growth without space-occupying character were named "en plaque" (n = 6) (Fig. 2). The third group consisted of tumors which showed additional intradural space-occupying growth (n = 10) (Fig. 3). Regarding the operative approach, we distinguished between intradural and intracavernous tumor removal. In cases of intracavernous tumor removal (n = 11), the dura of the medial temporal fossa was opened and we tried to remove as much of the tumor as possible while sparing the cranial nerves and the carotid artery. In cases of intradural tumor removal (n = 10), the intradural parts of tumors were removed as extensively as possible and, in addition, the dura of the tentorial fold was coagulated by low intensity bipolar coagulation and remnants of tumor tissue were scratched off. The cranial nerve deficits that existed upon the patients' admission were compared with the postoperative

Edited by H. Dietz, M. Brock, and M. Klinger

state upon discharge (mean 11 ± 5 days postoperatively) and with the late postoperative results obtained upon reexamination in the outpatient clinic (mean 22 ± 18 months postoperatively).

Results

Preoperatively, 48 out of the 105 cranial nerves which could have been involved showed impairment with different degrees of severity (Table 1): most often the oculomotor (n = 15,71% of possible involvement, PI) and the abducens nerve (n = 11,52% PI) were involved. They were followed by the trigeminal (n = 9,43% PI) and the optic nerve (n = 8,38% PI). Trochlear nerve palsy was observed in five patients (27% PI). In intracavernous and en plaque types of tumor, the frequency of cranial nerve deficit (56%, 57% PI) was similar (Table 2). In tumors of the space-occupying type, fewer cranial nerve deficits (30% PI) were observed preoperatively. Fifty-three percent (PI, n = 27) of cranial nerves were involved in patients who had undergone intracavernous tumor removal. In patients with intradural tumor removal, 21 (42% PI) cranial nerves were involved (Table 3).

Postoperatively, additional lesions of cranial nerves, none of which existed preoperatively, were observed in two cases. One oculomotor palsy followed intradural removal of a tumor of the space-occupying type. In the other patient, sensory loss of the face appeared following intracavernous removal of a tumor of the same type. One year later these lesions had completely regressed. Forty percent of the preoperatively affected cranial nerves showed additional impairment postoperatively, which turned out to be permanent in 25% (n = 12) (Table 4). The oculomotor nerve proved to be the nerve most often additionally impaired (67%), followed by the trigeminal nerve (45%). Additional impairment to the trigeminal nerve was permanent in only one case (11%); in oculomotor nerves, the operation improved the impairment of nerve function in only 27% (n = 4). Additional impairment of the abducent nerve was observed in only one case (9%) and proved to be permanent. Immediate postoperative improvement of preexisting cranial nerve deficits occurred rather seldom (n = 9,19%). The late results showed an improvement of deficits compared with the preoperative condition in 40% (n = 19). The best prognosis was obtained in the abducens (n = 7, 64%) and trochlear (n = 2, 40%) as well as in the oculomotor nerves (n = 6, 40%). However, in oculomotor nerves improvement was accompanied by aberrant regeneration in four cases.

Regarding the type of the tumor, the best results were obtained in intracavernous tumors, whereas in tumors of the space-occupying type less favourable results could be observed. Accordingly, intracavernous tumor removal resulted more often in improvement and less often in additional impairment of the involved cranial nerves.

In the follow-up examinations in two cases, an additional lesion of the trigeminal nerve was found, probably due to ongoing tumor growth, since in these patients no impairment of this nerve was found postoperatively.

There was no operative mortality.

Table 1. Cranial nerve deficit in tumors of the tentorial edge: results after surgery

	Preop.	Postoperative results			Late results		
		Improved	Unchanged	Worse	Improved	Unchanged	Worse
N. opticus	8 (38%)	1 (13%)	4 (50%)	3 (37%)	1 (13%)	4 (50%)	3 (37%)
N. oculomotorius	15 (71%)	1 (7%)	4 (27%)	10+1 (67%)	6 (40%)	3 (20%)	6 (40%)
N. trochlearis	5 (24%)	-	4 (80%)	1 (20%)	2 (40%)	2 (40%)	1 (20%)
N. trigeminus	9 (43%)	3 (33%)	2 (22%)	4+1 (45%)	3 (33%)	5 (56%)	1+2 (11%)
N. abducens	11 (52%)	4 (36%)	6 (55%)	1 (9%)	7 (64%)	3 (27%)	1 (9%)
Total	48 (46%)	9 (19%)	20 (42%)	19 (40%)	19 (40%)	17 (35%)	12 (25%)

Table 2. Cranial nerve deficit in tumors of the tentorial edge: results according to type of tumors

	Preop.	Postoperative results			Late results		
		Improved	Unchanged	Worse	Improved	Unchanged	Worse
Intracavernous (n = 5)	14 (56%)	5 (36%)	7 (50%)	2 (14%)	9 (64%)	4 (29%)	1 (7%)
En plaque (n = 6)	17 (57%)	2 (12%)	6 (35%)	9 (53%)	8 (47%)	4 (24%)	5+1 (29%)
Space occupying (n = 10)	17 (30%)	2 (12%)	6 (35%)	9+2 (53%)	2 (12%)	9 (53%)	6+1 (35%)

Table 3. Cranial nerve deficit in tumors of the tentorial edge: results according to the operative approach

	Preop.	Postoperative results			Late results		
		Improved	Unchanged	Worse	Improved	Unchanged	Worse
Intradural tumor removal (n = 10)	21 (42%)	2 (10%)	7 (33%)	12+1 (57%)	3 (14%)	10 (48%)	8+1 (38%)
Intracavernous tumor removal (n = 11)	27 (53%)	7 (26%)	12 (44%)	8+1 (30%)	16 (59%)	7 (26%)	4+1 (15%)

Table 4. Cranial nerve deficit in tumors of the tentorial edge: postoperative increase of the deficit

	Transient	Aberrant regeneration, III. nerve	Permanent
N. opticus	-	-	3 (37%)
N. oculomotorius	4 (27%)	4 (27%)	6 (40%)
N. trochlearis	-	-	1 (20%)
N. trigeminus	4 (44%)	-	1 (11%)
N. abducens	-	-	1 (9%)
	8 (13%)		12 (25%)
Intracavernous	1 (7%)	1	1 (7%)
En plaque	4 (24%)	2	5 (29%)
Space occupying	3 (18%)	1	6 (35%)
Intradural tumor removal	4 (18%)	2	8 (38%)
Intracavernous tumor removal	4 (15%)	2	4 (15%)

Discussion

Neurological deficits of ocular nerves and the trigeminal nerve are usually the major symptoms in tumorous lesions within the cavernous sinus (4, 5, 7), which are rather rare in neurosurgical practice (11). The primary location of the tumor determines which nerves will be involved first. Patients with tumors of Meckel's cave mainly complain of facial pain or numbness of the face (8, 13), but the sixth nerve may also be involved primarily (9). Primary aberrant regeneration of the oculomotor nerve is said to be a typical sign of meningioma of the cavernous sinus (10). As our results show, the third nerve seems to be the most sensitive one, since preoperatively it was often impaired and it was also the nerve which most often showed postoperative worsening. If a deficit of the third nerve was worsened by the operation and followed by improvement, no full functional recovery occurred and, in most cases, aberrant regeneration took place, which is typical for this cranial nerve (1, 6, 12). The reason for this observation may be the high number of ocular muscles innervated by this nerve and its superficial course within the cavernous sinus. On the other hand, the sixth nerve, which is the innermost nerve of the tentorial fold and which innervates only one external ocular muscle, proved to have the best prognosis.

Surprisingly, depending on the type of lesion, preexisting cranial nerve deficits in cases of tumors located entirely within the cavernous sinus had the best prognosis. This may be due to the fact that two of these tumors were of soft consistency and could be removed by curettage and suction. One of the space-occupying lesions of this type was a thrombosed aneurysm, which was left untouched. But the oculomotor nerve was neurolized. This operation resulted in rapid and complete recovery from the preoperatively existing oculomotor palsy. The other two tumors had been well demarcated meningiomas of the angioblastic type. Tumors of the en plaque type and the space-occupying type may have more infiltrating growth properties. In these cases sparing the cranial nerves during tumor removal from outside the cavernous sinus may become difficult but not impossible, as it is said to be (2). Venous bleeding (14) has not been a problem in any of these cases. Regarding the operative approach, better results were obtained when intracavernous tumor removal was attempted.

Depending on the indication for the operation on tumors of the tentorial edge, tumors of the space-occupying type have to be removed by operation regardless of cranial nerve deficits, since their space-occupying character will make them life threatening. Tumors located entirely within the tentorial fold may be operated on, since the postoperative prognosis of cranial nerve deficit in these tumors is favorable. In tumors of the cavernous sinus with an additional flat intradural part, the indication for operation remains questionable. An increase of preexisting cranial nerve deficit due to the operation will occur in one-third of the involved cranial nerves. Postoperative improvement of deficits will be obtained in only one-half of the preoperatively impaired cranial nerves. Therefore, the operation on these tumors will be of only little benefit for the patient. On the other hand, tumors of this type tend to creep along the basal dura. They are thus able to involve both optic nerves. If involvement of one optic canal is suspected clinically or by computerized tomography, surgery should not be delayed. Nevertheless, in each type of tumor of the tentorial edge, if surgery is indicated, removal of intracavernous parts of the tumor should be attempted.

Conclusions

- The majority of tumors of the tentorial edge are benign lesions which can be operated upon by a transsylvian route with low mortality and morbidity, with the exception of the cranial nerves.
- Surgery because of lesions or life-threatening growth of a tumor is seldom necessary.
- The pure intradural removal of the tumor is of practically no advantage in the treatment of cranial nerve lesions.
- Surprisingly, the best results are obtained by removing intracavernous tumors.

References

1. Bender, M.B., Fulton, J.F.: Functional recovery in ocular muscles of the chimpanzee after section of oculomotor nerve. Neurophysiology 1, 144-151 (1938)
2. Bonnal, J., Brotchi, J., Born, J.: Meningiomas of the lateral portion of the sella turcica. Acta Neurochir. (Suppl.) 28, 385-396 (1979)
3. Cabanis, E.A., van Effenterre, R., Iba-Zizen, M.T., Danicel, V., Salvolini, V.: Computerized tomography in parasellar space-occupying lesions and therapeutic decision. Acta Neurochir. (Suppl.) 28, 329-333 (1979)
4. van Effenterre, R., Bataini, J.P., Cabanis, E.A., Iba-Zizen, M.T.: High energy radiotherapy in the treatment of meningiomas of the cavernous sinus. Acta Neurochir. (Suppl.) 28, 464-467 (1979)
5. Godtfredsen, E., Ledermann, M.: Studies on the cavernous sinus syndrome. 2. Diagnostic and prognostic roles of ophthalmoneurological signs and symptoms in malignant nasopharyngeal tumors. Acta Neurochir. Scand. 41, 53 (1965)
6. Holland, G.: Elektromyographische Untersuchungen bei Fehlleitung regenerierender Nervenfasern nach Okulomotoriusparese. Klin. Monatsbl. Augenheilkd. 144, 686-696 (1964)
7. Jefferson, G.: Concerning injuries, aneurysms and tumors involving the cavernous sinus. Trans. Ophth. Soc. UK 73, 117-152 (1953)
8. Nijensohn, D.E., Araujo, J.C., Maccarty, C.S.: Meningiomas of Meckel's cave. J. Neurosurg. 43, 197-202 (1975)
9. Sakalas, R., Harbison, J.W., Vines, F.S., et al.: Chronic sixth nerve palsy. Arch. Ophthalmol. 93, 186-190 (1975)
10. Schatz, N.J., Savino, P.J., Corbett, J.J.: Primary aberrant oculomotor regeneration. Arch. Neurol. 34, 29-32 (1977)
11. Vidovzky, T., Beniost, G.: Comparative study of trigeminal neurinomas and parasellar meningiomas. Acta Neurochir. (Suppl.) 28, 397-401 (1979)
12. Walsh, F.B.: Third nerve regeneration, a clinical evaluation. Br. J. Ophthalmol. 41, 577-598 (1957)
13. Weinberger, L.M., Adler, F.H., Grant, F.C.: Primary pituitary adenoma and the syndrome of the cavernous sinus. Arch. Ophthalmol. 24, 1197-1236 (1940)
14. Zozulia, Y.A., Romodanon, S.A., Patsko, Y.V.: Diagnosis and surgical treatment of benign craniobasal tumours involving the cavernous sinus. Acta Neurochir. (Suppl.) 28, 387-390 (1979)

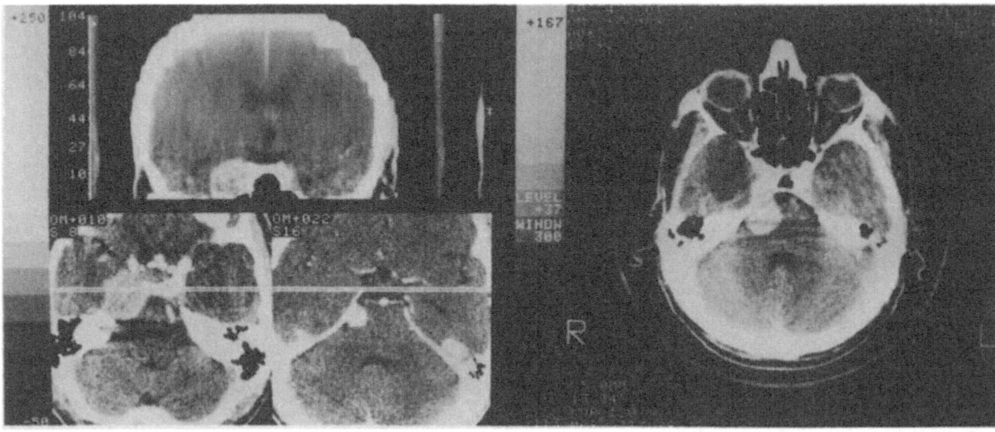

Fig. 1. Meningioma of the tentorial edge, intracavernous type. *Left:* preoperatively; *right:* two years following removal of the intracavernous part, before operation on the infratentorial part

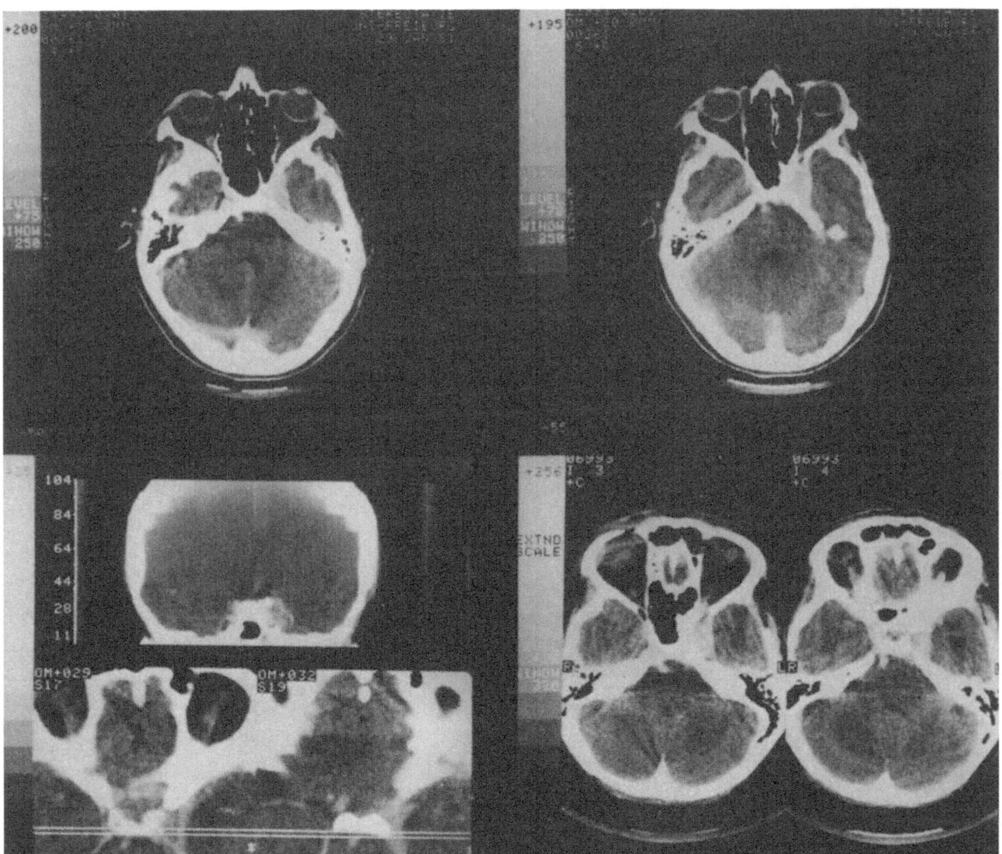

Fig. 2. Legend see p. 202

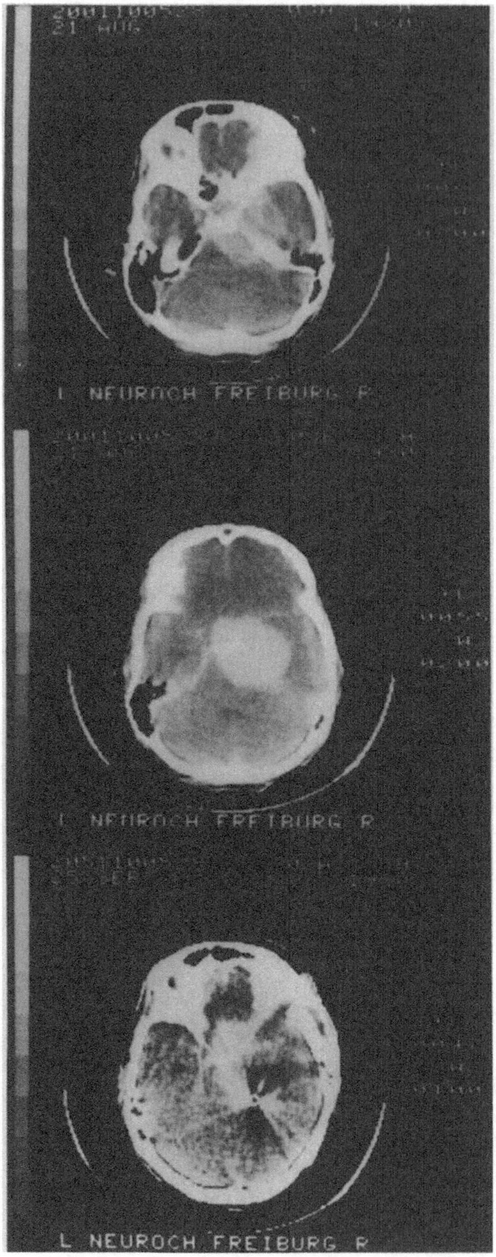

Fig. 3. Meningioma of the tentorial edge, space-occupying type. *Top and middle:* preoperatively; *bottom:* one month following partial intradural tumor removal

Fig. 2. Meningioma of the tentorial edge, en plaque type. *Upper row:* preoperatively; *bottom left:* 19 months following intradural tumor removal; *bottom right:* 33 months following operation. Ongoing tumor growth cannot be observed

The Advantages of Laser Therapy in the Region of the Tentorial Edge

O. J. Beck
Neurochirurgische Universitätsklinik, Klinikum Großhadern, Marchioninistraße 15, D-8000 München 70

Examples of the advantages of laser therapy are:

1. Excellent coagulation in the presence of highly vascularized tumors.
2. Adequate delineation of tumors due to different tissue absorption properties (Figs. 1, 2).
3. Surgery markedly facilitated due to laser-induced shrinkage of tumors (Figs. 3, 4).
4. Precise denaturation of tumor tissue with a predictable depth effect.

The necrotization of the tumor base in the area of the petrosal bone as well as the denaturation of tumors involving the transversal sinus are the most important factors for preventing the recurrence of tumors.

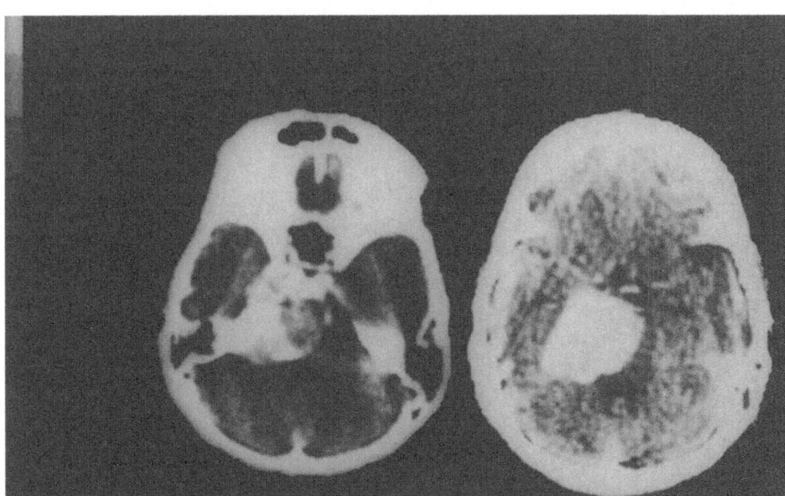

Fig. 1. Cerebellopontine angle meningioma on the left side

Advances in Neurosurgery, Vol. 13
Edited by H. Dietz, M. Brock, and M. Klinger

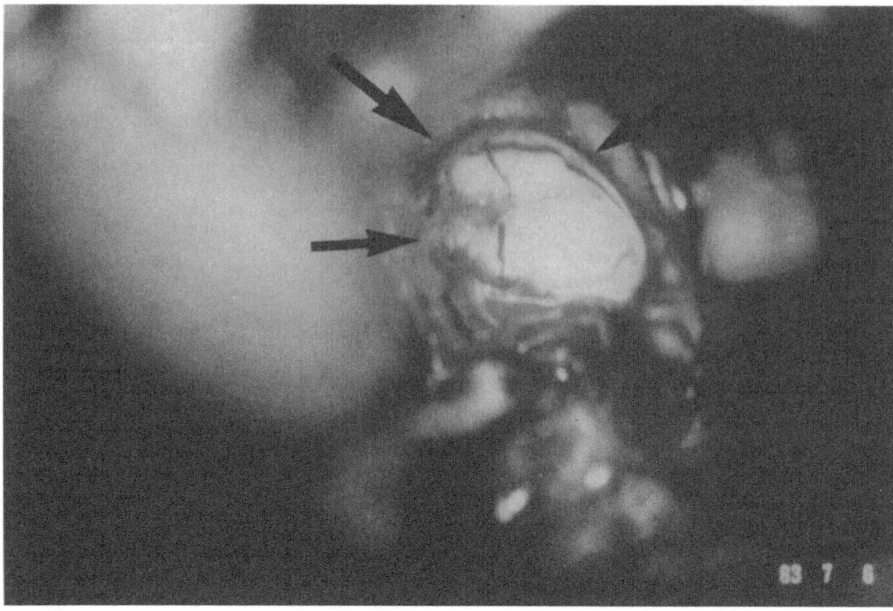

Fig. 2. Notch within brain-stem after removal of tumor

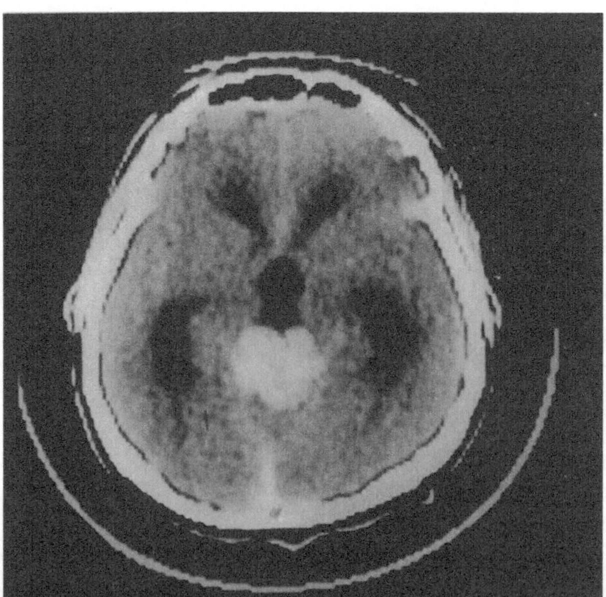

Fig. 3. Tumor in the pineal region

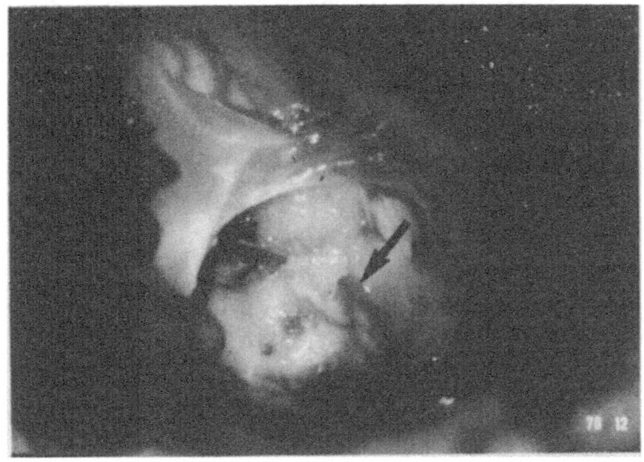

Fig. 4. Laser-induced shrinkage of tumor in the pineal region

The Surgical Anatomy of the Cavernous Sinus

R. Ramina, M. Samii, H. Baumann, and P. C. Warnke
Neurochirurgische Klinik, Krankenhaus Nordstadt, Haltenhoffstraße 41, D-3000 Hannover

Introduction

Following the advent of microsurgery and bipolar coagulation, extensive lesions of the skull base and within the cavernous sinus have been operated on (3, 8, 9, 11, 13). In the last six years, 31 patients with tumors invading the cavernous sinus (CS) were operated on in our clinic (Table 1). The most frequent tumors found in this series were skull base meningiomas. The surgical removal of tumors invading the CS is difficult and requires precise knowledge of the microanatomy of this region.

An anatomical study of the CS was carried out in 30 cadaveric specimens in our laboratory.

Table 1. Tumors infiltrating the cavernous sinus (1978-1984)

Meningiomas	16
Pituitary adenomas	6
Carcinomas	3
Trigeminal neurinomas	3
Epidermoid tumors	2
Esthesioneuroblastoma	1
Total	31

Material and Methods

Thirty cadaveric specimens consisting of the sellar and parasellar regions with the CS and its contents (Fig. 1) were dissected under microsurgical techniques.

Numerous anatomical studies of the cavernous sinus have been reported on (1, 2, 4, 6, 7, 10, 12, 18). The cavernous sinus has classically been described as a large trabeculated venous channel around the internal carotid artery and the abducent nerve (1, 4, 15, 16). According to the concept of TAPTAS (17), PARKINSON (10) (derived from corrosion studies), and HAMBY (5), the cavernous sinus is a plexus of various sized veins. This allows the exposure of the ICA and the VIth cranial nerve without entering the venous lumen. The cavernous sinus connects

 Advances in Neurosurgery, Vol. 13
Edited by H. Dietz, M. Brock, and M. Klinger

anteriorly with the superior and inferior orbital veins and with the sphenoparietal sinus. Posteriorly it connects with the superior and inferior petrosal sinus and with the sinus running down the dorsum sellae and the clivus, termed the basilar sinus. Both cavernous sinuses connect together through the anterior and posterior intracavernous sinuses. In some cases there are some connections below the pituitary gland, which may cause some problems for the transsphenoidal approach to pituitary tumors.

The varying course of the intracavernous portion of the ICA is of supreme importance in respect to the surgical treatment of lesions concerning the cavernous sinus (11) (Fig. 2). Contradictory descriptions regarding the course of the ICA within the sinus as well as its relationship to the lateral wall of the sinus have been reported (2, 11). In 12 of our 30 specimens this vessel ran extremely close to the lateral wall of the sinus. These variations may be due to arteriosclerotic alterations of the arterial wall (11). In seven cases the artery was very medial, close to the wall of the sella. In the remaining 11 specimens the course of the ICA was in the middle of the sinus cavity.

A profound knowledge of the intracavernous branches of the ICA is also very important, because they can enlarge as tumor feeding vessels (Fig. 3). The meningohypophyseal artery originating at the level of the dorsum sellae is the most constant branch: It was observed in all of our specimens (Fig. 3) and was also found in 100% of the cases dissected by DAY and RHOTON (2). The next most constant branch observed was the inferior lateral trunk of the cavernous sinus. It arises laterally from the horizontal portion of the ICA. This branch was present in 25 of our 30 cases. The capsular artery of McConnel originates from the medial side of the ICA and distally to the inferolateral trunk; it was noted in eight of our specimens.

An intracavernous origin of the ophthalmic artery was seen on three occasions.

The lateral wall of the cavernous sinus is formed by two layers: a superficial sheet of dura mater and a deep sheet of the dura containing the nerves III, IV, and V1, 2.

The course of these nerves was constant in our cases. The IIIrd cranial nerve was more medial than the IVth and more superior than the Vth 1, 2 (Fig. 4). These nerves presented a sheath of dura mater accompanying their penetration into the sinus wall (Fig. 4). The abducens nerve runs within the cavernous sinus and lateral to the ICA (Fig. 2). This nerve may be split into two or more branches. Its relationship to the lateral wall depends on the course of the ICA within the cavernous sinus.

Sympathetic fibers from the superior sympathetic ganglion initially run with the sixth nerve and then join the first division of the fifth cranial nerve (10).

According to PARKINSON (10), an operative approach to this space should be tried only if a radical removal of the lesion can be anticipated. In our 31 operated cases, total extirpation was possible in ten patients (30%). We had a mortality of 10%. Most of these lesions were approached by a frontotemporal craniotomy. For a better view of the anterior portion of the cavernous sinus and the origin of the ophthalmic artery, the anterior clinoid process is drilled out. The sinus is entered between the optic nerve and the lateral sinus wall. Another possibility is to expose the sinus through Parkinson's triangle between nerves III and IV and the first branch of the trigeminal nerve (Fig. 4). The attachment of the tumor to the dural sheets of the nerves running in the lateral sinus wall presents special technical difficulties for a total excision. With a microsurgical technique and high magnification these nerves are dissected free from the tumor. A radical excision of the lesion with preservation of all cranial nerves in this region is very difficult to achieve.

The possibility of a postoperative palsy and its meaning should be explained to patients presenting no palsy of the ocular nerves preoperatively. Reconstruction of the cranial nerves within the cavernous sinus may be attempted (14). However, the results of this procedure are dubious. If the ICA is surrounded by the tumor, high magnification is employed while peeling it out. Special attention must be paid to the branches of the ICA, which can be abnormally enlarged. Tumoral infiltration of the arterial wall represents a limitation to radical removal. In these cases the following procedure could be tried: An extra-intracranial anastomosis is performed prior to the ligature of the ICA in the neck. The supraclinoidal portion of the ICA is occluded proximal to the posterior communicating artery to avoid backflow. Finally the infiltrated portion of the ICA is resected. The cavernous sinus is usually filled with tumor. If venous bleeding from the remaining portion of the sinus does occur, it is controlled with fibrin sponges.

Conclusion

The total removal of tumors invading the cavernous sinus remains a challenge. Experience with microneurosurgery and good knowledge of its anatomy are required. The most important anatomical variations concerning the surgical approach to this region are reported in this paper.

References

1. Bedford, M.A.: The "cavernous" sinus. Br. J. Ophthalmol. 50, 41-46 (1966)
2. Day, A.L., Rhoton, A.L., Jr.: Aneurysms and arteriovenous fistulae of the intracavernous carotid artery and its branches. In: Youmans, J.R. (ed.) Neurological surgery, Chap. 51, pp. 1764-1785. Saunders, Philadelphia 1982
3. Dolenc, V.: Direct microsurgical repair of intracavernous vascular lesions. J. Neurosurg. 58, 824-831 (1983)
4. Gray, H.: Anatomy of the human body, p. 692. Lea & Febiger, Philadelphia 1973
5. Hamby, W.B.: Carotid cavernous fistulae. Thomas, Springfield, Ill. 1966
6. Harris, F.S., Rhoton, A.L., Jr.: Anatomy of the cavernous sinus. J. Neurosurg. 45, 169-180 (1976)
7. Lang, J.: Gehirn- und Augenschädel. In: Lang, J., Wachsmuth, W.: Praktische Anatomie, Vol. I, Part 1 B. Springer, Berlin Heidelberg New York 1979
8. Parkinson, D.: Transcavernous repair of carotid cavernous fistula: case report. J. Neurosurg. 26, 420-424 (1967)
9. Parkinson, D.: Carotid-cavernous fistula: Direct repair with preservation of the carotid artery. J. Neurosurg. 38, 99-106 (1973)

10. Parkinson, D., West, M.: Lesions of the cavernous plexus region. In: Youmans, J.R. (ed.) Neurological surgery, Chap. 94, pp. 3004-3023. Saunders, Philadelphia 1982

11. Ramina, R., Samii, M., Baumann, H.: Anatomical correlation between the structures of the cavernous sinus and the approach to the medial sphenoid ridge tumors. Presented at the 7th European Congress of Neurosurgery, Brussels, Belgium, Aug. 28 - Sept. 3, 1983

12. Rhoton, A.L., Jr., Harris, F.S., Renn, W.H.: Microsurgical anatomy of the sellar region and cavernous sinus. Clin. Neurosurg. Chap. 8, 54/85 (1977)

13. Samii, M., von Wild, K.: Operative treatment of lesions in the region of the tentorial notch. Neurosurg. Rev. 4-3-10 (1981)

14. Sandvoss, G., Cervas-Navarro, J., Yasargil, M.G.: Intracranial repair of the oculomotor nerve in cats. Presented at the 7th European Congress of Neurosurgery, Brussels, Belgium, Aug. 28 - Sept. 3, 1983

15. Taptas, J.N.: La loge du sinus caverneux. Rev. Otoneuroophtalmol. 21, 193-199 (1949)

16. Taptas, J.N.: Etiologie et pathogênie des exophtalmies d'origine vasculaire dites exophtalmies pulsaties. Arch. Ophtal. (Paris) 10, 22-50 (1950)

17. Taptas, J.N.: The so-called cavernous sinus: A review of the controversy and its implications for neurosurgeons. Neurosurgery 11/5, 712-717 (1982)

18. Umansky, F., Nathan, H.: The lateral wall of the cavernous sinus. J. Neurosurg. 56, 228-234 (1982)

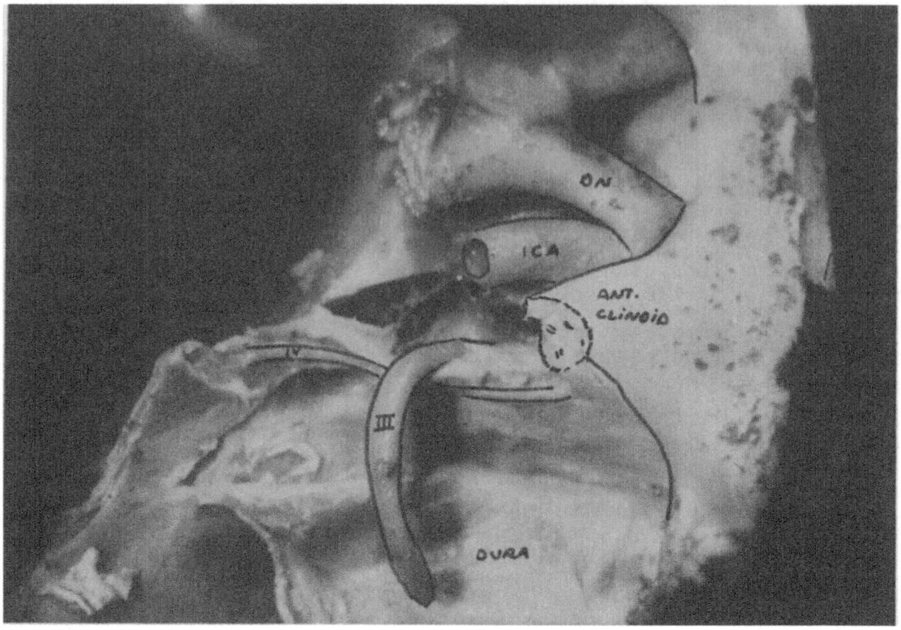

Fig. 1. Sellar and parasellar region with the cavernous sinus and its contents

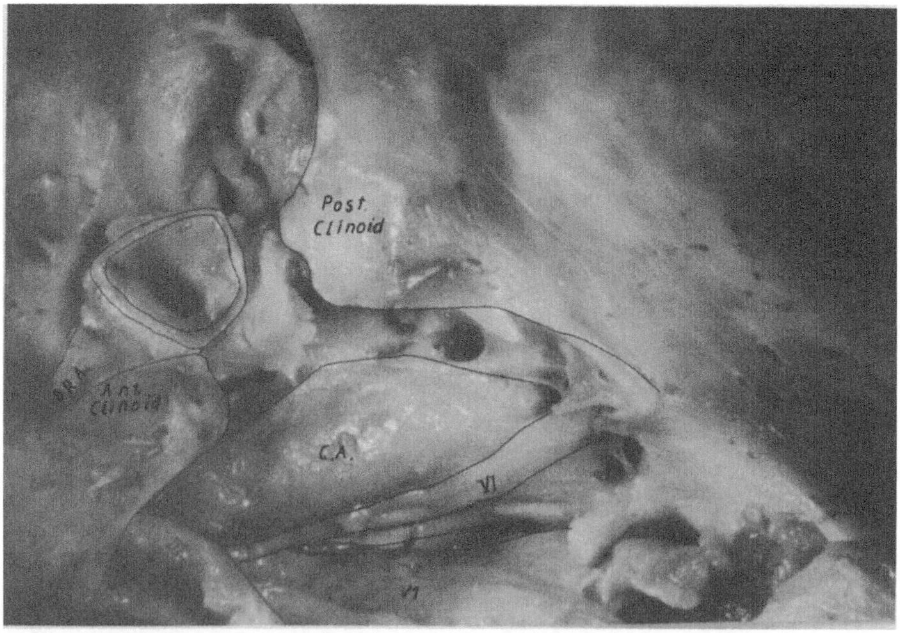

Fig. 2. Atypical course of the cavernous sinus (*C.A.*)

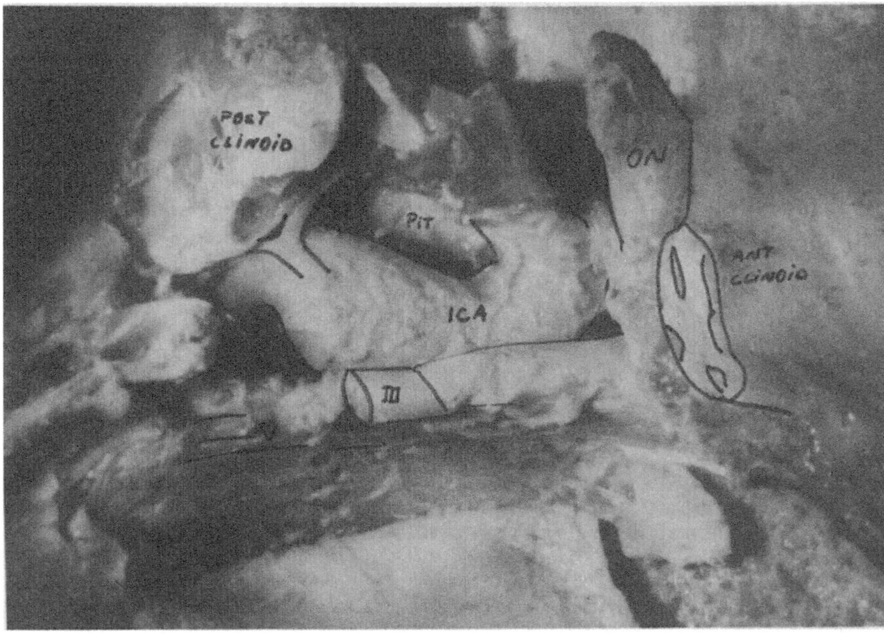

Fig. 3. Position of the internal carotid artery in relation to the posterior clinoid process

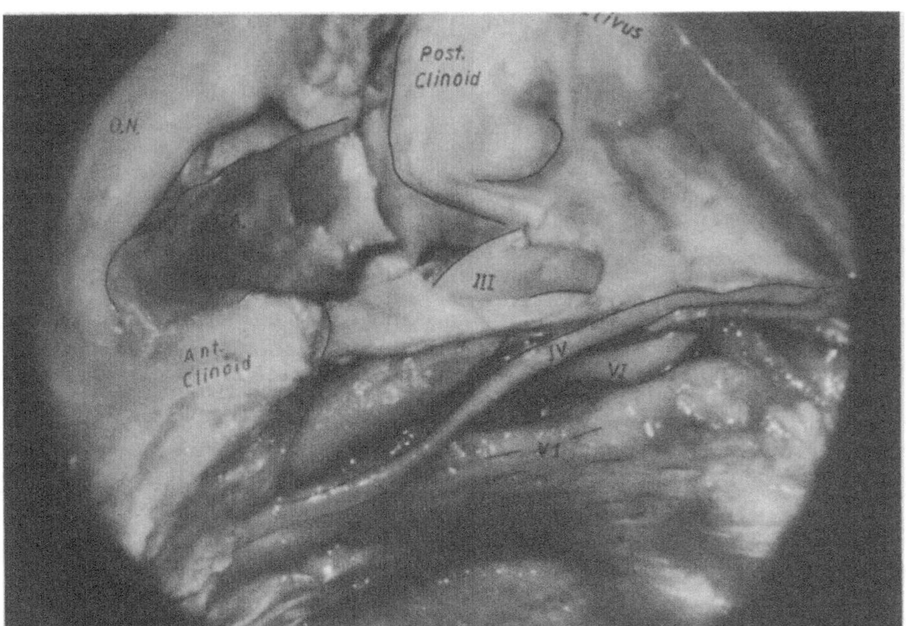

Fig. 4. The course of the III., IV., and VI. cranial nerves in relation to each other in the cavernous sinus

Evoked Potentials for Therapy Control During Operations at the Tentorial Margin

P. C. Warnke[1,3], R. Lorenz[2], M. Samii[1], and R. Ramina[1]

[1] Neurochirurgische Klinik, [2] Neurologische Klinik, Krankenhaus Nordstadt, Haltenhoffstraße 41, D-3000 Hannover

[3] The Evanston Hospital, Division of Neurology, 2650 Ridge Avenue, Evanston, IL 60201, USA

Introduction

Evoked potentials (EPs) were introduced into clinical practice by CALVET et al. (3). For the neurosurgeon EPs are usefel tools in the surgical management of tumors around the brain stem which by themselves or as a result of the necessary surgical approach cause brain stem compression. Up-to-date studies on intraoperatively recorded EPs (1, 4, 6) have been based on the neurotopical concept of BUCHWALD and HUANG (2). Recent findings of direct recordings of acoustic evoked responses (AERs) in humans by MØLLER and JANNETTA (9) gave rise to a new concept. According to MØLLER, wave II of the AER is generated by the acoustic nerve itself and not by the cochlear nucleus as has been believed up to now. Besides our interest in monitoring brain stem function during operation, the aim of our study was to examine whether the findings of MØLLER could be reproduced in the state of brain stem compression and how much time it takes for the brain stem to recover.

Material and Methods

Seven patients with tumors at the tentorial margin were monitored by EPs. Six had a tumor arising from the cerebellopontine angle (four acoustic neurinoma, one meningioma, one cholesteatoma), while one had a prepontine tumor (chondrosarcoma).

AERs were recorded by scalp electrodes placed on the forehead and mastoid. The potentials were obtained using a Nicolet CA 1000 averager and were filtered through a bandpass of 150 Hz to 3 KHz. The stimuli were click sounds of 85 dB intensity and 150 µs duration at a stimulus rate of 11.3/s. For averaging, 1000 samples were used. The analysis time was 10 ms. Somatosensory evoked potentials (SSEPs) were recorded from the scalp by electrodes placed at C3 and C4 according to the 10-20 system. Stimuli were presented by transcutaneous electrical stimulation of the median nerve at a stimulus rate of 2.9/s and 100 µs duration. Stimulus intensity was 4 mA above the motor threshold. A bandpass of 30 Hz to 1.5 KHz and a Nicolet CA 1000 averager were used. 250 samples each were analyzed with a sweep time of 60 ms. All patients underwent identical anesthesia.

Results

Brain stem compression by surgical retraction could be evaluated in all cases of posterior fossa tumors (Fig. 1). Even in the case of severe changes of AERs, no significant shift of latency or amplitude of SSEPs occurred during operations.

 Advances in Neurosurgery, Vol. 13
Edited by H. Dietz, M. Brock, and M. Klinger

Recovery of brain stem function could be studied within minutes after completion of surgical retraction (Fig. 2). In two cases with electrophysiological evidence of brain stem compression, a constant, non-shifted wave II of the AER could be evaluated (Fig. 2). In another two cases of acoustic neurinoma, functional preservation of the acoustic nerve could be controlled.

Discussion

As in other studies (5, 6), we were able to evaluate intraoperative brain stem compression by AERs, which showed a latency shift and depression of amplitude. Recovery of brain stem function was as easily detected as by other groups (1, 4). In the case of mere surgical retraction of the brain stem without a primary lesion of the acoustic nerve, no shift in wave II of the AER could be noticed. This supports the concept of MØLLER and co-workers (8, 9) and stresses that experimental findings in cats (7) are not representative for humans because of a quite different neural organization of the cochlear nucleus and the superior olivary complex of cats and primates (10, 11).

Conclusion

Acoustic evoked responses are a valuable tool to the neurosurgeon in order to control brain stem function throughout the operation.

References

1. Allen, A., Starr, A., Nudleman, K.: Assessment of sensory function in the operating room utilizing cerebral evoked potentials: study of fifty-six surgically anesthesized patients. Clin. Neurosurg. 28, 457-481 (1981)
2. Buchwald, J., Huang, C.: Far-field acoustic response: origins in the cat. Science 189, 382-384 (1975)
3. Calvet, J., Chatala, H.P., Coutamin, F., Hirsch, J., Scherrer, J.: Potentials evoquées corticaux chez l'homme. Etude analytique. Rev. Neurol. 95, 445-452 (1956)
4. Grundy, B.L.: Monitoring of sensory evoked potentials during neurosurgical operations: methods and application. Neurosurgery 11(4), 556-575 (1982)
5. Grundy, B.L.: Intraoperative monitoring of sensory evoked potentials. Anesthesiology 58, 72-87 (1983)
6. Hashimoto, I., Ishivama, Y., Totsuka, G., Mizutani, H.: Monitoring brain stem function during posterior fossa surgery with brain stem auditory evoked potentials. In: Lancaster, B.C. (ed.) Evoked potentials, pp. 377-390. MTP Press, 1980
7. Klug, N.: Personal communication
8. Møller, A.R., Jannetta, P., Bennett, M., Møller, M.B.: Intracranially recorded responses from the human auditory nerve: new insights into the origin of brain stem evoked potentials. Electroencephalogr. Clin. Neurophysiol. 52, 18-27 (1981)
9. Møller, A.R., Jannetta, P.: Interpretation of brain stem auditory evoked potentials: results from intracranial recordings in humans. Scand. Audiol. 12, 125-133 (1983)

10. Moore, J., Moore, R.: A comparative study of the superior olivary complex in the primate brain. Folia Primat. 16, 35-46 (1971)

11. Snider, R.S., Niemer, W.T.: A stereotaxic atlas of the cat brain. University of Chicago Press, Chicago 1961

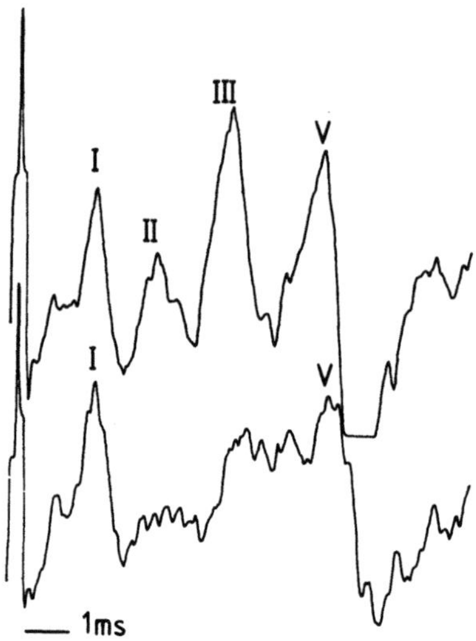

Fig. 1

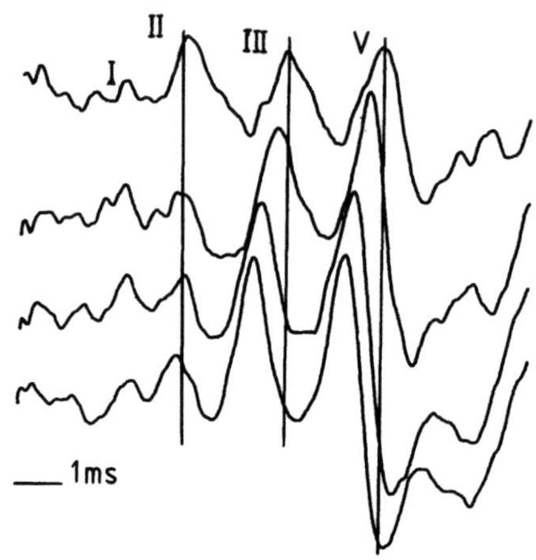

Fig. 2

Fig. 1. Patient R., meningioma of the right cerebellopontine angle. Intraoperative recording of AERs is shown. The upper recording has been obtained without surgical retraction; the lower recording with surgical retraction. Note loss of wave II and latency shift of wave V after onset of retraction

Fig. 2. Patient K., cholesteatoma of the right cerebellopontine angle. Intraoperatively recorded AERs are shown after the surgical retractor has been removed. The period covered from the first recording *(top)* to the last *(bottom)* is 45 min. Note brain stem recovery as indicated by latency shift of waves III and V, whereas wave II remains unchanged

New Research

Primary and Secondary Hypothalamus and Brain Stem Lesions

H. W. Pia
Neurochirurgische Universitäts-Klinik, Klinikstraße 29, D-6300 Gießen

Life means regulation and modulation, death means loss of regulation and modulation.

Lesions of the hypothalamo-hypophyseal system and the brain stem occur as direct primary and indirect secondary involvement by trauma and space-occupying lesions, mostly associated with raised intracranial pressure (19, 20). In contrast to morphological and clinical findings [in Germany by SPATZ (101), TÖNNIS (103), and ZÜLCH (124) and their co-workers], the accompanying vegetative, metabolic, and humoral disturbances were largely unknown and uncertain when my personal interest started 35 years ago (73-77). This led to clinical and experimental examinations and became the central research program with the foundation of the Neurosurgical Clinic in Giessen 30 years ago. Together with my neurosurgical co-workers, including neuroradiologists, neuropathologists, neurophysiologists, neurochemists, and a mathematician, in the first period (over nearly 20 years) I studied the central vegetative disturbances of respiration, circulation, and temperature, the central metabolic and endocrine disturbances of water and electrolyte, protein-amino acid, and glucose-fatty acid regulation, and the central disturbances of motor activity.

The concept of *central dysregulation* (Pia) has been elaborated elsewhere (76-83), and several syndromes of acute and chronic irritation and paralysis of vegetative and metabolic disturbances in different levels of the hypothalamo-hypophyseal system and brain stem have been described, revised, or integrated (Table 1) by BAUER (8-12), BANNO (7), EGGERT (22), GROTE (25-29), ITO (38, 39), LAUSBERG (50-59), LORENZ (60-69), PIA (76-83), SCHEPELMANN (92-95), SEEGER (30, 98-100), and WESEMANN (5, 6, 109-118).

With the recent progress in evaluating hypothalamo-hypophyseal and brain stem function in man in clinical conditions, the second period of our clinical and experimental research program started five years ago. Modern methods permit quite precise localization of the brain stem lesion, its extent, its dynamics, and to certain degree its nature. All data are continuously compared with clinical, experimental and post mortem findings to study the effect of hypothalamo-hypophyseal and brain stem dysfunction upon vegetative and neuroendocrine function. Our final aim is to understand better the mechanisms leading to integration and disintegration of the function of the hypothalamus, hypophysis, and brain stem and to acquire better knowledge of factors responsible for compensation and decompensation of this complex neurogenic and humoral system.

Some of the results of our past and main present studies will be discussed (1-3, 13-18, 21, 23, 25-29, 31-37, 40-49, 71, 72, 81-91, 96, 97, 104-123).

Advances in Neurosurgery, Vol. 13
Edited by H. Dietz, M. Brock, and M. Klinger

Table 1. Central dysregulation

Hypothalamic-pituitary syndromes
Acute irritation syndromes
Chronic defect syndromes
Acute paralysis syndromes
"Central hypothalamic death"
Mesencephalic syndromes
Acute irritation syndromes
Decerebration syndromes
Synchronous reactions and rhythms
Acute paralysis syndromes
"Central mesencephalic death"
Bulbar syndromes
Acute irritation syndromes
Acute paralysis syndromes
"Central bulbar death"

Syndromes of the Hypothalamo-Hypophyseal System

In contrast to the well-known findings in the brain stem due to raised intracranial pressure, lesions of the hypothalamo-hypophyseal system are less known and studied due to cisternal herniation and the enlargement of the third ventricle. They occur primarily and secondarily by displacement, rotation, and compression of the structures and the inherent vascular system of the hypothalamus, the hypophyseal stalk, and the anterior and posterior lobe of the hypophysis, resulting in slight or severe disturbances involving hemorrhages and infarctions (Fig. 1a). They may be accompanied by corresponding lesions of the adrenal cortex (91) (Fig. 1b). In all lethal cases with direct and indirect lesions and clinical signs, changes of different magnitude of the hypothalamus, the supraoptic and paraventricular nuclei, the neurosecretory system of the stalk, and both the posterior and the anterior lobes of the hypophysis were present.

In the case of a 16-year-old boy with bilateral traumatic brain lacerations there were hemorrhagic lesions around and inside the pituitary stalk. The neurosecretory pathways were loosed and the stalk showed diffuse extravasation of erythrocytes (Fig. 2a). Two patients with processes of the posterior fossa had similar lesions. In a 19-year-old girl, a diffuse vascular lesion of the cerebellum was accompanied by marked upward herniation of the cistern of Galen und multiple perivascular hemorrhagic and edematous foci of the hypothalamus and diffuse necrosis of the anterior lobe (Fig. 2b).

So far neuroradiology has made only a small contribution to the diagnosis of secondary hypothalamo-pituitary disturbances. The first findings of a complete blockage of the basal cistern were described by LAUN and HILDEBRANDT (31, 46). Out of 11 traumatic cases with diabetes insipidus, eight had an occluded basal cistern (Fig. 3).

Consequently disturbances of the autonomous, the hypothalamo-adenohypophyseal, and the hypothalamo-neurohypophyseal systems and of adrenal glands and kidneys are to be expected. Depending on the intensity and acuteness, irritation and paralysis syndromes with hyper- and hypoactivity occur (Table 2).

Table 2. Hypothalamic-pituitary syndromes

Acute irritation syndromes	*Acute paralysis syndromes*
Vasodilatation	Vasodepression and vasoparalysis
Diencephalic attacks:	Circulatory failure
Increase: vegetative parameters	Attacks of cardiac arrest
Decrease: venous blood pressure	Hypothermia
Increase: catabolic processes, protein, amino acids	Central diabetes
	Diabetes insipidus
Hyperglycemia	Pituitary failure
Polyuria	"Central hypothalamic death"
Respiratory alkalosis	
Chronic hypothalamic defect syndromes	
Decrease: vegetative parameters	
Metabolic rate	
Respiratory quotient	
Anterior pituitary hormones	
Lack of regulation and adjustment	

In acute irritation syndromes diencephalic attacks or crises are found, as analyzed by LORENZ (60). They are expressed by acute vasodilatation with coma, dilated unreacting pupils, increased perspiration, lacrimation, salivation, tracheal excretion, flushing, and a synchronous rise of all vegetative parameters except for central venous pressure, which decreases. Apart from the rare diencephalic attacks, changes in the pulse rate and the ECG were observed. Besides periodic alterations of the pulse rate and a corresponding increase in the P-wave and flattening of the T-wave, and vice versa, there were a considerable number of different ECG changes. These indicate irritation of the ergotropic and tropotropic areas of the hypothalamus. Systematic examinations are lacking.

The acute vegetative paralysis syndromes are governed by vasodepression and vasoparalysis with hypotension, attacks of cardiac arrest, circulatory failure, and hypothermia. The vegetative syndromes are combined with characteristic metabolic and humoral disturbances. Besides predominant catabolic reactions and still unclear changes of the protein and lipid metabolism and dissociations of the amino acid pool (10, 11), hyperglycemia is typical.

The *central hypothalamic hyperglycemia* (Fig. 4a) described by GROTE (26) is associated with hyperinsulinemia and hyperglucagonemia, resistance to insulin, lack of ketonuria, and low levels of cortisol and HGH. The normal stimulation of glucose by the Conard test is inhibited.

Experimental studies (114, 117) may explain this inappropriate secretion and ineffectiveness of insulin and glucagon. In experimental brain edema there is an intracellular deficit of glucose. Glucose marked with C_{14} does not enter the zone of edema. This is due to the blockage or lack of all the enzymes responsible for the glucose metabolism, the enzymes included in the Embden-Meyerhoff chain, the citric acid circle, and the respiratory chain. Twelve enzymes of the chain that were checked, beginning with the first link, hexokinase, and ending with the last, cytochromoxidase, showed the same result (Fig. 4b). In central hypothalamic hyperglycemia the hypothalamic *glucose level sensors* blocked by destruction or edema react as in intracellular glucopenia in spite of the extreme hyperglycemia.

Fourteen years ago, at the congress in Freiburg in 1970, GROTE, PIA, and WESEMANN (27, 28) described a *hypothalamic syndrome* characterized by extreme hyperglycemia, hyperthermia, diabetes insipidus, and secondary aldosteronism.

In a patient with a temporal glioblastoma and the clinical signs of hypothalamus and midbrain herniation, massive diuresis started, with fluid output of 9.5 liters/day, and blood sugar rose from 120 mg% to 970 mg%. Despite balancing of water and electrolytes, increasing hypernatremia and hypokalemia occurred, together with a mixed metabolic-respiratory acidosis. The blood sugar rose to 2000 mg% and could not be lowered by administration of 300 units of insulin. The patient died after two days because of circulatory failure.

Disturbances of water and electrolyte metabolism have been studied in the intervening period, especially using improved diagnostic devices, by HILDEBRANDT and RAP (31, 86, 89-91). Sixteen acute secondary cases (11 traumatic with four survivors, and five spontaneous lethal cases) had a syndrome of diabetes insipidus, arterial hypotension, and hypothermia. In four cases with death during the first day the syndrome was characterized by oliguria, hypotension, and hypothermia. The clinical diagnosis made in nearly all cases was that of a *bulbar syndrome*; the severe disturbances of water and electrolyte metabolism, however, favored severe disturbances of the hypothalamo-pituitary axis.

The *vasopressin test*, with a normal rise in ACTH, gluco-, and mineralocorticoids, was negative in all lethal cases and proved the clinical diagnosis of a breakdown of the hypothalamo-pituitary connections. The vasopressin test was normal in the few surviving cases. The connection and correlation between polyuria and oliguria are complex and unclear. The 19-year-old girl whose morphological findings were related above showed the expected relationship between dysregulation of the water metabolism and ADH. During the first 24 hours the water output was reduced and correlated with the increased ADH. Parallel with the decreasing ADH during the third day polyuria developed, together with hypernatremia, hypotension, and hypothermia (Fig. 5).

In six out of seven patients with ADH, examination (Fig. 6) has shown primary or secondary raised values with a subsequent decrease. None of them showed a good correlation between water output and ADH level. Two cases showed a dissociation of the ADH-osmolality relation. In one oliguric case, the ADH-level was extremely low. The normal serum osmolality reaction on the hypothalamus seems to be blocked, so that the ADH reacts independently. Our present findings in severe acute lesions have demonstrated excessive disturbances of the system with the following syndromes:

A primary irritation syndrome with a rise in ADH and oliguria followed by ADH lowering or a dissociation of the ADH-osmolality relation and primary or secondary polyuria. As long as hypotension and hypothermia are mild and there is normal vasopressin stimulation, it is compatible with survival. *The acute secondary paralysis syndrome* is characterized by a negative vasopressin test. *In acute paralysis syndrome* oliguria is combined with marked depression of all vegetative parameters and complete dissociation. The last two syndromes are the substrate of *acute hypothalamo-hypophyseal death* – a special and specific form of central death. The clinical relevance has been proved by pathological disturbances of the hypothalamus, stalk, and hypophysis without changes in the brain stem and the medulla oblongata.

Chronic Hypothalamo-Hypophyseal Defect Syndromes

Chronic lesions, as benign tumors of the suprasellar region with direct involvement of the hypothalamo-hypophyseal system, seem to have no or only little effect upon the regulatory system. The vegetative and basal endocrine and metabolic parameters may be normal or lowered, i.e., low HGH, ACTH, and cortisol levels. In most cases loading tests prove the lacking stimulation and regulation, i.e., of the mentioned hormones, or an increased sensitivity of glucose levels against insulin. They also demonstrate a slight disturbance in the hypothalamo-pituitary transmission. Most important is the largely preserved adaptation and compensation.

An exceptional case (H.U.H. 260251261) may demonstrate involvement and the course of a chronic hypothalamo-hypophyseal defect syndrome. In 1979 extirpation and radiotherapy of a cerebellar arachnoid sarcoma were carried out following a shunt operation for hydrocephalus. No recurrence occurred. In 1982 there was extirpation and radiotherapy of multiple spinal metastases without recurrence. In July 1983 a large metastasis of the hypothalamus was diagnosed (Fig. 7). After radiotherapy the tumor was eliminated. The last examination was performed in October 1983. The course of the vegetative parameters during the four clinical treatments was characterized by a progressive decrease in blood pressure, pulse rate, and temperature, particularly during the period with the manifest hypothalamic tumor, and reduced modulation in comparison with the first periods.

The lowered *mean temperature* of 36.5°C decreased during cooling. A normal thermoregulatory reaction concerning the metabolic rate and electric muscle activity did not take place before a temperature below 35.5°C. After irradiation the thermogenetic threshold had normalized. During the heating period up to 55°C there was no evaporative heat loss up to a core temperature of 39.5°C. After radiation the reaction remained abnormal; however, the heating period had to be stopped (Fig. 8). The loading test showed a cold disturbance of the thermoregulation, with displacement of the threshold with normal regulation and no reaction against heating with partial normalization after elimination of the tumor.

Low basal values of STH, FSH, LH, TSH, and cortisol, with no or reduced stimulation, as well as diabetes insipidus with hypernatremia, high serum osmolality, low ADH, low urine osmolality, an increase in serum osmolality, and no rise in ADH after the Conard test demonstrated marked disturbances of the hypothalamo-adeno- and neurohypophyseal system. The radiation normalized the hypothalamo-neurohypophyseal transmission nearly totally; the signs of anterior lobe insufficiency, however, were less influenced.

ADH may be normal, reduced, or concerning the serum osmolality, relatively lowered; most important are the loading tests with natrium chloride, dehydration, and water excess. The normal ADH reaction is lacking in chronic cases (Fig. 9). It is to be supposed that the supraoptic nuclei are directly blocked. In two cases the ADH osmolality was displaced into the hyperosmolarity part. The vasopressin test is usually positive in chronic cases, and signifies a much better prognosis.

Examinations of the *circadian rhythm* by continuous EEG recording and checking of hormones and neurotransmitters provide a new access to the complex regulatory mechanisms. In the case of a 50-year-old man with a giant suprasellar adenoma there was no circadian, no sleep-wake rhythm. The only findings were special rhythms with slow wave periods of 80-100 min; they occurred in the total EEG spectrum and as isolated frequencies (Fig. 10). In the most severe cases (Fig. 11) and in acute irritation there is a decrease in the core temperature to 35.5°C, in metabolic rate to 1000 cal/day (4200 Joule), and in the respiratory quotient. During lowering of the ambient temperature by 6°C the core temperature decreases (104, 105); there is no reaction of the metabolic rate.

Chronic hypothalamo-pituitary defect syndromes may be latent; however, they may be revealed by loading tests with lacking or reduced stimulation, adaptation, and modulation. All or some partial function of the hypothalamus and the anterior and posterior lobes of the hypophysis may be involved. The findings mean a reduced capacity of compensation and the danger of a latent or imminent decompensation.

Brain Stem Syndromes

The diagnosis of primary and secondary lesions of the brain stem has been improved by special CT techniques, NMR studies, and multimodality evoked potentials (1-4, 18, 23, 41, 43, 44, 46-48, 96, 97, 119, 120). When these investigations are combined with clinical examinations, special animal experiments, morphological examinations, and mathematical correlations (15, 33-37, 42, 87, 104-108, 121, 122), the site, extent, type, and to a certain degree etiology, course, and prognosis can be evaluated quite exactly and correlated with the vegetative and metabolic disturbances.

By means of CT even small lesions can be detected, i.e., small direct hemorrhages as hyperdense lesions as well as infarcts or tumors as hypodense or mixed lesions. The cisterns are open. In secondary lesions with raised intracranial pressure herniation of the cisterns with partial or complete occlusion and secondary hypodense lesions of the brain stem are characteristic. Their type and intensity, influenced by site, acuteness, and age, can be detected much better than lesions of the brain stem itself (17, 46-49, 96, 97). At the end, with central death, the brain becomes uniformly hypodense and structureless.

In the case of a right-sided intracerebellar hematoma one sees transtentorial herniation of the cerebellar apex with occlusion of the cistern of Galen and the posterior part of the supratentorial and total infratentorial sections of the ambient cistern. The cerebellar tonsils are displaced downward to the level of the foramen magnum (Fig. 12).

In the most severe cases of acute herniations, medial and paramedial hemorrhages of the mesencephalon and upper pons and hemorrhagic infarcts of the herniated brain and the occipital lobe can be identified. The important differences between the supra- and infratentorial compartment are illustrated by a case of basilar artery occlusion involving a normal mesencephalon and complete infarction of the pons, the first described CT correlate of a "locked-in-syndrome" (Fig. 13).

In comparable experiments by ZIERSKI and RAP (87, 122, 123) with short-lasting intermittent cerebral compression by means of an inflatable balloon, marked disturbances of the blood-brain barrier without morphological findings occurred in two limited zones in front of and behind the tentorium with involvement of (a) the thalamic and hypothalamic and (b) the mesencephalic and upper pontine structures, respectively (Fig. 14a). After repeated ICP increases we find herniations of the cisterns and structural changes of the hypothalamus, brain stem, and occipital lobe, the site of frequent secondary infarcts in man.

Regional CBF measurements by microspheres (122) (Fig. 14b) after balloon inflation and CSF infusion with hydrocephalus demonstrate a progressive fall in CBF, mostly in the supratentorial and only later and slightly in the infratentorial structures, including the lower brain stem. In the group with tentorial herniation a distinct compartmentalization occurred, with a significant difference and rate of CBF change between supra- and infratentorial structures. The infusion group without herniation showed no compartmentalization. The findings underline the significance of mesencephalic herniation and the early and marked appearance of reduced circulation of the hypothalamic and upper midbrain structures.

Comparable measurements of intracranial pressure in men and experiments demonstrate the direct significant correlation between perimesencephalic cisternal herniations, cerebral blood flow, and intracranial pressure. With ICP above 30 mmHg the cisterns are occluded nearly completely. Both parameters directly parallel the prognosis (Fig. 15).

Mesencephalic Syndromes

In view of the morphological and pathophysiological results, mesencephalic syndromes play an important role (Table 3). They have been checked intensively and several syndromes identified.

Table 3. Mesencephalic syndromes

Acute irritation syndromes	*Acute paralysis syndromes*
Disinhibition and increase of vegetative parameters Peripheral vasoconstriction	Apallic syndromes:
Increase of vegetative parameters, energy and protein metabolism, CO_2 stimulation of respiration	Lability of vegetative parameters "Central mesencephalic death" Circulatory insufficiency Loss of modulation
Decerebration syndromes	
Synchronous reactions and rhythms: vegetative parameters, muscle tonus and activity, ICP	

Acute irritation syndromes are an expression of an extreme ergotropic reaction with peripheral vasoconstriction, an increase in all vegetative parameters, and disinhibition of respiration centers against CO_2. A loss of evaporative heat loss seems to occur (55, 59).

In acute paralysis syndromes these symptoms are aggravated; central temperature may rise to 43°C, and the normal pulse rate modulation of 5-30 beats/min goes up to 50-80 and sometimes even to 100 beats/min. At the same time there is an extreme rise in all metabolic and neuroendocrine parameters. The irritation becomes life-threatening. The decompensation becomes manifest by way of a breakdown in the arterial blood pressure and machine-like respiration without any modulation (24, 64, 81-83) and causes the specific *mesencephalic death*. Thanks to modern treatment – today we would call this therapeutic complex brain protection – it occurs only exceptionally.

In mesencephalic defect syndromes, as in the persistent vegetative state, the so-called *apallic status*, there is lability with certain compensation. The basal values are normal, especially under the conditions of intensive care. Signs of dysregulation and decompensation are always present when the patient is subjected to stress or loading tests.

Synchronous Reactions and Rhythms

Synchronous reactions and rhythms as well as decerebration syndromes are specific phenomena of irritation and disinhibition of the mesencephalon itself. They are isolated from the modulating and inhibiting influences of the cortex and subcortex and exposed completely to the internal and external sensoric afferent stimuli.

Synchronous reactions and rhythms (Table 4) occur besides and without decerebration in midbrain lesions. Various synchronous reactions, periodicity, and rhythms were observed in 70% of our patients (64, 65, 98, 99).

Synchronous reactions may concern all vegetative parameters or single ones. They are characterized by a spontaneous synchronous rise and fall with or without periodicity. The combination with a synchronous decrease in respiration rate – as in lower decerebration – is observed exceptionally.

Cheyne-Stokes respiration, Biot's respiration, periodic undulations, and other periodic rhythms may be connected with synchronous rhythms of *motor activity* (Fig. 16a) (92-95), but more frequently the latter occur alone. The neuronal disintegration at midbrain level concerns the time-control mechanism too. Traube-Hering-Meyer *blood pressure waves*

Table 4. Mesencephalic rhythmic phenomena

Respiratory rhythms:	
Cheyne-Stokes	
Biot	
Machine respiratory	
Combined with rhythms of motor activity	
Blood pressure waves:	
(Traube-Hering-Meyer waves)	
Intact brain stem:	5-6/min. waves
Midbrain disturbances:	3-4/min. waves
Combined with:	
Cheyne-Stokes rhythms	
Uniform respiratory rhythms	
Delta wave outbursts	
Slowing of pulse rate	
Left bundle block with atrioventricular rhythms	
ICP outbursts and pressure waves	
Bulbar disturbances:	1-2/min. rhythms

(Fig. 16b) are found in 5-6, 3-4, and 1-2 per minute rhythms. Lesions of the oral brain stem show 3-4 per minute rhythms, isolated or combined with rhythms of the cardiac circulatory system, respiration, ICP, and outbursts of delta waves in the EEG. One to two per minute waves indicate the complete loss of central regulation. They are found in central death and are probably of spinal origin (66).

Besides the described rhythmic phenomena in second and minute frequencies, TONN (102) observed first time ultradian rhythms of hourly frequency. A 16-year-old boy with a traumatic hematoma at the pontomesencephalic level showed a marked alpha-band in the EEG power spectrum and at the same time a second delta activity. There was no circadian rhythm. Thirty-six hours later the alpha-activity ceased for 90 min (three cessations during six hours). There is no explanation at present for this unusual and unknown type of ultradian rhythm (Fig. 17).

Decerebration Syndromes

Decerebration syndromes belong to the rhythmic synchronous phenomena of the mesencephalon and upper pons. Induction and stimulation via afferent stimuli as algic, thermic, acoustic, and optic stimuli produce a great multiplicity and variety of syndromes. LORENZ (65) described two types. Most frequently there exists a syndrome with a synchronous rise in respiration rate, heart rate and arterial blood pressure with lowering of venous pressure and outbursts of slow wave activity in the EEG. A second, similar, syndrome showed a synchronous decrease in respiration rate and no delta activity. Whether the interpretation of these syndromes as *upper and lower decerebration* is correct, remains uncertain (Table 5).

Table 5. Decerebration syndromes

Upper decerebration	*Lower decerebration*
Synchronous increase	Synchronous increase
Pulse rate	as in upper decerebration
Arterial and venous blood pressure	Synchronous decrease
Respiration rate	Respiration
EEG: Slow wave outbursts	EEG: No outbursts
Motor activity	Motor activity
ICP	ICP
Synchronous reactions and rhythms	

More detailed experiments by SCHEPELMANN (93, 94) and KLUG, HOFFMANN, and ZIERSKI (41, 42) led to new findings concerning the level, site, and type of lesions and especially the relationship between cisternal herniation, intracranial pressure, and provocation.

In cases with *occluded perimesencephalic cisterns*, spontaneous and provoked decerebration episodes are characterized by a nearly synchronous rise in respiration and heart rate, motor activity (integrated EMG), arterial blood pressure, and intracranial pressure, and a decrease in central venous pressure. Normalization takes place variously (Fig. 18a). High plateau waves of intracranial pressure are sometimes associated with a high frequency of fits.

With *free perimesencephalic cisterns* the same syndrome occurs with no or slightly increased ICP. Induced episodes showed a lowering of ICP (Fig. 18b). There was no strong correlation between decerebration and level of ICP.

In spite of their complexity and the many unsolved questions, there is no doubt that lesions of the upper brain stem at the level of the tentorial notch and especially those with perimesencephalic herniations and raised intracranial pressure lead to excessive neuronal activation. The characteristic signs are increased modulation, and spontaneous and induced synchronization and rhythmicity of different intensity, frequency, and time sequence (in second, minute, and hourly bands, sometimes with machine-like uniformity and regularity). The latter can be explained by a common mechanism of disinhibition alone.

Pontine and Bulbar Syndromes

Diagnosis and follow-up of acute pontine and especially bulbar lesions may be difficult using CT and NMR for technical and practical reasons, respectively. In chronic lesions the application of improved CT techniques and NMR mark a new era.

Evoked potentials (acoustic, visual, short latency, and cortical somatosensoric EVPs and blink reflex) have resulted in the most important progress in terms of precision of diagnosis and prognosis of brain stem lesions, being introduced into our clinical and experimental research by N. KLUG and G. CSECSEI.

In a patient with right-sided infarction at the mesencephalopontine level the brain stem acoustic evoked potentials were present only on the left side with the first three components up to the superior olivar nucleus in the lower pons. There was no reaction from rostral components: the lateral lemniscus, inferior colliculus, and lateral geniculate body. These findings correspond to those of blink reflex with lack of both of the second responses (R 2) bilaterally (Fig. 19a). Visual evoked potentials and left-sided somatosensoric evoked potentials were normal; the absence of the latter on the right side was caused by an older infarct of the middle cerebral artery territory (Fig. 19b). Evoked potentials in our pressure experiments demonstrate the dependency and the rostrocaudal course of pressure-induced brain stem lesions. During rising ICP after a short period of decreased latency and increased amplitude indicating transient neuronal activation, the latency of rostrally generated potential components of acoustic evoked potentials is increased (Fig. 20a), followed by disappearance of the peaks in a rostrocaudal direction. The abolition of P V corresponds clinically to midbrain herniation and dilatated pupils. Another pressure rise leads up to 110 mmHg to the abolition of AEP and central death. An additional localized and pressure dependent reaction is demonstrated by the responses of the blink reflex (Fig. 20b). Between 40 and 50 mmHg R 2 is abolished, corresponding with pupillary and respiratory disturbances. With a further increase the latency of R 1 is prolonged and the amplitude diminished. Loss of R 1 means the collapse of central regulation and severe functional damage of the lower brain stem. Normalization of ICP followed by a repeated increase produces changes of R 1 at lower levels. R 2 remains abolished (18). These few examples demonstrate the present-day possibilities of localizing lesions in the brain stem and correlating them with the complex neurogenic and neurohumoral findings.

Corresponding findings can be observed in human pathology and demonstrate the progression of a clinical and vegetative midbrain syndrome via a pontine into a bulbar syndrome.

In a patient with severe head trauma (Fig. 21) there was an initial moderate increase in ICP (35 mmHg) with occasional synchronous increases of blood pressure, heart rate, and ICP with normal perfusion pressure. A large pressure wave (80 mmHg) leads to a drop in perfusion pressure without changes in heart rate and blood pressure. Cerebral perfusion pressure recovers slightly with the fall in ICP, but the next increase lowers it permanently. Shortly before bulbar death ICP reaches values around 100 mmHg; the mean arterial pressure is 50 mmHg, and the CPP negative. There is no modulation, and only 0.15/min pressure waves are seen. Corresponding to the loss of regulation and modulation, the relationship between the change in mean ICP and the amplitude of ICP is abolished (35, 37, 122).

Acute bulbar irritation syndrome (Table 6) is characterized by irregularity, lack of coordination, and ataxia of all vegetative functions. There is no synchronization, no episodes or rhythms, no regularity, and no Cushing reflex (17, 18), with a rise in arterial pressure and a decrease in heart rate. The differentiation between midbrain and bulbar syndromes is best demonstrated by respiratory disturbances. The reactivity of respiration areas to CO_2 is diminished or abolished, and is chemically directed by O_2 deficit. Additionally, O_2 supply may be dangerous. Muscle tonus and muscle activity are reduced.

Acute bulbar paralysis syndromes are also more complex than is supposed on the basis of the findings in central bulbar death after arrest of spontaneous respiration during artificial ventilation. Our contribution concerns the syndrome of hypothermia with total poikilothermia (51, 55, 59) and the fact that the hypothalamo-hypophyseal system may be at least partially intact, maintaining hormone excretion and positive reactions to stimulation (26). The fundamental observation is that normal modulation of vegetative and metabolic functions is lost, with resulting continuous "straight curves" (see Fig. 21).

Table 6. Bulbar syndromes

Acute irritation syndromes	*Acute paralysis syndromes*
Lability, irregulatory, uncoordination and ataxia of vegetative functions	Arrest of respiration
No reactivity of respiratory center to CO_2, directed by O_2 deficit	Artificial respiration: Decrease and loss of modulation of vegetative parameters, hypothermia with total poikilothermia
Irregular respiratory periods	"Central bulbar death"
	Loss of function of brain with "normal" reactions of HGH and cortisol and stimulation

Summary

In our present state of knowledge any attempt to differentiate acute or especially chronic syndromes of central dysregulation is problematic and open to criticism. However, in the past 35 years we have succeeded in describing some syndromes of neuronal disinhibition, irritation, and paralysis of the hypothalamo-hypophyseal system and brain stem.

Our recent findings with improved CT technique, multimodality evoked potentials, and improved methods of measuring neurohormones, hypophysotropic hormones, and metabolic disturbances have provided greater access to the two complexes of central dysregulation – the central hormonal-humoral dysregulation of the hypothalamo-hypophyseal system and the central neurogenic dysregulation of the brain stem. There are still many white spots on the map of the central regulation areas. We have to study in man the neuroreceptors, neurotransmitters, and neuromodulators, their flow and integration, and the mechanisms of adaptation, compensation, and decompensation. The aim of our endeavors is to recognize and understand disturbances of these vital structures earlier and better in order to correct them or to avoid their progression, as *life means regulation and modulation*, and *death means loss of regulation and modulation*, or, to use the words of Claude Bernard regarding homoeostasis: "La fixité du milieu interne est la condition de la vie libre".

References

1. Agnoli, A.L., Busse, O., Laun, A., Wirbatz, A., Schock, P., Feistner, H.: Prognostic significance of subarachnoid CSF spaces abnormalities in CT. In: Anatomy – Physiology in CT. Kugler Medical Publications, Amstelveen 1980
2. Agnoli, A.L., Cristante, L., Busse, O., Feistner, H.: Brain herniation by cranial computer tomography: Clinical radiological correlations. In: Anatomy – Physiology in CT, pp. 113-118. Kugler Medical Publications, Amstelveen 1980
3. Agnoli, A.L., Feistner, H., Busse, O., Cristante, L.: Comparative clinical and neuroradiological findings in brain stem infarctions. In: Anatomy – Physiology in CT, pp. 147-151. Kugler Medical Publications, Amstelveen 1980
4. Agnoli, A.L., Laun, A., Busse, O., Schoch, P.: Computerized tomography in brain stem haemorrhage, diagnostic and prognostic aspects. In: Anatomy – Physiology in CT. Kugler Medical Publications, Amstelveen 1980
5. Baethmann, A., Koczorek, K.H.R., Reulen, H.J., Wesemann, W., Hofmann, H.F., Angstwurm, A., Brendel, W.: Die Beeinflussung des traumatischen Hirnödems durch Aldosteron, Aldosteron-Antagonisten und Dexamethason im Tierexperiment. In: Postoperative Störungen des Elektrolyt- und Wasserhaushaltes, pp. 259-285. Schattauer, Stuttgart New York 1968
6. Baethmann, A., Wesemann, W., Brendel, W.: Enzymaktivität in der Großhirnrinde von adrenalektomierten Ratten und ihre Beeinflussung durch Aldosteron und Dexamethason. Pflügers Arch. Ges. Physiol. 300, 37 (1968)
7. Banno, T., Lorenz, R.: Störungen des Säure-Basen-Haushaltes bei neurochirurgischen Patienten. Anästhesiol. Info. 17, 76-89 (1976)

8. Bauer, B.L.: Parenterale Ernährung in der Neurochirurgie. Anaesth. Resusc. 13, 124-130 (1966)

9. Bauer, B.L.: Probleme bei der postoperativen und posttraumatischen Ernährung von neurochirurgischen Patienten. Acta Neurochir. (Wien) 11, 96-108 (1966)

10. Bauer, B.L.: Protein and amino acid metabolism in central dysregulation. In: Pia, H.W., Grote, E., Mundinger, F., Gleave, J.R.W. (eds.) Modern aspects of neurosurgery, Vol. I. Proc. Ann. Meetings Deutsche Gesellschaft für Neurochirurgie, 1969 and 1970, pp. 148-171. Excerpta Medica, Amsterdam 1971

11. Bauer, B.L.: Untersuchungen über das Verhalten von N-Metaboliten und Aminosäuren bei zentralen Regulationsstörungen. Habil.-Schrift, Gießen 1973

12. Bauer, B.L., Schultis, K.: Posttraumatische Katabolie und parenterale Ernährung. Actuelle Chirurgie 1, 281-286 (1966)

13. Behr, R.: Veränderungen der thermogenetischen Schwellentemperaturen nach hypothalamischen Mikroinjektionen von 6-Hydroxydopamin (6-OHDA) bei verschiedenen adaptierten Meerschweinchen. Inaugural-Dissertation, Gießen 1984

14. Behr, R., Zeisberger, E., Merker, G.: Response of the guinea-pig to external cooling after aminergic denervation of the anterior hypothalamus. J. Therm. Biol. 8, 125-128 (1983)

15. Behr, R.: Personal communication

16. Braunsdorf, W., Christophis, P., Rap, Z.M., Pia, H.W.: The role of cerebral veins in the genesis of secondary lesions in the occipital lobe. In: Auer, L.M., Loew, F. (eds.) The cerebral veins, pp. 293-298. Springer, Wien New York 1983

17. Calatayud, V.: Cisternal herniations in raised intracranial pressure. Inaugural-Dissertation, Gießen 1984

18. Csécsei, G., Klug, N., Rap, Z.M.: Effect of increased intracranial pressure on blink reflex in cats. Acta Neurochir. 68, 85-92 (1983)

19. Cushing, H.: Concerning a definite regulatory mechanism of the vasomotor center which controls blood pressure during cerebral compression. Bull. Johns Hopkins Hosp. 12, 290-292 (1901)

20. Cushing, H.: Physiologische und anatomische Beobachtungen über den Einfluß auf den intrakraniellen Kreislauf und über einige damit verwandte Erscheinungen. Mitt. Grenzgeb. Med. Chir. 9, 773-808 (1902)

21. Dolinski, A.: Untersuchungen zum Metabolismus von Alanin bei Glucose-Haushaltsstörungen bei Hirnläsionen. Habil.-Schrift, Lodz/Polen 1981. Neur. Neurochir. Pol. 13, 177-182 (1977)

22. Eggert, H.R.: Tierexperimentelle Untersuchungen zur Behandlung der Elektrolytverteilungsstörungen beim kältetraumatischen Hirnödem mit Mineralcorticoiden, Glucocorticoiden und Aldosteron-Antagonisten. Inaugural-Dissertation, Gießen 1971

23. Feistner, H., Busse, O., Agnoli, A.L.: Vergleichende klinische und CT-Befunde bei Hirnstamminfarkten. Nervenarzt 75, 163-166 (1981)

24. Frowein, R.A.: Zentrale Atemstörungen bei Hirnverletzungen und Hirntumoren. In: Monographien Gesamtgebiet Neurol und Psychiat. Springer, Berlin Göttingen Heidelberg 1963

25. Grote, E.: Der Einfluß des Zentralnervensystems auf die Glucosehomöostase beim Menschen. Habil.-Schrift, Gießen 1977

26. Grote, E.: The CNS control of glucose metabolism. Acta Neurochir. (Suppl.) 31, Springer, Wien New York 1981

27. Grote, E., Pia, H.W., Wesemann, W.: The influence of hypothalamic lesions on metabolism and peripheral organization. Acta Neurochir. (Suppl.) 28, 463 (1979)

28. Grote, E., Pia, H.W., Wesemann, W.: Dysregulation of glucose metabolism in patients with brain tumour and injuries. In: Advances in Neurosurgery, Vol. 7, pp. 318-326. Springer, Berlin Heidelberg New York 1979

29. Grote, E., Lorenz, R., Vuia, O.: Clinical and endocrinological findings in ectopic pinealoma and spongioblastoma of the hypothalamus. Acta Neurochir. 53, 87-98 (1980)

30. Guerndt, W., Kasper, G.: CO_2-Atemantrieb bei gerichteter Hirnkompression und bei meningealer Reaktion. Inaugural-Dissertation, Gießen 1972

31. Hildebrandt, G.: Personal communication

32. Hildebrandt, G., Lorenz, R.: Influence of oxygen supply upon vegetative functions during increased intracranial pressure. Acta Neurochir. 60, 169-181 (1982)

33. Hoffmann, O.: Mathematische Modelle zur Untersuchung der Liquordynamik. Inaugural-Dissertation, Gießen 1980

34. Hoffmann, O.: Ein mathematisches Modell zur Simulation der Liquordynamik. In: Informatik-Fachberichte 56, Simulationstechnik, pp. 343-350. Springer, Berlin Heidelberg New York 1982

35. Hoffmann, O., Zierski, J.: Analysis of ICP pulse pressure relationship as a function of arterial blood pressure. Clinical validitation of a mathematical model. Acta Neurochir. 66, 1-21 (1982)

36. Hoffmann, O., Kurzaj, E., Zierski, J., Winkler, B.: Blood flow in the brain stem during acute cerebral compression. In: Advances in neurotraumatology. Int. Congr. Ser. 612, pp. 334-336. Excerpta Medica, Amsterdam Oxford Princetown 1983

37. Hoffmann, O., Zierski, J.: Analysis of the intracranial pulse pressure relationship by simultaneous application of a mathematical model and comparison with clinical data. In: Proc. of the First European Simultation Congress (Congress ESL 83), pp. 488-503. Springer, Berlin Heidelberg New York 1983

38. Ito, A., Lorenz, R.: Duration of respiratory periods of uniform respiratory rhythms in 35 patients with neurosurgical diseases. Acta Neurochir. 43, 77-91 (1978)

39. Ito, A., Lorenz, R.: Variability of the respiratory phase, respiratory pause and numbers and durations of respiration during periodic breathing. Acta Neurochir. 43, 263-274 (1978)

40. Klug, N.: Brainstem auditory evoked potentials in syndromes of decerebration, bulbar syndromes and in central death. J. Neurol. 227, 219-228 (1982)

41. Klug, N.: Funktionsuntersuchungen des Hirnstamms im akuten Mittelhirnsyndrom unter Berücksichtigung vegetativer Meßgrößen während der Dezerebration. Habil.-Schr., Gießen 1984

42. Klug, N., Hoffmann, O., Zierski, J., Buss, K.: Intracranial pressure and muscle activity in patients with decerebrate rigidity. Acta Neurochir. 60, 155-167 (1982)

43. Klug, N., Csécsei, G., Rap, Z.M.: Evoked potentials and blink reflex in acute midbrain syndromes. Clinical and experimental find-

ings. In: Advances in neurotraumatology. Intern. Congr. Ser. 612, pp. 207-209. Excerpta Medica, Amsterdam Oxford Princetown 1983

44. Klug, N., Csécsei, G., Hoffmann, O.: Der Verlauf der frühen akustisch evozierten Potentiale (AEHP) im Dezerebrations- und Bulbärhirnsyndrom sowie beim zentralen Tod. Ideggyógyászati Szemle 36, 134-144 (1983)

45. Koźniewska, E., Rap, Z.M., Skolsińska, K.: Cerebrovascular effect of vasopressin on CBF. In: Gotoh, H. et al. (eds.) Cerebral blood flow and metabolism. Acta Neurolog. Scand., Suppl. 72, 602-603 (1979)

46. Laun, A.: Acute lesions of the brain stem – a clinical and morphological examination. Habil.-Schrift, Gießen 1985

47. Laun, A., Agnoli, A.L.: Brain stem haemorrhage. In: Pia, H.W., Langmaid, C., Zierski, J.: Spontaneous intracerebral haematomas, pp. 197-201. Springer, Berlin Heidelberg New York 1980

48. Laun, A., Agnoli, A.L., Rap, Z.M., Schönmayr, R., Villagrasa, J.: Morphological and CT findings in traumatic brainstem haemorrhage. In: Advances in Neurotraumatology. Int. Congr. Ser. 612, pp. 16-24. Excerpta Medica. Amsterdam Oxford Princetown 1983

49. Laun, A., Busse, O., Calatayud, V., Klug, N.: Cerebellar infarcts in the area of supply and their surgical treatment. Acta Neurochir. 71, 295-306 (1984)

50. Lausberg, G.: Der Verlust der Temperaturregulation beim zentralen Tod – reversibel? Dtsch. Med. Wschr. 24, 1301-1303 (1970)

51. Lausberg, G.: Temperaturregulation bei intrakranieller Drucksteigerung. Acta Neurochir. (Wien) 23, 172-173 (1970)

52. Lausberg, G.: Die prognostische Bedeutung zentraler Temperaturregulationsstörungen bei Mehrfachverletzungen mit cerebralem Schwerpunkt. In: Gauthier-Lafaye, J.-P., Otteni, J.C.: XXe Congr. Français d'Anesthésie – Réanimation, pp. 203-209. Strasbourg 1970

53. Lausberg, G.: Störungen der Temperaturregulation nach schweren gedeckten Schädelhirnverletzungen. Zbl. Chir. 95, 1655 (1970)

54. Lausberg, G.: Posttraumatische zentrale Hyperthermie und Hypothermie. Actuelle Chirurgie 5, 353-358 (1970)

55. Lausberg, G.: Disorders of central temperature regulation. In: Pia, H.W., Grote, E., Mundinger, F., Gleave, J.R.W.: Modern aspects of neurosurgery, Vol. 1-2, pp. 111-115. Excerpta Medica, Amsterdam 1971

56. Lausberg, G.: Die Bedeutung zentraler Temperaturregulationsstörungen für Therapie und Prognose schwerer gedeckter Schädelhirnverletzungen. Hefte Unfallheilk. 107, 209-213 (1971)

57. Lausberg, G.: Das Verhalten der Körpertemperatur nach schweren gedeckten Schädel-Hirn-Verletzungen im Kindesalter. Münch. Med. Wschr. 113, 725-726 (1971)

58. Lausberg, G.: Das Temperaturverhalten im Schock aus neurochirurgischer Sicht. Z. Wiederbelebung-Organersatz-Intensivmedizin (Suppl.) 2, 96-101 (1971)

59. Lausberg, G.: Zentrale Störungen der Temperaturregulation. Acta Neurochir. (Wien) Suppl. 19 (1972)

60. Lorenz, R.: Überwachung von Vitalwerten Schwerkranker auf einer neurochirurgischen Wach- und Intensivpflegestation. Elektromedika (Erlangen) 36, 1-5 (1968)

61. Lorenz, R.: Automatische Blutdruckmessungen nach Riva-Rocci-Korotkoff. Dtsch. Med. Wschr. 93, 690-694 (1968)

62. Lorenz, R.: Zur Frage der automatischen Erfassung vegetativer Regulationsgrößen. Zbl. Neurochir. 30, 1-28 (1969)

63. Lorenz, R.: Diagnose und Therapie der zentralen Regulationsstörungen. Hefte Unfallheilk. 99, 66-71 (1969)

64. Lorenz, R.: Cardiac and circulatory regulation in the presence of raised intracranial pressure. In: Pia, H.W., et al. (eds.) Central dysregulation. Int. Congr. Ser. 242, pp. 26-34. Excerpta Medica, Amsterdam 1971

65. Lorenz, R.: Wirkungen intrakranieller raumfordernder Prozesse auf den Verlauf von Blutdruck und Pulsfrequenz. In: Acta Neurochir. (Suppl.) 20. Springer, Wien New York 1973

66. Lorenz, R.: Rhythmic phenomena of blood pressure in neurosurgical patients. In: Umbach, W., Koeppchen, H.P. (eds.) Central rhythmic and regulation, pp. 301-306. Hippocrates, Stuttgart 1974

67. Lorenz, R.: Central disturbances of respiratory drive caused by brain damage in man. 19. Intern. Congr. Neurovegetative Research, Berlin, March 1984

68. Lorenz, R., Pia, H.W.: Moderne Möglichkeiten per- und postoperativer Überwachung in der Neurochirurgie. Beitr. Neurochir. 13, 108-113 (1966)

69. Lorenz, R., Ito, A.: The definition of Cheyne-Stokes rhythms. Acta Neurochir. 43, 61-76 (1978)

70. Mohr, P., Lorenz, R.: The effect of experimentally produced intracranial haematoma upon ICP. In: Intracranial pressure IV, pp. 207-210. Springer, Berlin Heidelberg New York 1980

71. Mueller, H.W., Binz, K.: Glass capillary gas chromatography of the serum acid fraction via automatic injection of lipid extracts. J. Chromatogr. 228, 75-93 (1983)

72. Mueller, H.W., Loeffler, E., Schmandt, W.: On the storage, shipping, and extraction of serums lipids for the gas chromatographic analysis of the fatty acid fraction. Clinica Chimica Acta 124, 343-349 (1982)

73. Pia, H.W.: Die Verquellung der Cisterna basalis und ambiens im Hirngefäßbild. Acta Neurochir. (Wien) 3, 315-328 (1953); Zbl. Neurochir. 14, 283-285 (1954)

74. Pia, H.W.: Die Pathogenese der Gefäßschäden der Occipitallappen bei gesteigertem Hirndruck. Proc. II. Int. Congr. Neuropathology, pp. 317-319. Excerpta Medica, Amsterdam 1955

75. Pia, H.W.: Die Einwirkung der Hirndrucksteigerungen auf den Hirnstamm, ihre Klinik und Behandlung. Münch. Med. Wschr. 98, 1609-1612 (1956)

76. Pia, H.W.: Die Schädigung des Hirnstammes bei den raumfordernden Prozessen des Gehirns. Acta Neurochir., Suppl. 4, Springer, Wien 1956

77. Pia, H.W.: Neue Erkenntnisse auf dem Gebiet der Hirndrucksteigerung und moderne Behandlungsmaßnahmen. Klin. Wschr. 35, 900-903 (1957)

78. Pia, H.W.: Klinische Einklemmungssyndrome. Acta Neurochir. (Wien) (Suppl.) VII, 471-483 (1961)

79. Pia, H.W.: Zentrale Regulationsstörungen bei kindlichen Hirnverletzungen und ihre Behandlung. Acta Neurochir. (Wien) 21, 71-92 (1969)

80. Pia, H.W.: Koma und intrakranielle Drucksteigerung. In: Notfall: Bewußtlosigkeit, pp. 52-63. Thieme, Stuttgart 1974

81. Pia, H.W.: Central dysregulation. Z. Neurol. 204, 1-21 (1973)

82. Pia, H.W.: Central dysregulation in brain stem lesions. In: Recent Progress in Neurological Surgery. Int. Congr. Series No. 320, pp. 290-299. Excerpta Medica, Amsterdam 1974

83. Pia, H.W.: Vegetative and metabolic syndromes in hypothalamus and brain stem lesions. 19. Intern. Congress of Neurovegetative Research, Berlin, March 1984

84. Rap, Z.M.: Inhibitory effect of antidiuretic hormone on the outflow of cerebrospinal fluid during vasogenic brain edema induced by cold lesions. In: Cervos-Navarro, Fritzka (eds.) Cerebral microcirculation and metabolism, pp. 171-175. Raven Press, New York 1981

85. Rap, Z.M.: Influence of damage of hypothalamo-hypophyseal neurosecretory system and adrenalectomy on blood brain barrier alteration during intracranial hypertension. Acta Neuropath. (Berlin), Suppl. VII, 10-12 (1981)

86. Rap, Z.M., Chwalbińska-Moneta, J.: Vasopressin in the blood during acute short-term intracranial hypertension in cats. In: Cervos-Navarro, J., Betz, E., Ebhard, G., Ferszt, R., Wüllenweber, R. (eds.) Advances in Neurology, Vol. 20, pp. 381-388. Raven Press, New York 1978

87. Rap, Z.M., Csécsei, G., Klug, N., Zierski, J., Pia, H.W.: Morphological analysis of experimental decerebration after acute epidural compression. In: Auer, L.M., Loew, F. (eds.) pp. 299-304. Springer, Wien, New York 1983

88. Rap, Z.M., Kózniewska-Koloziejska, E., Skolsińska, K.: Effect of vasopressin on the cerebral blood flow and cerebrospinal fluid outflow. In: Pathophysiology and pharmacotherapy of cerebro-vascular disorders, pp. 12-14. Witzenstrok, Baden-Baden Köln New York 1980

89. Rap, Z.M., Kròlicki, L., Skolasińska, K.: The role of the hypothalamo-hypophyseal neurosecretory and adrenergic system in Cushing reflex. In: Schulmann, K., et al. (eds.) Intracranial pressure IV, pp. 340-343. Springer 1980

90. Rap, Z.M., Straszewski-Barczak, J.: Adrenergic response and morphological changes in the neurosecretory system and adrenal cortex during intracranial hypertension in cats. In: Pathophysiology and pharmacotherapy of cerebro-vascular disorders, pp. 12-14. Witzenstrok, Baden-Baden Köln New York 1980

91. Rap, Z.M., Zaremba, J.: Pathomechanism of secondary morphological lesions in the hypothalamo-hypophyseal system in case of increased intracranial pressure. Pol. Med. J. 1, 187-207 (1971)

92. Schepelmann, F.: Untersuchungen über das Verhalten der motorischen Aktivität des Menschen nach Schädigungen des Zentralnervensystems. Habil.-Schrift, Gießen 1975

93. Schepelmann, F.: Human motor activity in decerebrate states and their sequelae. Acta Neurochir. (Wien) 46, 185-217 (1979)

94. Schepelmann, F.: Rhythmic pattern of motor activity after lesions of the central nervous system. Acta Neurochir. (Wien) 49, 153-189 (1979)

95. Schepelmann, F., Eggert, H.: Relations of motor activity and respiration following cerebral lesions in man. EEG and Clin. Neurophysiol. 43, 514-518 (1977)

96. Schönmayr, R.: Chronic brain stem lesions – a clinical and morphological examination. Habil.-Schrift, Gießen 1985

97. Schönmayr, R., Agnoli, A.L.: Brain stem tumours. Diagnosis and surgical treatment. Neurosurg. Rev. 6, 57-65 (1983)

98. Seeger, W.: Atemstörungen bei intrakraniellen Massenverschiebungen. Acta Neurochir. (Wien) (Suppl.) XVII. Springer, Wien New York 1968

99. Seeger, W.: The central regulation of respiration in raised intracranial pressure. In: Pia, H.W., et al. (eds.) Modern aspects of neurosurgery, Vol. 1, pp. 64-71. Central dysregulation. Excerpta Medica, Amsterdam ICS 242, 1970

100. Seeger, W., Lorenz, R.: Methodische Besonderheiten und Fehlermöglichkeiten bei der Erfassung zentraler Atemstörungen. Beitr. Neurochir. 15, 302 (1968)

101. Spatz, H., Stroescu, G.J.: Zur Anatomie und Pathologie der äußeren Liquorräume des Gehirns. (Zisternenverquellung beim Hirntumor.) Nervenarzt 7, 425-437, 481-498 (1934)

102. Tonn, J.: Personal communication

103. Tönnis, W.: Pathophysiologie und Klinik der intrakraniellen Drucksteigerung. In: Handbuch der Neurochirurgie, Vol. I/1. Springer, Berlin Göttingen Heidelberg 1959

104. Trojanowski, T.: Regional cerebral blood flow disturbances after subarachnoid haemorrhage. DFG-SFB 32, 214-219 (1980)

105. Trojanowski, T.: Blood brain barrier changes after experimental subarachnoid haemorrhage. Acta Neurochir. 60, 45-54 (1982)

106. Trojanowski, T.: Experimental subarachnoid haemorrhage. Part I. A new approach to subarachnoid blood injection in cats. Acta Neurochir. 62, 171-175 (1982)

107. Trojanowski, T.: Extravasation volume and dynamics of subarachnoid arterial bleeding in cats. Part II. Acta Neurochir. 64, 103-108 (1982)

108. Trojanowski, T.: Regional cerebral blood flow disturbances after subarachnoid haemorrhage. Habil.-Schrift, Lublin/Polen - Gießen 1982

109. Wesemann, W.: Zur Pathogenese und Therapie des Hirnödems (klinisch-chemische und tierexperimentelle Untersuchungen). Habil.-Schrift, Gießen 1972

110. Wesemann, W., Pia, H.W.: Aldadiene-Kalium in der Neurochirurgie. In: Postoperative Störungen des Elektrolyt- und Wasserhaushaltes, pp. 259-270. Schattauer, Stuttgart 1968

111. Wesemann, W., Grote, E.: Diabetes mellitus and insipidus: a syndrome of hypothalamic dysregulation. Excerpta Medica, Congr. Series No. 242, pp. 208-212. Amsterdam 1970

112. Wesemann, W., Rohde, I.: Elektrolytstörungen und Säure-Basen-Gleichgewichtsverschiebungen bei neurochirurgischen Patienten. In: Hydrodynamik, Elektrolyt- und Säure-Basen-Haushalt im Liquor und Nervensystem, pp. 128-138. Thieme, Stuttgart 1970

113. Wesemann, W., Pia, H.W., Grote, E.: Regulation and dysregulation of glucose uptake and utilization in acute cerebral lesions. Acta Neurochir. 46, 325 (1979)

114. Wesemann, W.: Hyperglykaemien. Verlaufsbeobachtungen bei zerebralen Tumoren und Verletzungen. In: Behringer, A. (ed.) Diabetes mellitus, pp. 723-731. Maudrich, Wien München Bern 1973

115. Wesemann, W.: Dauerregistrierung des Leistungsumsatzes bei Patienten mit Schädel-Hirn-Trauma und Hirntumoren. Infusionstherapie 2, 365-376 (1975)

116. Wesemann, W.: Spezielle Probleme der enteralen und parenteralen Ernährung bei Patienten mit Hirnläsionen. In: Grundlagen und neue Aspekte der parenteralen und Sondenernährung, pp. 57-64. Thieme, Stuttgart 1978

117. Wesemann, W.: Der Kohlehydratstoffwechsel bei Schädelhirntraumen. In: Kohlehydratverwendung im Stress-Stoffwechsel, pp. 23-34. Thieme, Stuttgart New York 1980

118. Wesemann, W., Kayama, T.: Perioperative Ernährung – Spezielle Probleme in der Neurochirurgie. Akt. Ernährung 4, 131-140 (1979)

119. Zeisberger, E., Behr, R., Ewen, K., Merker, G.: Threshold changes for heat production and dissipation after intrahypothalamic administration of 6-hydroxydopamine. In: Environment, drugs and thermoregulation, pp. 58-61. Karger, Basel 1983

120. Zierski, J.: Intracranial pressure after posterior fossa tumour operations with particular reference to the decompensation after drainage. In: Advances in Neurosurgery, Vol. 5, pp. 203-208. Springer, Berlin Heidelberg New York 1978

121. Zierski, J.: Extradural, ventricular and subdural pressure recording. In: Intracranial pressure, Vol. IV, pp. 371-376. Springer, Berlin Heidelberg New York 1980

122. Zierski, J., Kurzaj, E., Hoffmann, O., Winkler, B.: Cerebral blood flow in the brain stem during increased ICP. In: Intracranial pressure, Vol. V. Springer, Berlin Heidelberg New York 1983

123. Zierski, J., Hoffmann, O., Klug, N.: Interrelationship between ICP and central dysregulation. In: Advances in neurotraumatology. Internat. Congr. Series 612, pp. 294-296. Excerpta Medica, Amsterdam 1983

124. Zülch, K.J.: Störungen des intrakraniellen Druckes. In: Handbuch der Neurochirurgie, Vol. I/1. Springer, Berlin Göttingen Heidelberg 1959

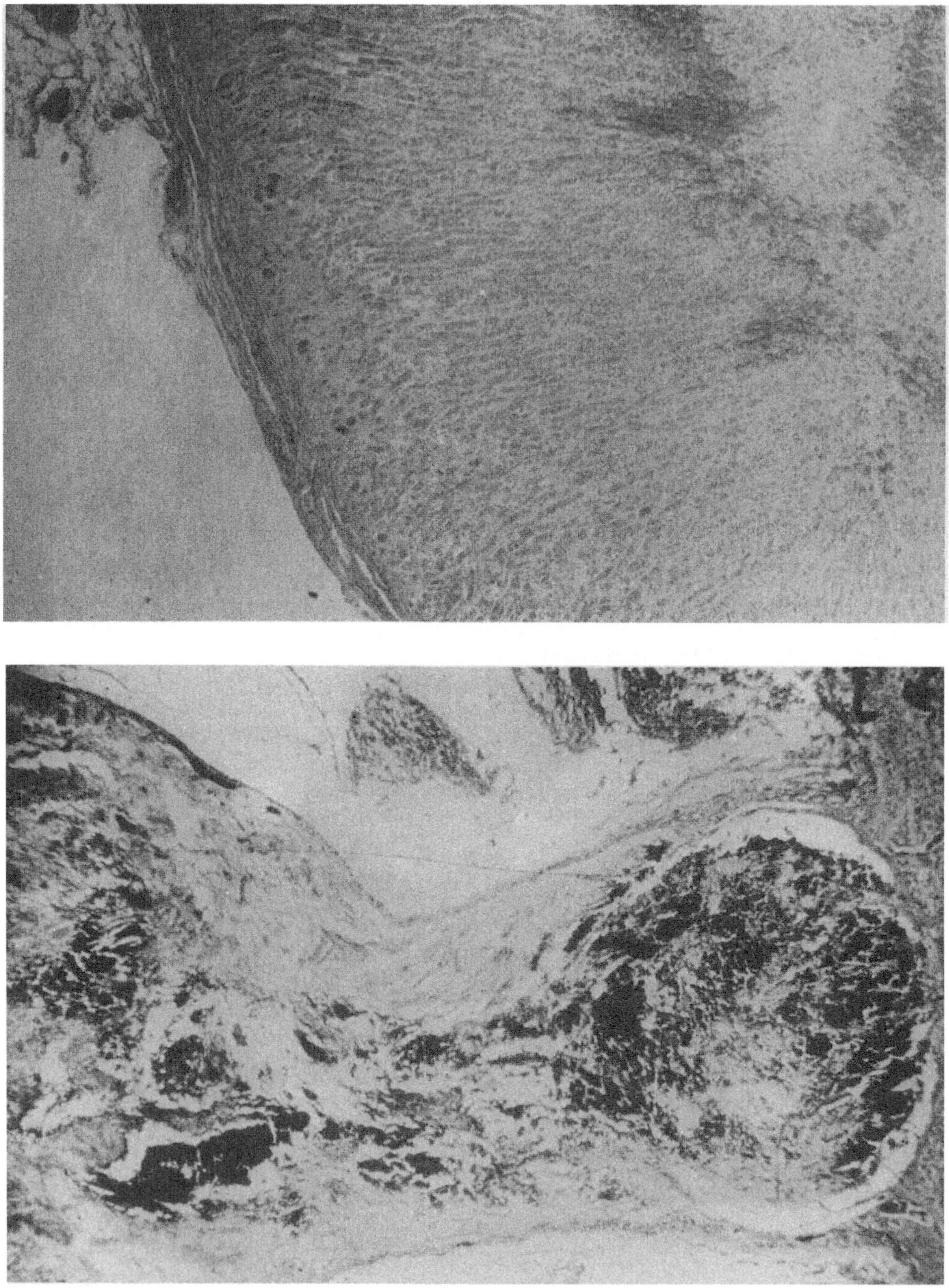

b

a

Fig. 1a,b. Acute subarachnoid hemorrhage. Central hypothalamo-hypophyseal death. Hemorrhages and hemorrhagic necrosis of a the hypothalamus, pituitary stalk, and hypophysis and b the adrenal cortex

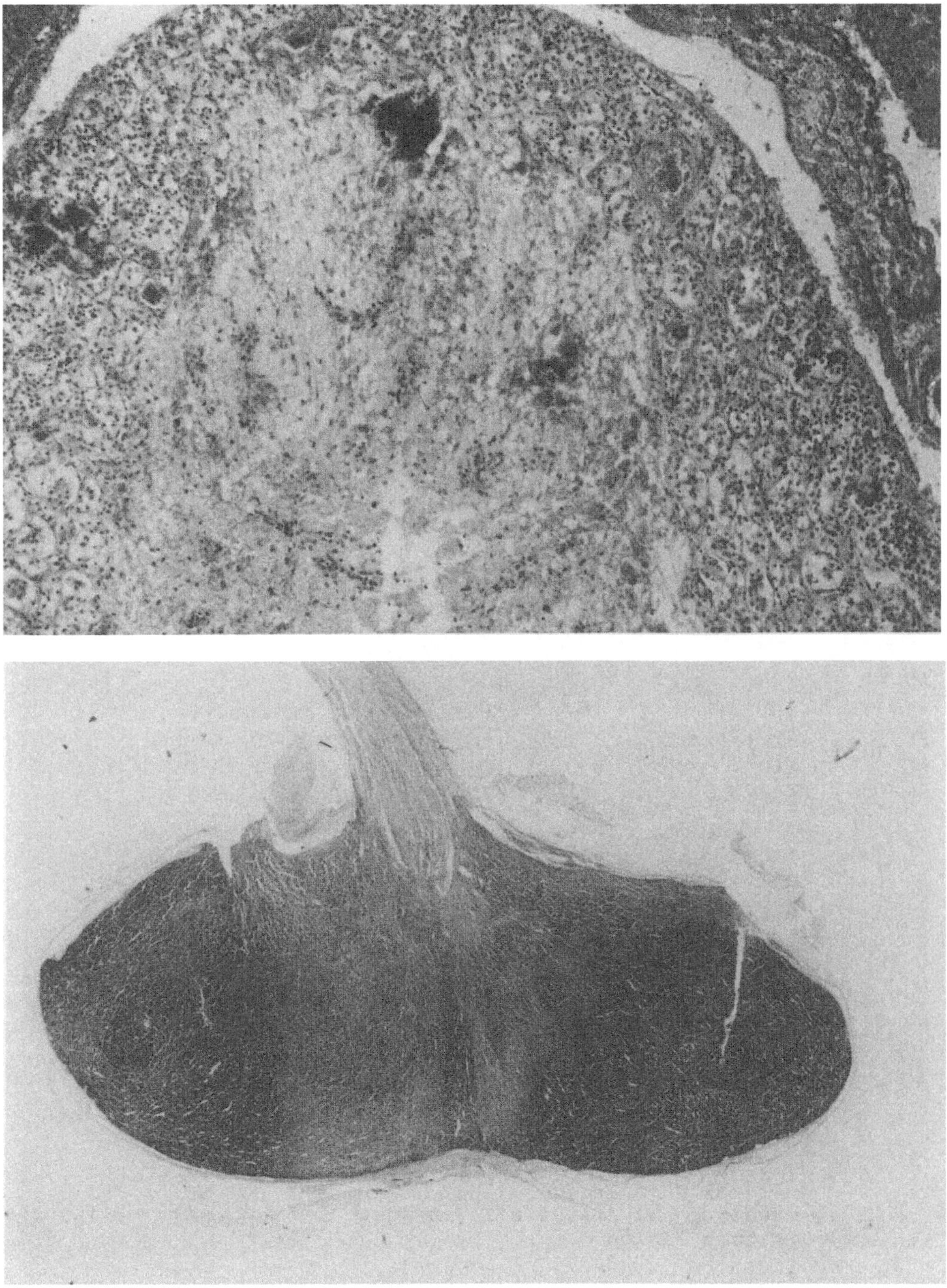

a

b

Fig. 2a,b. Morphological findings in secondary hypothalamo-pituitary lesions, with acute paralysis clinically. a Pituitary stalk with multiple erythrocyte extravasations and damage to neurosecretoric pathways. Male, 16 years, bilateral contusions. b Acute necrosis of central parts of the adeno-hypophysis. Female 19 years, cerebellar space-occupying vascular lesions. Diabetes insipidus

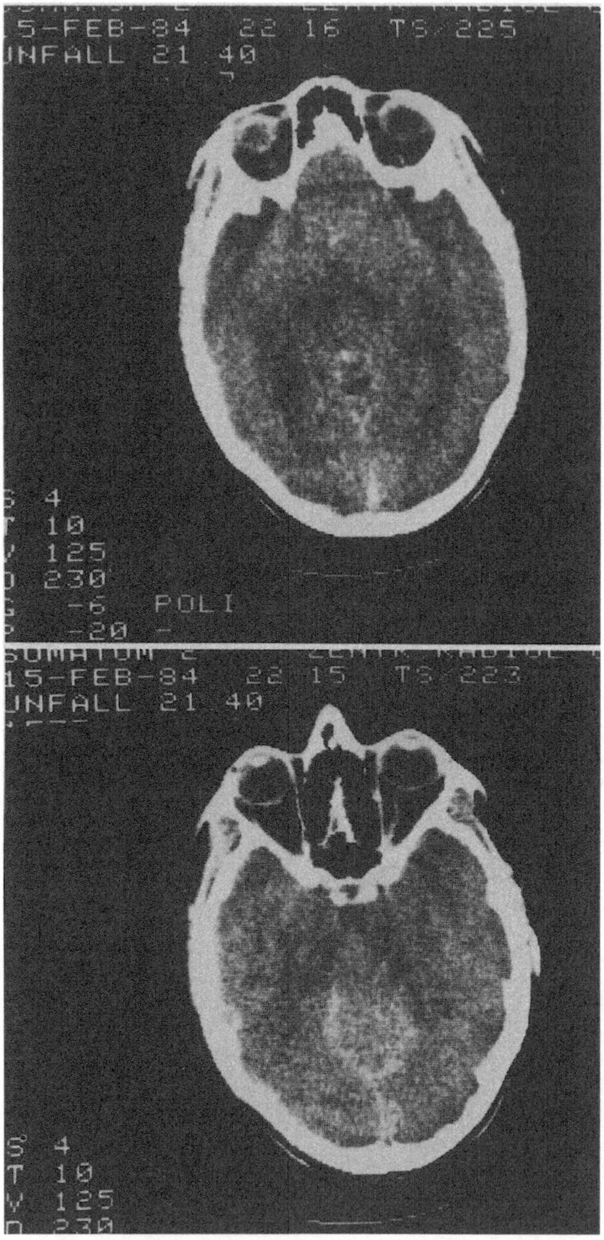

Fig. 3. Occluded basal cisterns in an acute secondary traumatic hypothalamo-pituitary lesion

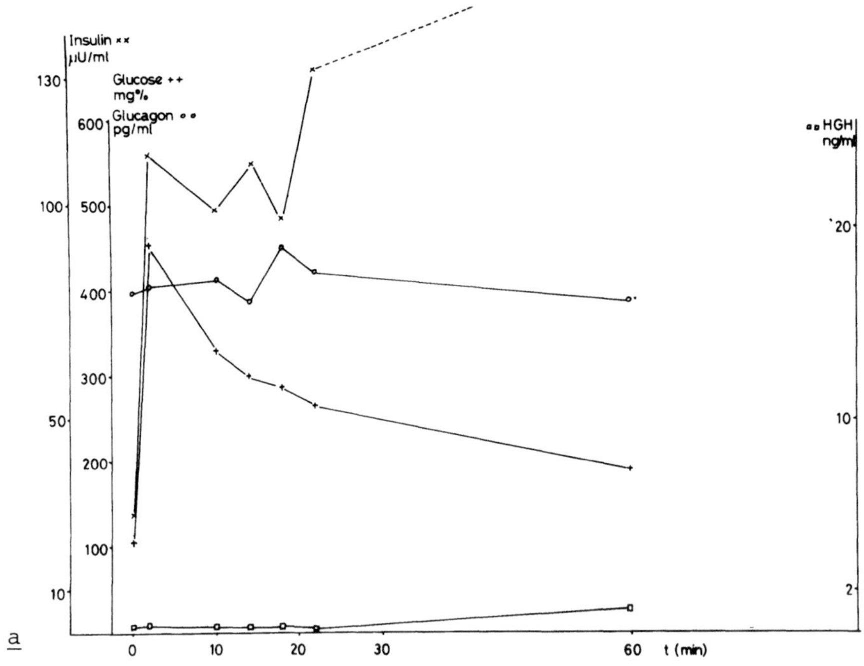

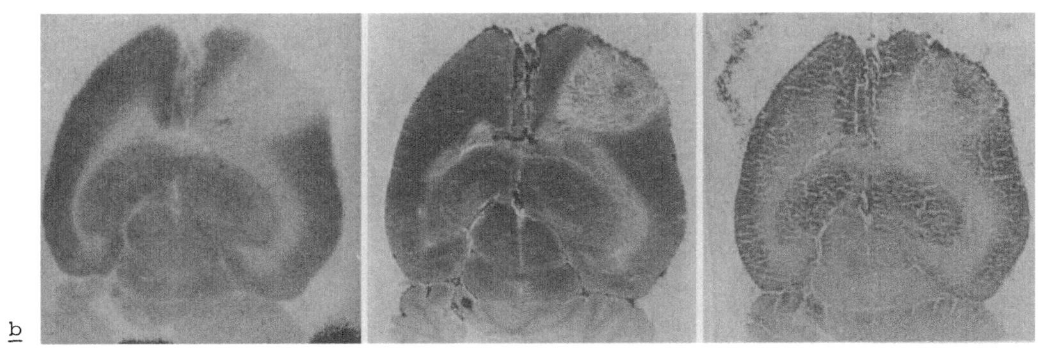

Fig. 4. a Bilateral olfactory meningioma with increased hyperinsulinemia, increased hyperglucagonemia, hyperglycemia, and constantly reduced HGH after loading with glucose. b Localized brain edema after electric trauma. Complete blockage of blood-brain barrier for glucose C^{14} *(left)*, hexokinase *(middle)*, and cytochromoxidase *(right)*

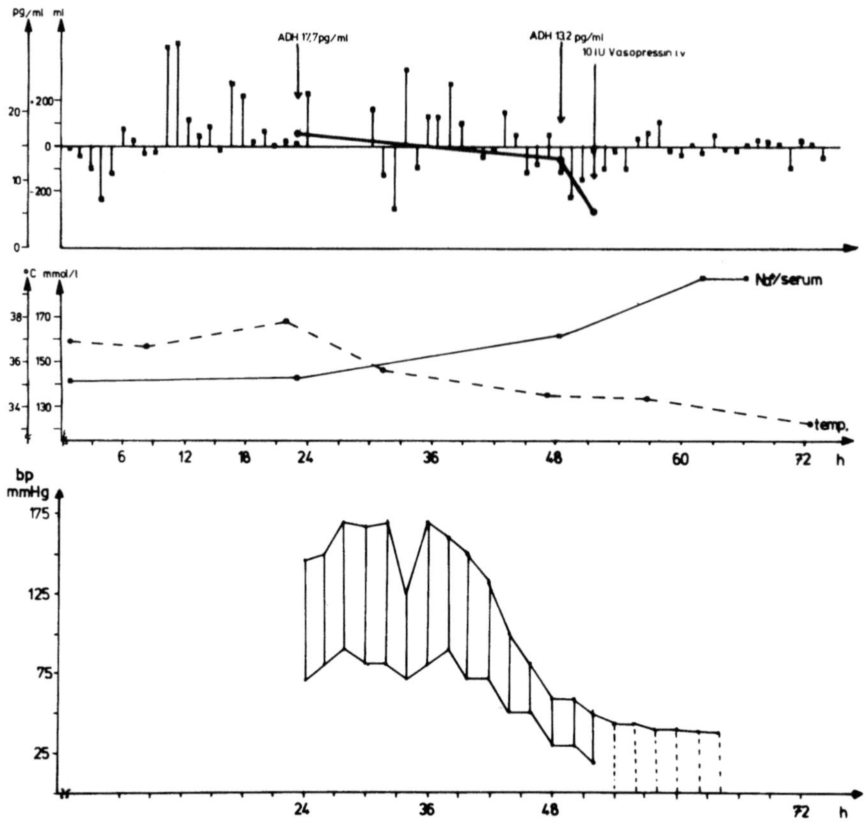

Fig. 5. Acute secondary hypothalamo-pituitary syndrome and death. Primary oliguria *(lines upward)* with raised ADH; polyuria *(lines downward)* with falling ADH, parallel with hypernatremia, arterial hypotension, and hypothermia

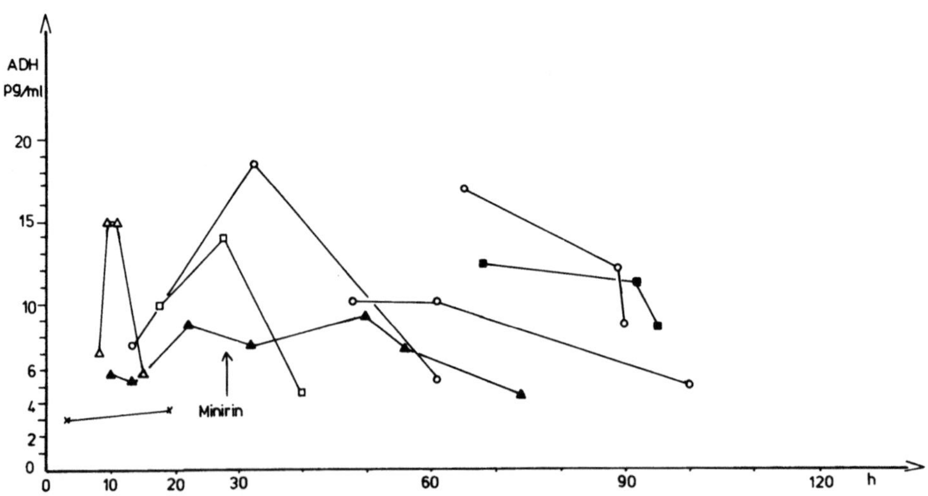

Fig. 6. ADH course in seven acute cases. Primary or secondary rise in ADH with a subsequent decrease in six cases with diabetes insipidus. In one case with oliguria, extremely lowered ADH

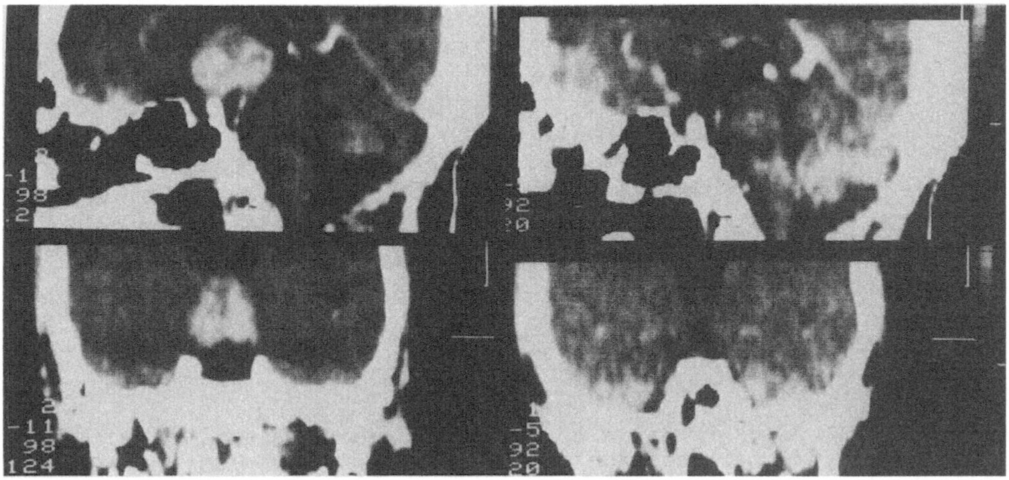

Fig. 7. HUH 260251261. Cerebellar arachnoid sarcoma with multiple secondary CSF metastases. CT with metastasis of the hypothalamus and obliteration after radiotherapy

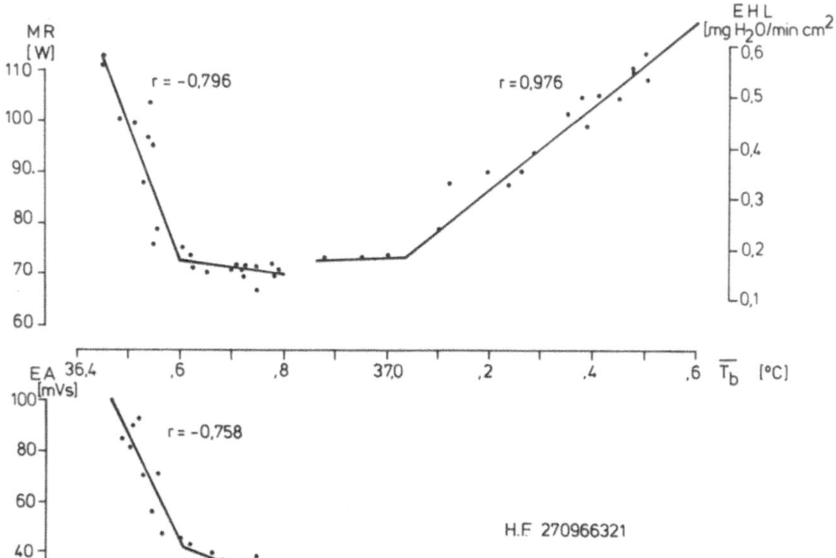

Fig. 8. Case shown in Fig. 5. Temperature loading. Before (———) and after (– – – –) radiation. Mean temperature *(Tb)* lowered with a lowered thermogenetic threshold before radiation and a normal threshold afterward. Normal thermogenetic reaction concerning metabolic rate *(MR)* and electric muscle activity *(EA)*. No evaporative heat loss *(EHL)* during the heating period *(right)*

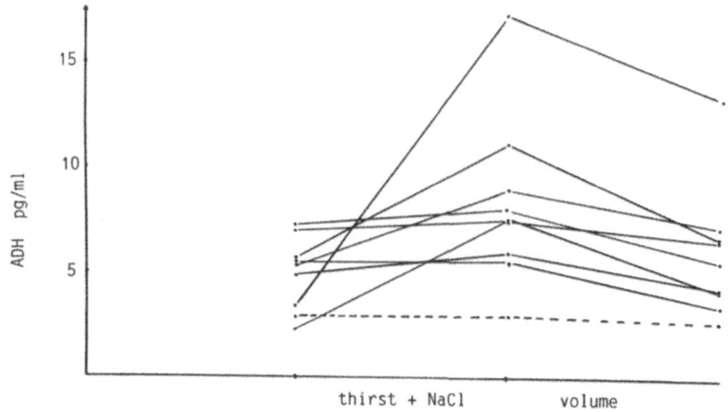

Fig. 9. ADH loading tests in normal cases and after peripheral operations. ———, normal reaction of ADH. No ADH response in chronic hypothalamic lesions (– – – –)

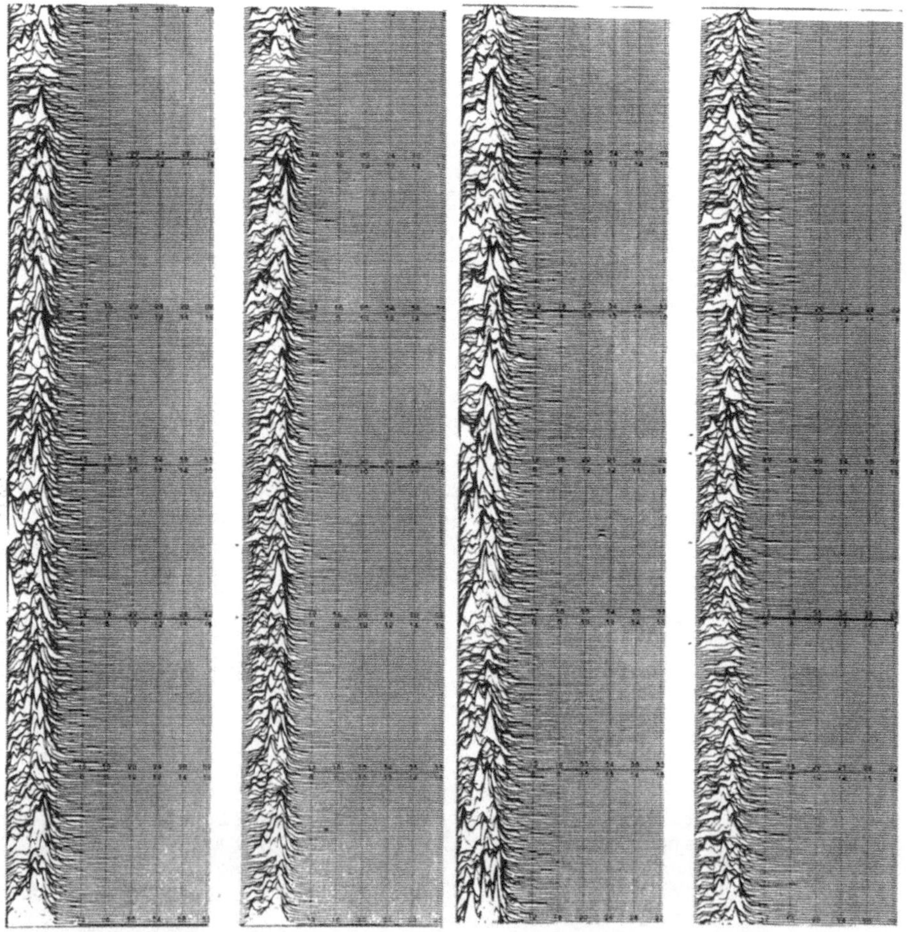

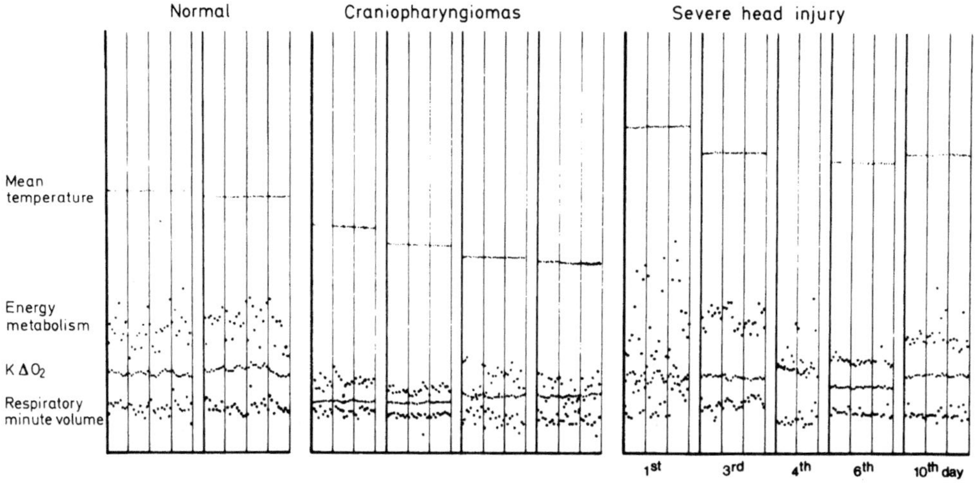

Fig. 11. Energy metabolism and temperature in normal *(left)*, acute *(right)*, and chronic *(middle)* hypothalamo-hypophyseal lesions. In chronic lesions, temperature and metabolic rate were extremely reduced, with lowering of core temperature after cooling and heating and no reaction of the metabolic rate. In acute cases (spontaneous course), central irritation of temperature and metabolism occurred

Fig. 10. Loss of circadian rhythm with slow wave ultradian rhythms (EEG power spectrum) in a suprasellar pituitary adenoma with chronic hypothalamo-pituitary defect syndrome

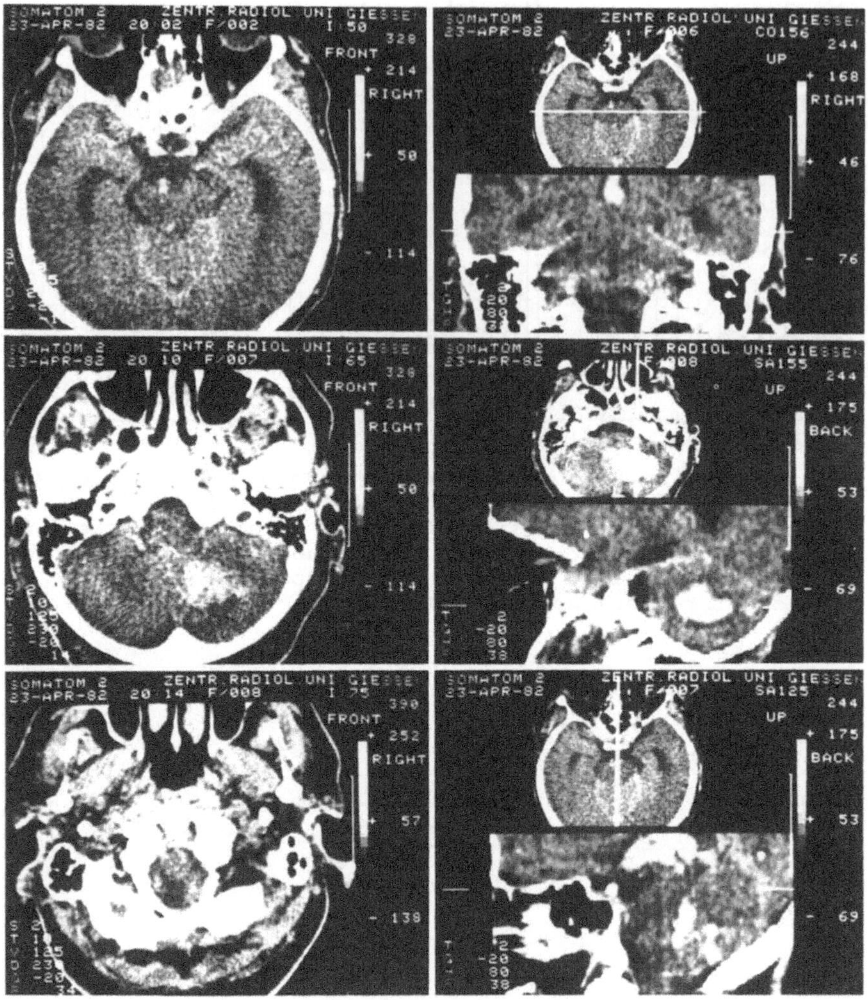

Fig. 12. Cisternal herniations of the cistern of Galen, parts of the ambient cistern, and the cerebellomedullary cistern in a case of right-sided cerebellar hematoma

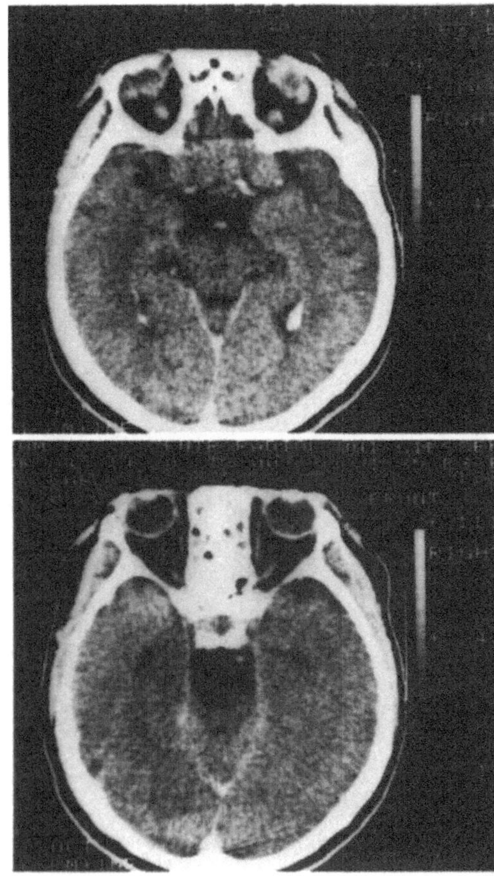

Fig. 13. Pontine infarct with locked-in-syndrome. Normal midbrain and complete infarct of pons

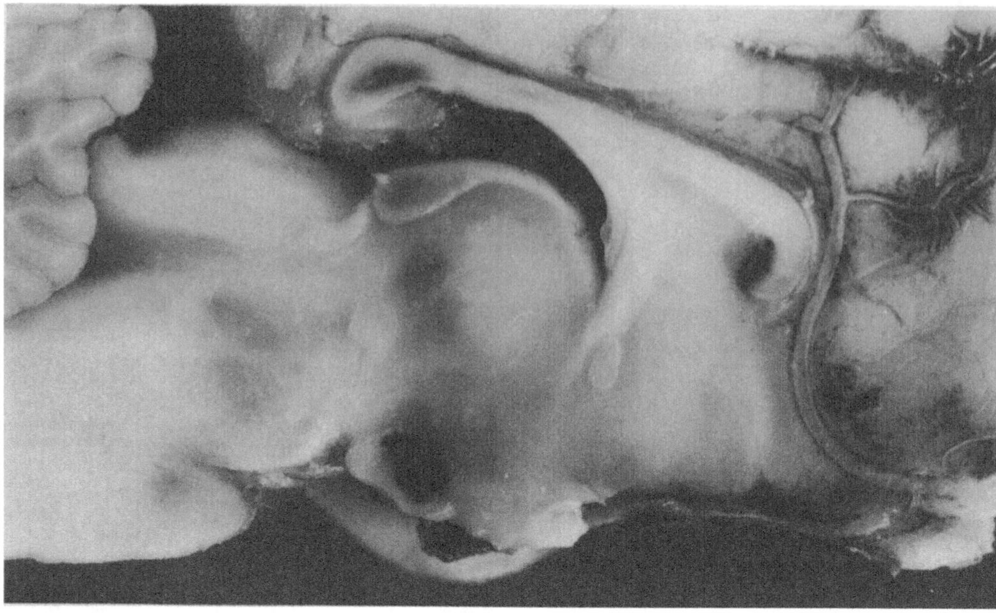

a

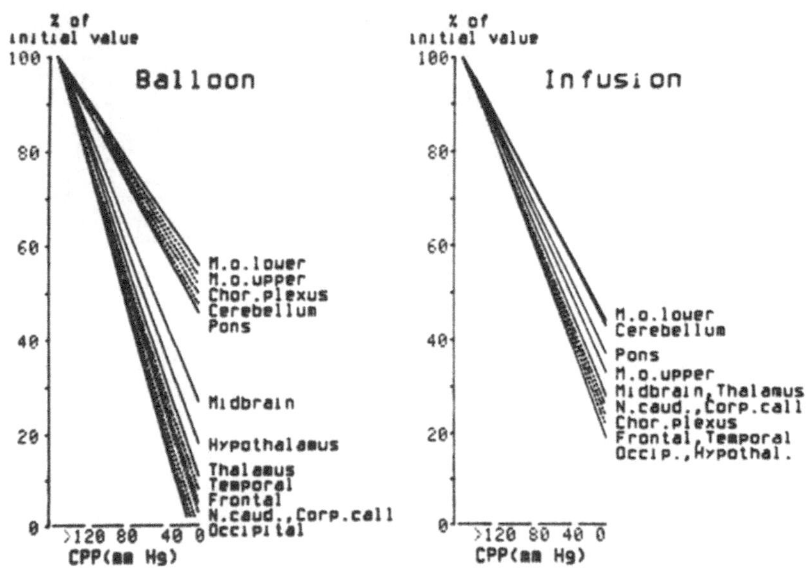

b

Fig. 14. a Severe disturbances of blood-brain barrier (Evans blue) after balloon brain compression in limited zones in front of and behind the tentorium, with marked involvement of the hypothalamus and midbrain and the upper pons region. b Regional CBF measurements. Reduced CBF with rising ICP – markedly with brain compression and mesencephalic herniation (balloon), and less pronounced in the infusion group without herniations. Compartmentalization *(left)* between supra- and infratentorial structures

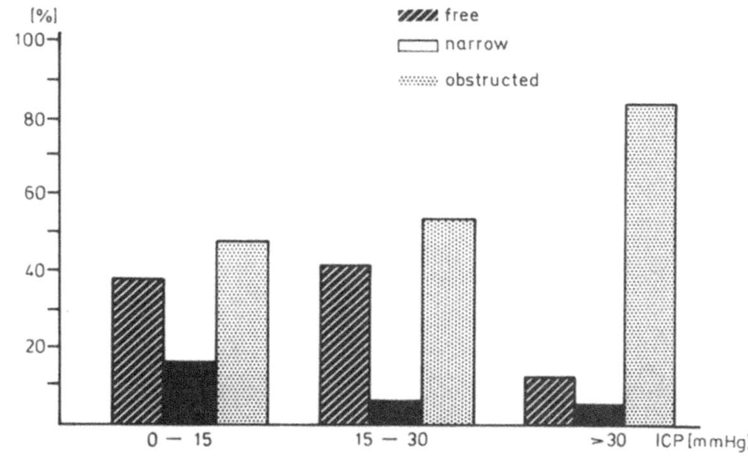

Fig. 15. Relation between ICP and cisternal herniation in acute mid-brain syndromes

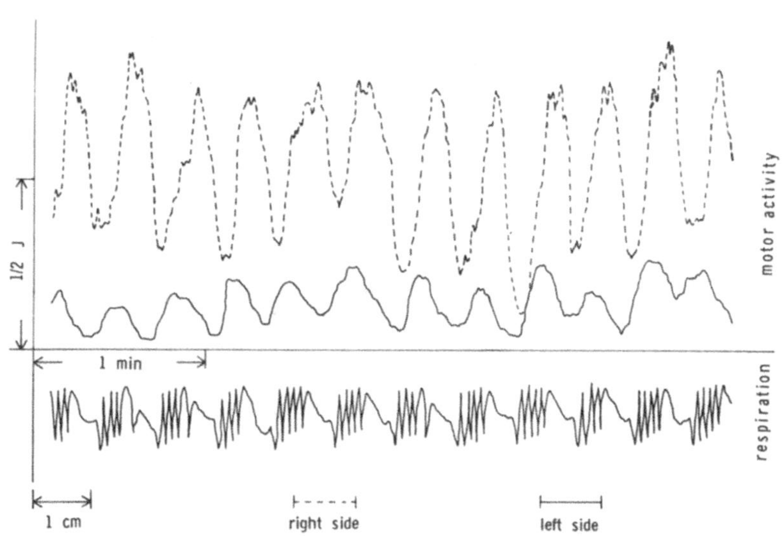

a

Fig. 16a,b. Mesencephalic rhythms. a Synchronous rhythms of motor activity and Cheyne-Stokes respiration. b Blood pressure waves of different frequency

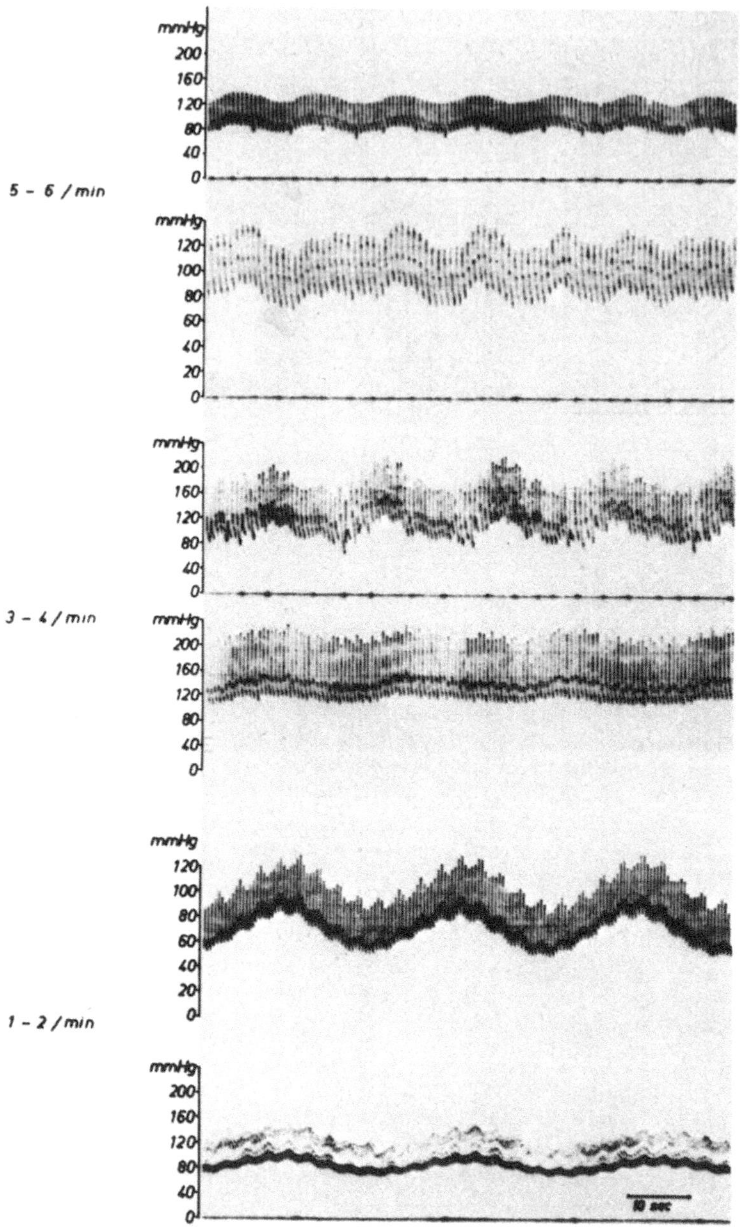

Fig. 16b. Legend see p. 247

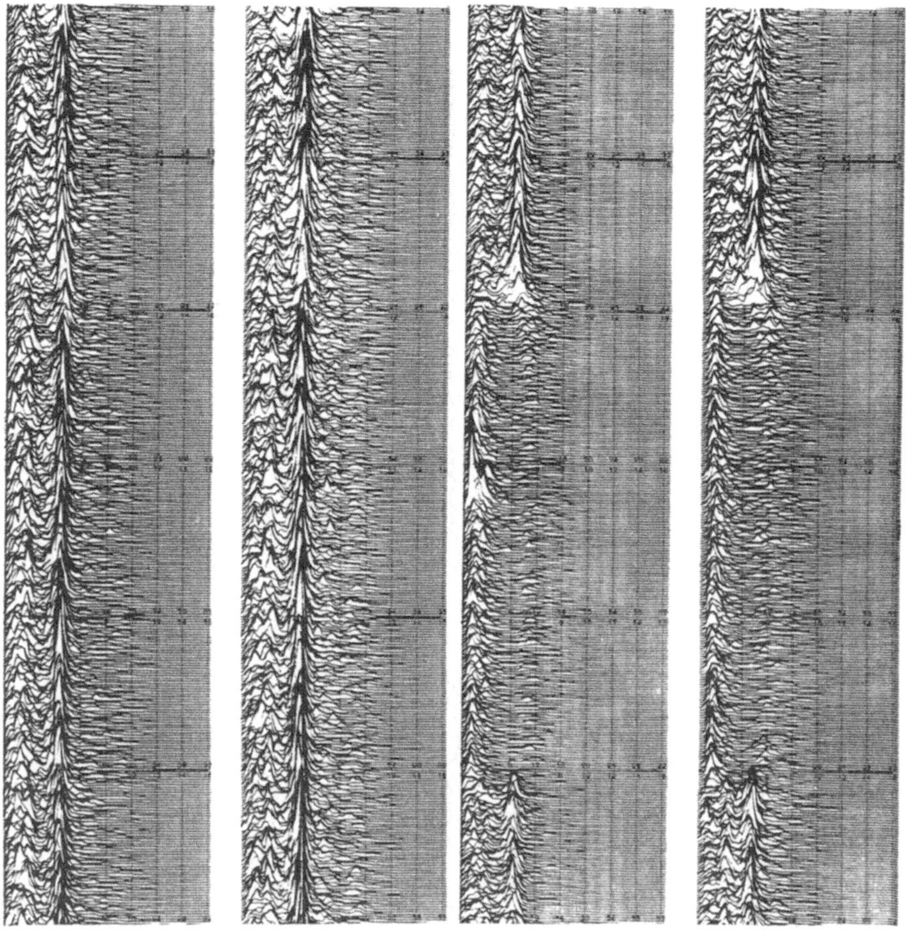

Fig. 17. EEG power spectrum in a case with traumatic pontine hemorrhage. Loss of circadian rhythm with marked delta and alpha frequences *(two columns on the left)*. Thirty hours later *(two columns on the right)*, three ultradian rhythms with loss of alpha activity for 90 min within 3 h

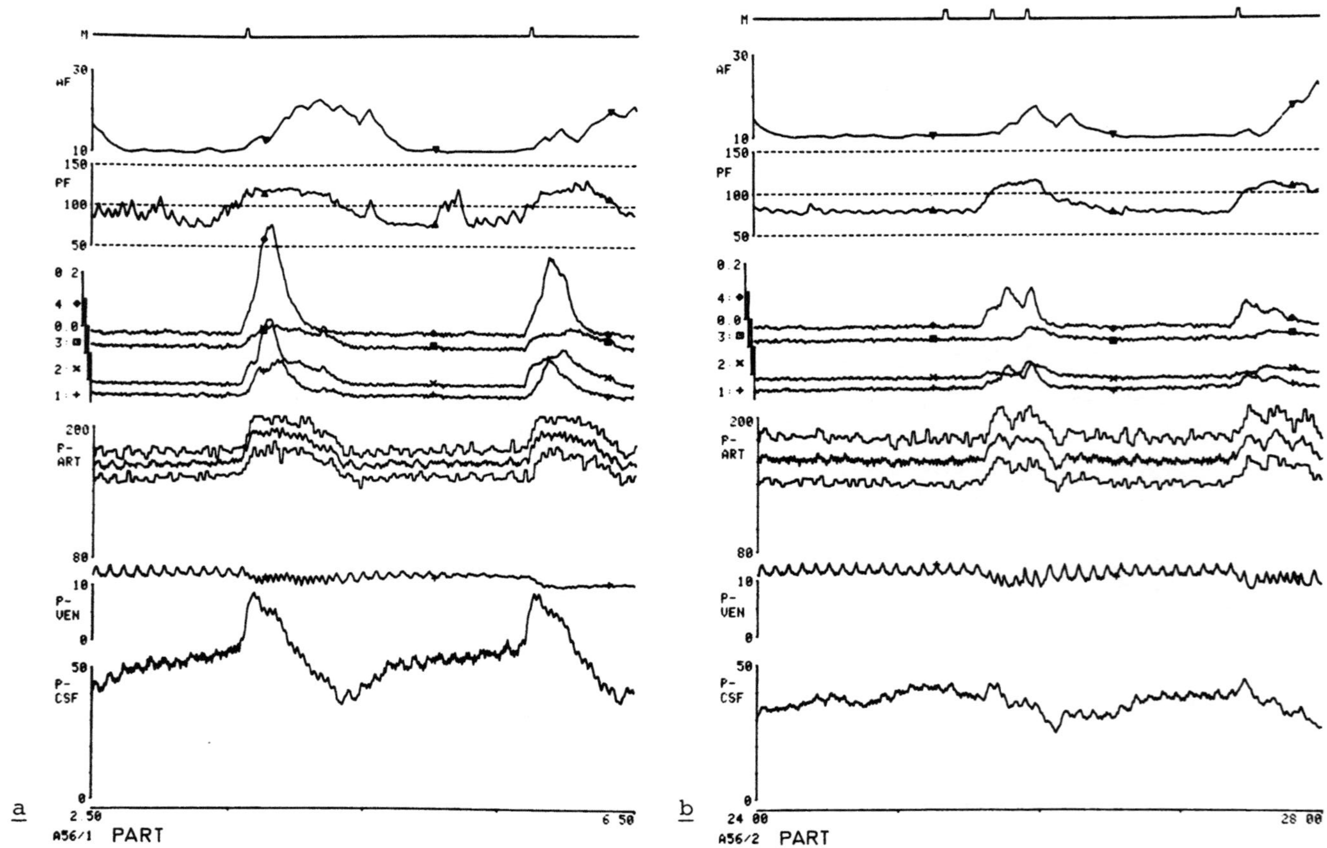

Fig. 18a,b. Spontaneous decerebration episodes and ICP. a Secondary lesions with mesencephalic herniation. Synchronous rise of respiration *(RF)*, pulse *(PF)*, muscle activity, arterial pressure *(P-ART)*, and ICP *(P-CSF)*, and lowering of venous pressure *(P-VEN)*. b Lesions without cisternal herniation; no correlation between episodes and ICP

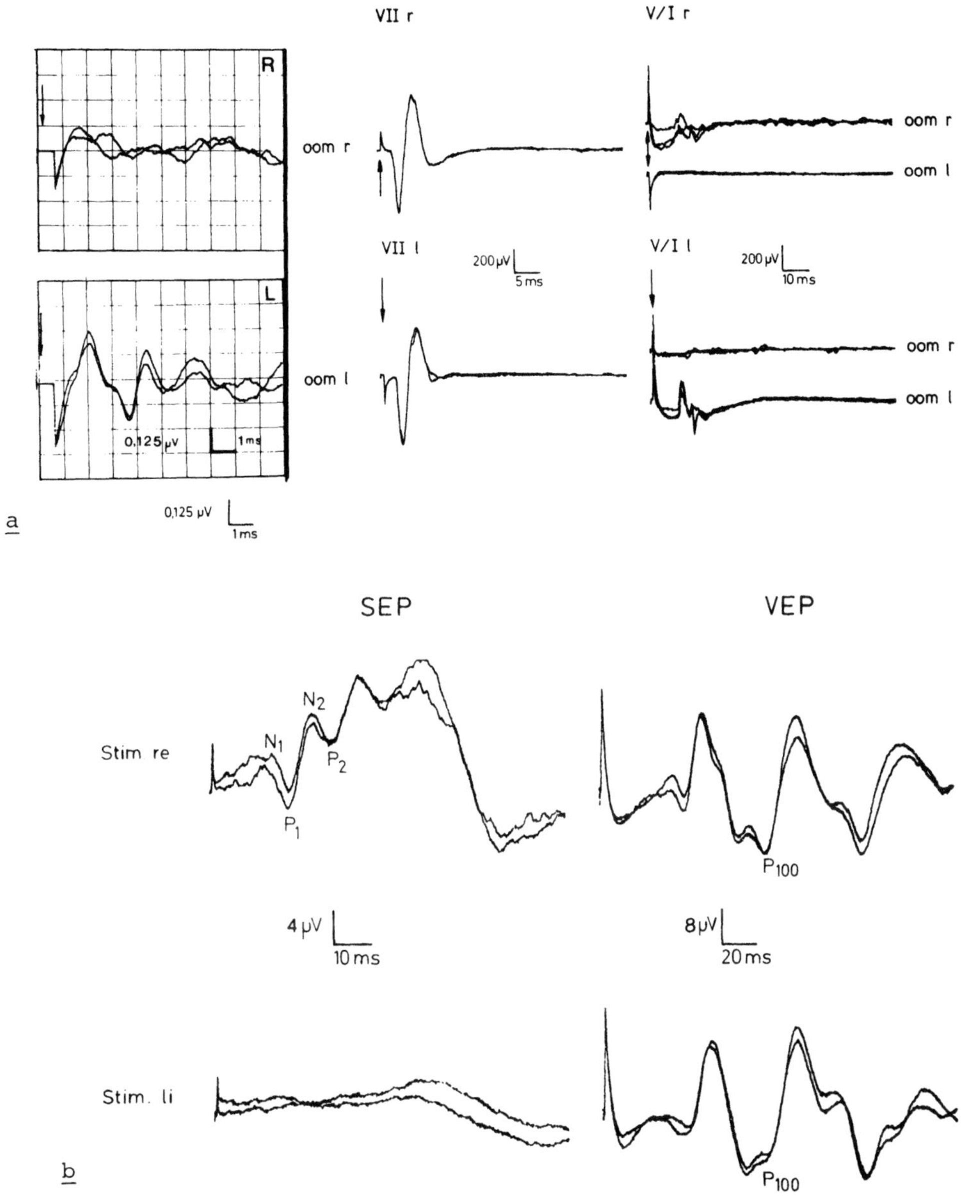

Fig. 19a,b. Right-sided mesencephalopontine infarct. Status after infarct of right middle cerebral artery territory. a Findings regarding acoustic evoked potentials *(right)* and blink reflex *(left)*. b Findings regarding somatosensoric evoked potentials *(left)* and visual evoked potentials *(right)*

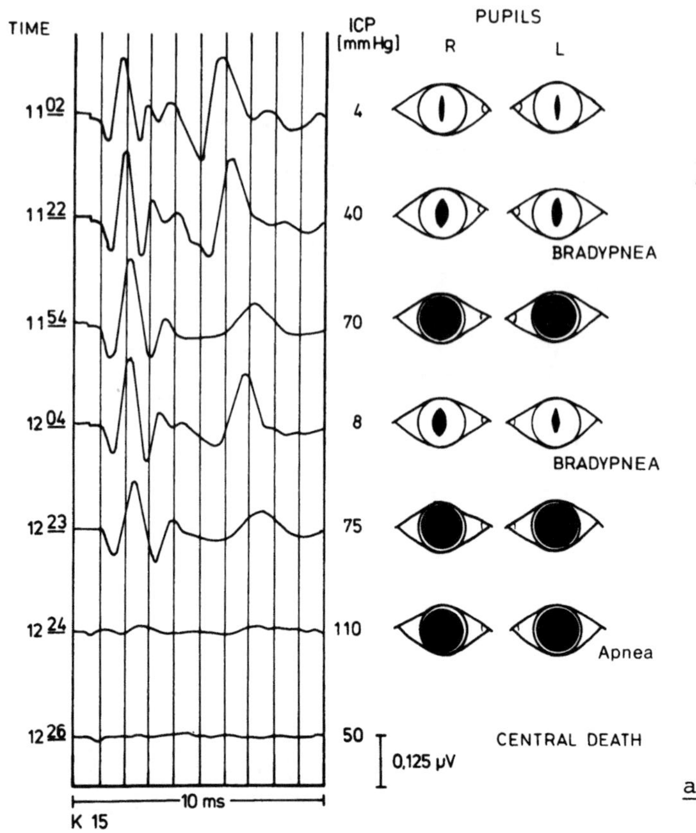

Fig. 20a,b. Cerebral balloon compression with mesencephalic herniation with repeated rise of ICP. a Acoustic evoked potentials; b blink reflex

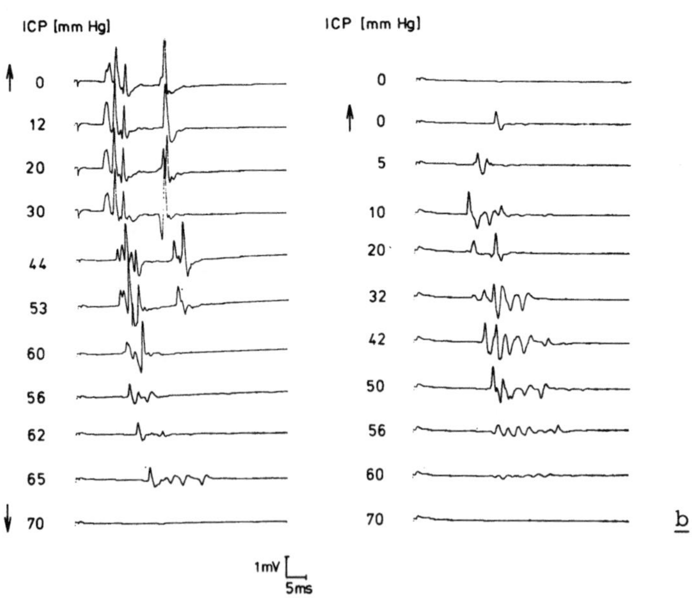

Fig. 20a,b. Cerebral balloon compression with mesencephalic herniation with repeated rise of ICP. a Acoustic evoked potentials; b blink reflex

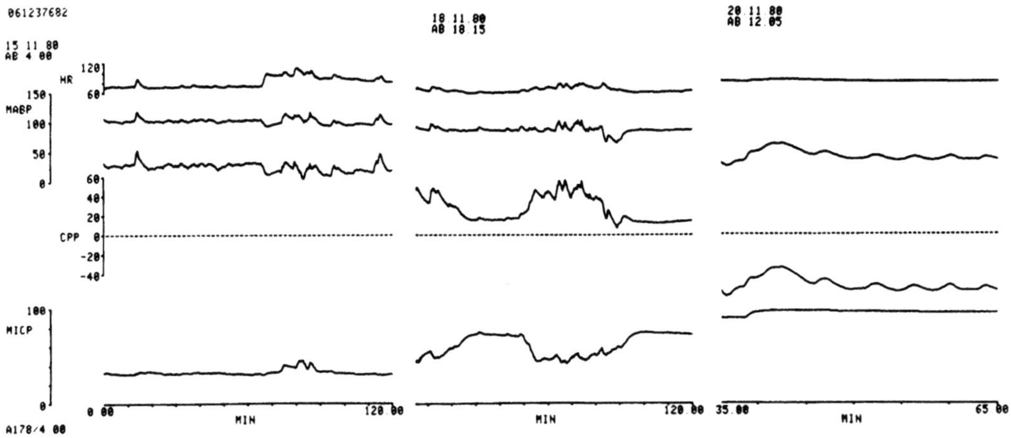

Fig. 21. Severe brain injury with progression from midbrain syndrome to bulbar death. Spontaneous course with registration of mean arterial blood pressure *(MABP)*, cerebral perfusion pressure *(CPP)*, and mean ICP *(MICP)*

Receptors of Steroid Hormones, Prolactin, and Somatotropin (Growth Hormone) in Human Pituitary Adenomas

O. Hey[1], K. Pollow[2], M. Schommer[2], G. Hoffmann[2], and J. Happ[3]
[1] Neurochirurgische Universitätsklinik, [2] Universitäts-Frauenklinik und Abteilung für Experimentelle Endokrinologie, D-6500 Mainz
[3] Abteilung für Nuklearmedizin der Universität, D-6000 Frankfurt

Introduction

It is generally accepted that hormone receptors are protein molecules which are not ubiquitous but are found in or attached to a target cell. In the interaction of a hormone with its receptor on target cell membranes, the initial step is the specific binding of the hormone with the receptor. The resulting phenomenon, which has been dealt with in a number of excellent articles (4, 6, 8-10), is termed the hormone-receptor complex.

The receptor molecule of proteohormones (prolactin and growth hormone) is membrane bound. The membrane-associated receptor-hormone complex is channeled via adenylate cyclase into the cell and produces, via a cascade of successive reactions, a specific effect (Fig. 1). In contrast to the receptors of proteohormones, the receptors of steroid hormones (estradiol and progesterone) are localized intracellularly in the cytoplasm. The steroid hormone-receptor complex channels into the nucleus to the chromatin and causes gene activation. This leads to synthesis of messenger RNA, which channels out of the nucleus and induces a specific cell function and structure (Fig. 2).

Materials and Methods

The biochemical analysis of hormone receptors is based on the above-described mode of action. The specific binding of labeled human prolactin, human growth hormone (HGH), and various steroid hormones was studied in 20 pituitary tumors (Fig. 3). The tissue was removed intraoperatively:

1. In three cases of prolactinomas treated preoperatively with bromocriptine
2. In four cases of prolactinomas without bromocriptine therapy
3. In six other hormone-producing tumors (five HGH adenomas and one ACTH adenoma with Nelson's syndrome) without prolactin secretion
4. In six cases of hormone inactive tumors
5. In one case of intrasellar metastasis of hypernephroma

The tumor tissue was collected from the operating room immediately after excision. Samples were kept at -70°C for up to four weeks before processing. After washing in ice cold buffer, the tumor tissue was homogenized. The cytosol fraction used for steroid hormone receptor characterization was prepared by ultracentrifugation of the homogenate (105 000 × *g* supernatant). The 105 000 × *g* pellet was retained for membrane-bound prolactin and growth hormone receptor examination.

 Advances in Neurosurgery, Vol. 13
Edited by H. Dietz, M. Brock, and M. Klinger

In order to compare the specific binding parameters for different steroid hormones (estradiol and progesterone), multiple point saturation analysis was performed by incubating cytosol overnight with varying concentrations of ^{3}H-labeled steroids. Furthermore, sucrose density gradient centrifugation and competition experiments were done.

Specific binding of prolactin and growth hormone was determined in enriched plasma membrane fractions obtained after fractionation of the 105 000 × *g* pellets by differential ultracentrifugation techniques. After incubation in triplicate with ^{125}I-labeled prolactin or growth hormone, the uptake of labeled hormones was calculated as specific binding, being the difference between counts bound in the absence and presence of excess unlabeled hormones expressed as a percentage of total counts added. In some cases where sufficient material was available, SCATCHARD analysis was used to quantitate binding capacity (6).

Results

Results summarized in Table 1 show that the estradiol receptors (ER) and progesterone receptors (PGR) were detectable in only a few tumor tissue samples. ER-positive tissue (≥ 20 fmol/mg cytosol protein) was found in one prolactinoma. ER-negative tissue (< 20 fmol/mg cytosol protein) was present in three cases: one prolactinoma, one HGH adenoma, and one nonsecreting adenoma (18, 10, and 17 fmol/mg protein, respectively). ER could not be detected in the remaining tumors.

Significant binding sites for progesterone were present in just one of 20 patients who showed prolactin receptors as well (28.4% specific binding/mg membrane protein). This patient had an intrasellar metastasis of hypernephroma.

Human growth hormone receptors (HGHR) were analyzed in seven patients. Four tumor tissue samples were HGHR-positive (≥ 3% specific binding/mg membrane protein) and three HGHR-negative (< 3% specific binding/mg membrane protein).

The analysis of prolactin receptors (PRLR) proves that the three prolactinomas treated with bromocriptine over a period of two years were PRLR-negative (< 3% specific binding). In contrast to these, the nontreated prolactinomas were PRLR-positive (≥ 3% specific binding) (Fig. 4). Prolactin receptors were also detectable in three HGH adenomas, three inactive adenomas without prolactin secretion, one Nelson's tumor, and one ACTH adenoma.

Discussion

So far there have been only a few reports on comparable results of hormone receptor analysis in human pituitary adenomas (2, 5). Previous examinations were performed in the form of in vitro studies in animals. Our data demonstrate that the majority of tumors are steroid receptor-negative. These tumors proliferate without having an influence on estrogen and progesterone. Our study further shows that prolactin receptors are detectable on the cells of HGH adenomas and inactive adenomas. An essential finding was that the three prolactinomas treated two years preoperatively with bromocriptine were prolactin receptor-negative. It is well known that bromocriptine inhibits prolactin secretion even when it is given to pituitary fragments in vitro or to pituitary biocytocultures (1, 3, 11). Consequently bromocriptine has a direct effect on the prolactin-producing cells. Prolactin cells are equipped with dopamine receptors of the type D_2 (7). By release of dopamine from

Table 1. Concentration of estradiol receptors (ER), progesterone receptors (PGR), prolactin receptors (PRLR), and human growth hormone receptors (HGHR) in human pituitary tumor cells (ND, not detectable)

No. of patients	ER	PGR	PRLR	HGHR
	Cytosol protein (fmol/mg)		% spec. binding/mg protein	
1	ND	ND	2.2	
2	ND		6.9	0.9
3	24		0.9	4.0
4	ND		2.0	
5	ND		5.0	
6	18		5.7	
7	ND		8.5	
8	ND		4.9	3.0
9	10		0.3	0.0
10	ND		0.8	
11	ND		13.0	
12	ND		1.5	
13	ND		3.0	2.7
14	ND		5.6	4.2
15	17		1.2	
16	ND		16.8	
17	ND		1.2	7.0
18	ND		-	
19	ND	↓	4.1	
20	ND	1.0	28.4	

the hypothalamus, prolactin secretion is inhibited. The effect of bromocriptine on the prolactin cell is like that of dopamine on these receptors.

An additional effect of bromocriptine on the membrane-bound receptors of prolactin cells in human pituitary tumors is probably provoked by a lesion of membrane. Whether this is a specific effect of bromocriptine has to be established by further examinations.

Conclusion

The steroid hormone receptors for estradiol and progesterone as well as the proteohormone receptors for prolactin and growth hormone have been determined in various human pituitary adenomas. Our findings were as follows: First, the tumor cells of most tumors have no receptors for estradiol and progesterone. Secondly, prolactin receptors are detectable in prolactinomas as well as in other pituitary tumors. Thirdly, in prolactinomas treated with bromocriptine before surgery, prolactin receptor-negative cells were present; this finding may well be explained by a lesion of the membrane of prolactin cells caused by this drug.

References

1. Kebian, J.W., Calne, D.B.: Multiple receptors for dopamine. Nature 277, 93-96 (1979)
2. Lüdecke, D.K., Trams, G., Saeger, W.: Sex hormone receptors in human pituitary adenomas. Acta endocrinologica 23, 104 (1983)
3. Mashiter, K., Adams, E., Beard, M., Holley, A.: Bromocriptine inhibits prolactin and growth hormone release by human pituitary tumors in culture. Lancet II, 197 (1977)
4. O'Malley, B.W., Schrader, W.T.: The receptors of steroid hormones. Scient. Am. 234, 32 (1976)
5. Pichon, M.F., Bression, D., Peillon, F., Milgrom, E.: J. Clin. Endocrinol. Metab. 51, 897 (1980)
6. Pollow, K.: Die Bedeutung von Hormonrezeptoren für die Behandlung maligner Erkrankungen. Therapiewoche 33, 6809-6825 (1983)
7. Rosenfeld, M.R., Makman, H.H., Ahn, H.W., Thal, L.J., Mishra, R.K., Katzmann, R.: Selective influence of ergot alkaloids on cortical and striatal dopaminergic and serotoninergic receptors. In: Goldstein, M., Calne, D.B., Liebermann, A., Thorner, M.O. (eds.) Ergot compounds and brain function. Neuroendocrine and neuropsychiatric aspects, pp. 83-93. Raven Press, New York 1980
8. Roth, J.: Metabolism 22, 1059 (1973)
9. Shin, R.P.C., Friesen, H.F.: Prolactin receptors. Meth. Mol. Biol. 9, 565-598 (1976)
10. Sutherland, E.W.: Zur Wirkungsweise der Hormone. Angew. Chem. 84, 11, 117 (1972)
11. Yanai, R., Nagasawa, H.: Effect of bromocriptine on pituitary synthesis and release of prolactin and growth hormone in rats. Horm. Res. 5, 1-5 (1974)

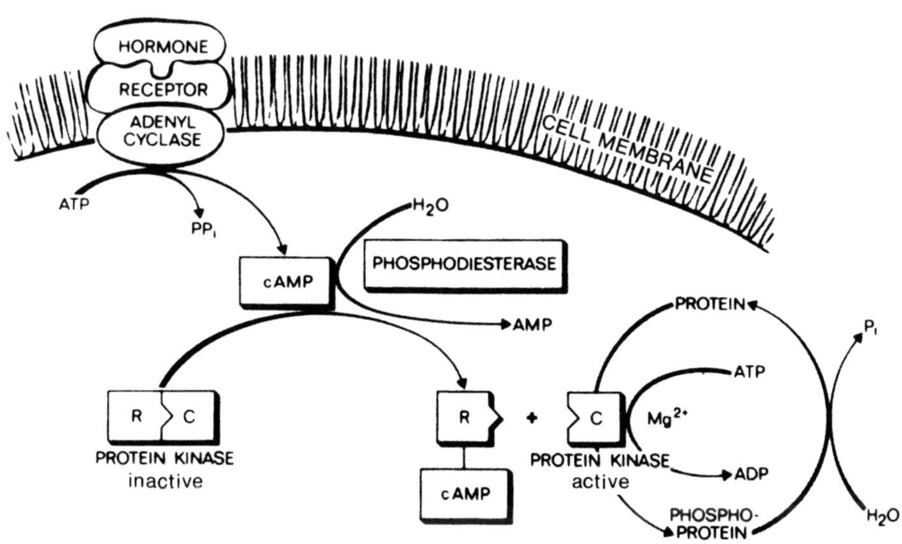

Fig. 1. Molecular mechanism of action of proteohormones on the adenylate cyclase system (6)

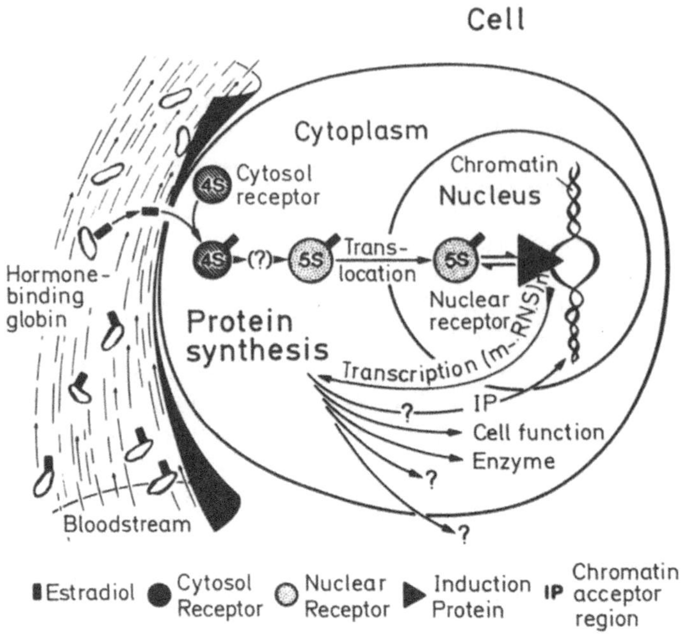

Fig. 2. Molecular mechanism of action of steroid hormones on receptor-hormone interaction and gene activation (6)

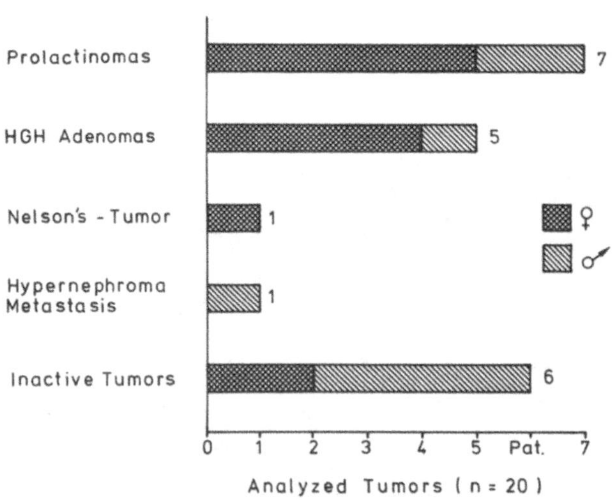

Fig. 3. Analysis of pituitary tumors for the determination of pituitary tumor cells

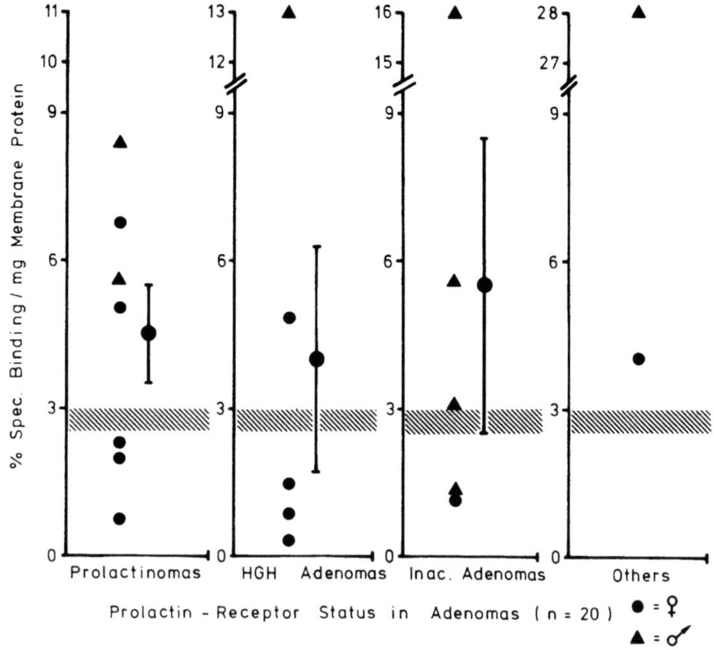

Fig. 4. Prolactin receptor concentration in human pituitary tumors. Receptor-positive: ≥ 3% specific binding/mg membrane protein. Receptor-negative: < 3% specific binding/mg membrane protein. Single values and $s_{\bar{x}}$ (standard deviation of mean value) are shown

Adenylate Kinase Isoenzymes in Intracranial Tumors

C. M. Luz[1], R. H. Schirmer[1], J. Hamer[2], and W. Sachsenheimer[2]
[1] Institut für Biochemie II, [2] Neurochirurgische Abteilung, Universität Heidelberg, Im Neuenheimer Feld, D-6900 Heidelberg

Introduction

Adenylate kinases (AK) catalyze the reaction ATP + AMP = 2 ADP (7). At least two genetically distinct isoenzymes have been identified in man, the chromosome 9-linked cytosolic AK1 and the chromosome 1-linked AK2, which is localized in the mitochondrial intermembrane space (1). The electrophoretic pattern of these isoenzymes is a useful marker for determining the stages of hematopoetic cell differentiation in certain leukemias (6). Furthermore, the balanced polymorphism of the AK1 subtypes AK1*1 and AK1*2 has been successfully applied for demonstrating the clonal origin of the Philadelphia translocation in chronic myeloid leukemia (11).

In the search for malignancy-associated enzyme changes and for stage-specific enzyme patterns in solid tumors, we started the analysis of AK activities and AK isoenzyme patterns in nontumorous brain tissue and in a number of intracranial tumors.

Material and Approach

Twenty-six intracranial tumors were studied. The following histologic types were present: one medulloblastoma, two astrocytomas of the cerebellum, one oligodendroglioma, two astrocytomas, five glioblastomas, one neurinoma, ten meningiomas, one hemangioblastoma, one gliosarcoma, one epidermoid, one metastasis from a lung tumor.

As soon as possible after excision, the tumors were taken up in 150 mM NaCl and frozen. They were stored for up to three months at -80°C; under these conditions the specimens did not lose AK activity. Prior to biochemical analysis, each sample was thawed rapidly and homogenized with three volumes of 2 mM EDTA-10 μM PMSF-150 nM pepstatin, pH 7.0 at 4°C. The suspensions were allowed to stand for about 30 min in an ice bath. After a clearing centrifugation at 2800 *g* for 20 min at 4°C, the AK activity of the extracts was assayed and described in ref. (2). Prior to determining the AK isoenzyme patterns, it proved to be essential to remove lipids by a clearing spin at 122 000 *g* for 15 min at 22°C (Fig. 2). Then samples containing 5-22 mU AK in 3-25 μl were subjected to electrophoresis on cellulose acetate gel (Cellogel from Chemetron) according to ref. (5); the gels were stained for AK activity afterwards, as shown in Figs. 1-4. It should be noted that 3%-5% of the AK activity after centrifugation at 2800 *g* and at 122 000 *g*, respectively, was due to AK2, as detected by specific inhibition of AK1 by di(adenosine-5')pentaphosphate (= AP_5A) (10).

 Advances in Neurosurgery, Vol. 13
Edited by H. Dietz, M. Brock, and M. Klinger

The specimens of nontumorous brain were analyzed immediately after excision.

Results and Discussion

The nontumorous brains which were examined did not form a homogeneous group (Table 1). In two brains from patients who died after chronic disease, AK activities were found to range from 0.6 U/g wet tissue to 1.5 U/g. The third brain, which was obtained from a patient who died of an acute event, presented activities from 11.9 U/g to 18.9 U/g.

Table 1. Adenylate kinase activities in nontumorous brain

Region	AK activity U/g w.t.[a]	U/g w.t.[b]	U/g w.t.[c]
Putamen	0.6	1.0	18.9
Cerebellum	0.9	0.6	17.4
Pons	1.5	1.0	14.5
Insula	0.9	0.9	12.6
Internal capsule	1.1	1.0	11.9

w.t., wet tissue

[a]Specimens obtained from a male patient who died of respiratory insufficiency during pulmonary edema

[b]Specimens obtained from a female patient who died of cardiac failure following coronary heart disease

[c]Specimens obtained from a female patient who died of pulmonary embolism

In two out of 26 tumors no AK activity could be detected (Table 2). The activities of the other 24 tumors, ranging from 0.3 U/g in the case of the medulloblastoma to 21.8 U/g in the case of the gliosarcoma, covered the scale of both types of nontumorous brain, filling up the gap between 2 U/g and 11 U/g.

The varying AK activities in the tumors have also to be assessed in the light of (a) difficulties in handling the specimens between extirpation and freezing and (b) their variable size and content of normal brain and necrotic tissue.

Thus, up to this point we noticed no clear indication of a specific change in the AK activity in intracranial tumors when compared with nontumorous brain, whereas other authors have found a correlation between the appearance of AK activity in the cerebrospinal fluid and the presence of (malignant) brain tumors (9).

The analysis of the AK isoenzyme patterns in the examined regions of nontumorous brain (Fig. 1) as well as in the intracranial tumors (Figs. 2-4) shows that AK 1 is present almost exclusively. Thus, in contrast to certain leukemias (6), there is no indication of tumor- or stage-specific AK isoenzymes or AK isoenzyme patterns; the differences in AK activity found in the tumors concern AK1 only.

Table 2. Adenylate kinase activities in intracranial tumors

RNo	Sex	Age	Histologic diagnosis	AK activity (U/g wet tissue)
2	M	43	Gliosarcoma/sarcoglioma	21.8
3	F	55	Glioblastoma multiforme	19.4
13	F	59	Meningioma, fibroblastic	13.6
5	F	57	Meningioma	13.1
14	M	53	Meningioma, endotheliomatous	9.2
4	F	70	Meningioma	6.8
19	F	35	Astrocytoma (Kernohan degree III)	5.2
16	M	52	Meningioma, endotheliomatous-transitional (degree II)	4.8
6	F	60	Glioblastoma fusiforme	4.7
20	F	36	Meningioma, endotheliomatous	3.9
26	M	51	Meningioma	3.9
15	F	50	Oligodendroglioma	3.1
10	F	49	Meningioma, transitional	2.9
8	M	40	Hemangioblastoma (Lindau's tumor) (recurrence)	2.5
22	F	51	Astrocytoma (Kernohan degree III-IV)	2.3
17	M	57	Epidermoid (recurrence)	2.0
1	M	10	Astrocytoma, pilocytic (Kernohan degree I)	1.7
18	F	21	Glioblastoma multiforme	1.6
12	F	48	Meningioma, angioblastic	1.0
11	F	45	Neurinoma Antoni A/B (recurrence)	0.9
21	F	24	Astrocytoma, pilocytic (Kernohan degree I)	0.5
24	M	47	Metastasis from a lung tumor	0.5
23	F	59	Meningioma, transitional	0.3
25	F	28	Medulloblastoma	0.3
7	M	64	Glioblastoma multiforme	n.d.a.
27	M	63	Glioblastoma/astrocytoma (Kernohan degree IV)	n.d.a.

The study of a larger number of tumors should prove whether AK1, because of its central role in the coordination of energy metabolism and biosynthetic pathways, is an enzyme which limits the rate of growth (4). In addition, the correlation of AK activity in intracranial tumors on the one hand and in cerebrospinal fluid (9) and blood on the other should be examined further in connection with anamnestic and clinical data.

Conclusions

Cellulose acetate gel electrophoresis is a powerful tool for isoenzyme analyses in certain types of leukemia (6). As described here, a modified form of the method is applicable in the case of solid tumors. However, in respect of intracranial tumors, the activity and isoenzyme pattern of adenylate kinase seem to have no diagnostic value; AK1 is the predominant isoenzyme in nontumorous brain and in all studied tumors, although the role of the enzyme in brain cells and in tumor cells may be different. It remains to be clarified whether AK, the only salvage enzyme for AMP (4, 7), limits the rate of growth (4) in certain tumors. In this case inhibitors of AK1 can be designed (3) as cytostatic drugs on the basis of the known three-dimensional structure of the enzyme (1, 8).

References

1. Frank, R., Trosin, M., Tomasselli, A.G., Schulz, G.E., Schirmer, R.H.: Mitochondrial adenylate kinase (AK2) from bovine heart. Homology with the cytosolic isoenzyme in the catalytic region. Eur. J. Biochem. (1984) (to be published)
2. Hamada, M., Okuda, H., Oka, K., Watanabe, T., Ueda, K., Nojima, M., Kuby, S.A., Manship, M., Tyler, F.H., Ziter, F.A.: An aberrant adenylate kinase isoenzyme from the serum of patients with Duchenne muscular dystrophy. Biochim. Biophys. Acta 660, 227-237 (1981)
3. Hampton, A., Kappler, F., Picker, D.: Species- or isozyme-specific enzyme inhibitors. 4. Design of a two-site inhibitor of adenylate kinase with isozyme selectivity. J. Med. Chem. 25, 638-644 (1982)
4. Lipmann, F.: The ATP-phosphate cycle. Curr. Top. Cell. Reg. 18, 301-311 (1981)
5. Meera Khan, P.: Enzyme electrophoresis on cellulose acetate gel: zymogram patterns in man-mouse and man-Chinese hamster somatic cell hybrids. Arch. Biochem. Biophys. 145, 470-483 (1971)
6. Meera Khan, P., Blankenstein-Wijnen, L.M.M., Wijnen, J.T., Geraedts, J.P.M., Willemze, R., van Kessel, A.G., Hagemeijer, A.G., de Bruyn, C.H.M.M., de Gast, G.C.: Adenylate kinase (AK) isozymes as leukemia markers. In: Knapp, W. (ed.) Leukemia markers, pp. 529-533. Academic Press, New York 1981
7. Noda, L.: Adenylate kinase. In: Boyer, P.D. (ed.) The enzymes, vol. 8, pp. 279-305. Academic Press, New York 1973
8. Pai, E.F., Sachsenheimer, W., Schirmer, R.H., Schulz, G.E.: Substrate positions and induced-fit in crystalline adenylate kinase. J. Mol. Biol. 114, 37-45 (1977)
9. Ronquist, G., Frithz, G., Ericsson, P., Hugosson, R.: Malignant brain tumours associated with adenylate kinase in cerebrospinal fluid. Lancet I, 1284-1286 (1977)
10. Sachsenheimer, W., Goody, R.S., Schirmer, R.H.: Elimination und Exkretion von Adenylatkinasen nach Zellschädigungen. Klin. Wschr. 53, 617-622 (1975)
11. van Kessel, A.H.M.G., von Agthoven, A.J., Hagemeijer, A.: Clonal origin of the Philadelphia translocation in chronic myeloid leukemia demonstrated in somatic cell hybrids using an adenylate kinase-1 polymorphism. Canc. Genet. Cytogenet. 6, 55-58 (1982)

Fig. 2 see p. 264

Fig. 2. Zymograms of AK isoenzymes in intracranial tumors. Lipids had not been removed prior to electrophoresis. Tumors no. 4 (channel 2), no. 5 (channel 3), no. 6 (channel 4), no. 8 (channel 5), no. 9 (channel 6), and no. 10 (channel 7). Channels 1 and 8 contain the standard mixture (see Fig. 1). For specification of the tumors, see Table 2

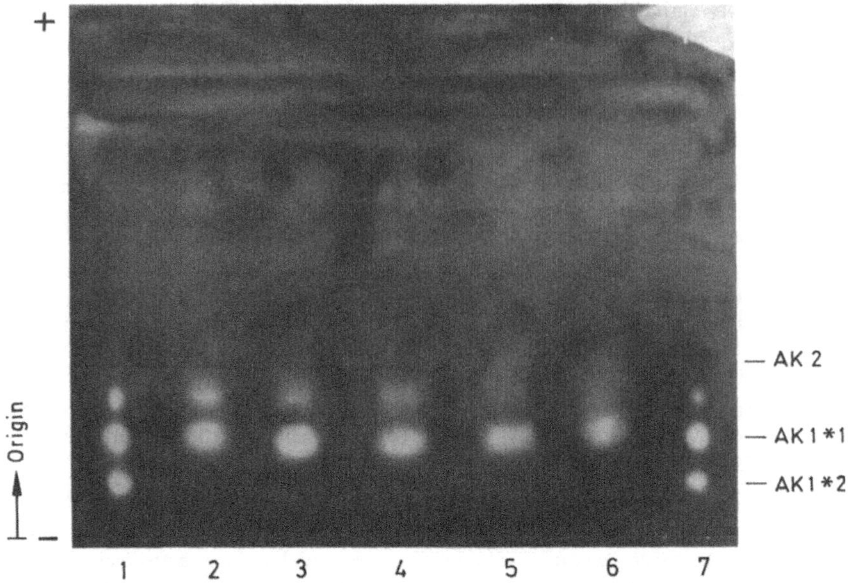

Fig. 1. Zymograms of AK isoenzymes in nontumorous brain. Lipids had been removed prior to electrophoresis. Putamen (channel 2), internal capsule (channel 3), insula (channel 4), cerebellum (channel 5), pons (channel 6). The first and last channels represent a standard which contains AK1*1 and AK1*2. In all channels, the band just above AK1*1 is caused by a modified form of AK1*1, whereas the most anodal band represents AK2

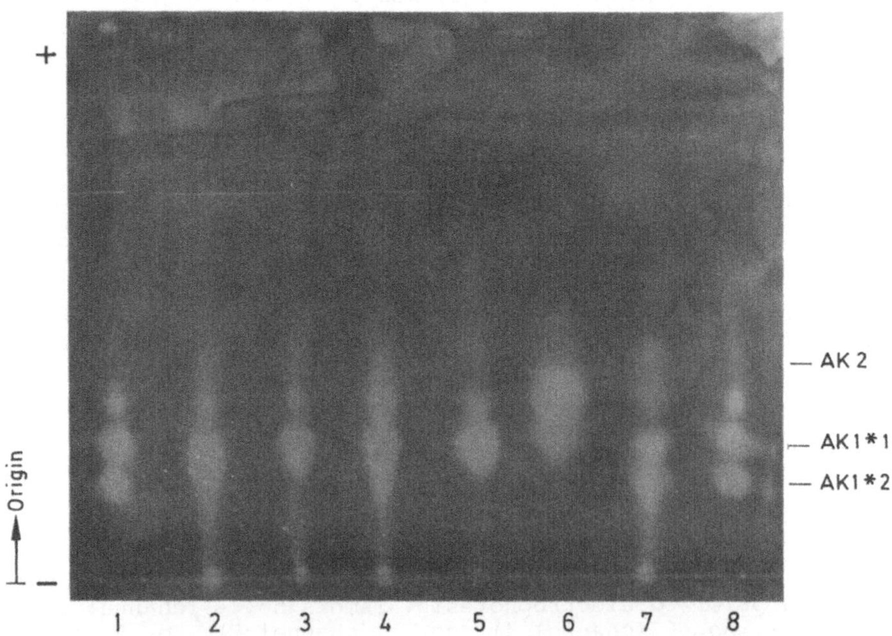

Fig. 2. Legend see p. 263

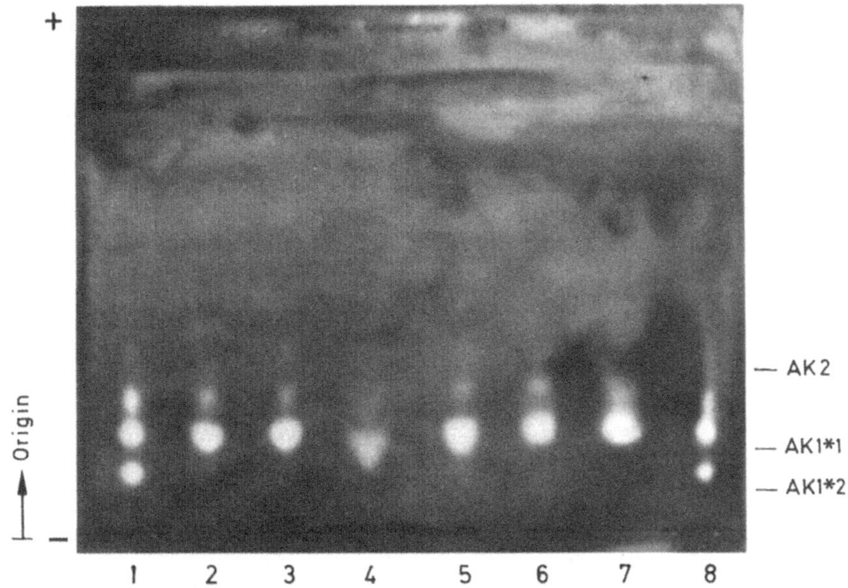

Fig. 3. Zymograms of AK isoenzymes in intracranial tumors. Lipids had been removed prior to electrophoresis. Tumors no. 2 (channel 2), no. 3 (channel 3), no. 11 (channel 4), no. 13 (channel 5), no. 14 (channel 6), and no. 15 (channel 7). Channels 1 and 8 contain the standard mixture (see Fig. 1). For specification of the tumors, see Table 2

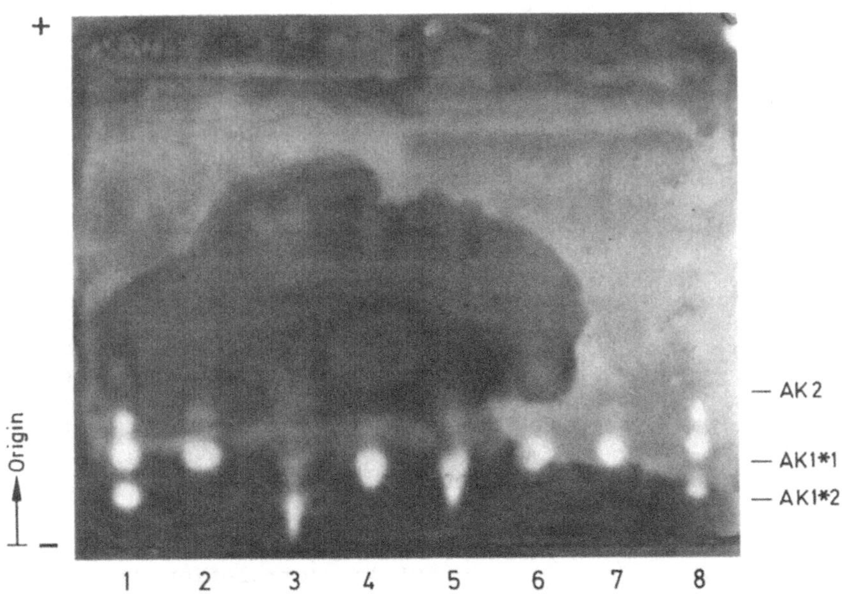

Fig. 4. Zymograms of AK isoenzymes in intracranial tumors. Lipids had been removed prior to electrophoresis. Tumors no. 16 (channel 2), no. 10 (channel 3), no. 19 (channel 4), no. 20 (channel 5), no. 22 (channel 6), and no. 26 (channel 7). Channels 1 and 8 contain the standard mixture (see Fig. 1). For specification of the tumors, see Table 2

Quantitative Immunohistochemical Evaluation of Tumor Edema in Brain Tumors

Th. Rommel[1], W. Bodsch[2], B. Grosse Ophoff[2], K.-A. Hossmann[2], and J. Menzel[1]

[1] Neurochirurgische Klinik der Städtischen Krankenanstalten Köln,
[2] Max-Planck-Institut für neurologische Forschung, Abteilung für Experimentelle Neurologie, Ostmerheimerstraße 200, D-5000 Köln 91

Introduction

The dynamic development of vasogenic brain edema is closely linked to the alterations of the brain tissue water content, the electrolyte concentration, and the extravasation of serum proteins. So far, quantitative detection of serum proteins has been possible in animal experiments on the basis of immunohistochemical investigations. This underscores the significance of protein extravasation in the genesis of brain edema (4, 7). The method introduced by Bodsch is now used in biopsies of glial and meningeal tumors as well as their peritumoral tissue.

Material and Methods

Samples of glioblastomas ($n = 10$), meningiomas ($n = 13$), and the peritumoral tissue were fixed intraoperatively with liquid nitrogen, and quantitative determinations of serum proteins and hemoglobin content of the biopsy material were performed. In principle, tissue homogenates of the samples were passed over a column containing I^{125}-labeled antihuman serum proteins or hemoglobin antibodies as a solid support. Serum proteins in the brain sample were retained on the column support by the antibody-antigen reaction while other proteins freely passed the column. The specifically absorbed serum proteins or hemoglobin could then be eluted quantitatively from the antibody support and measured by a radioimmunoassay. Cerebral blood volume (CBV) was calculated from the contents of serum proteins and hemoglobin in the brain and of serum proteins, hemoglobin, and hematocrit in the peripheral blood on the assumption that the hematocrit levels in the brain and the venous blood are the same. Water content and electrolytes were measured by the difference in wet and dry weight of tissue and by atomic absorption spectrophotometric measurements. The total tissue content of dexamethasone was determined by high performance liquid chromatography (HPLC).

Results

In the glioblastomas, a proportional correlation was found between extravasal serum protein content and the tissue water content (Figs. 1, 2). The serum protein concentration was between 8 and 47 mg/g d.w. The water content was between 82% and 86%. In the peritumoral tissue, the water content was 80%-82%. There was also a proportional correlation with the serum proteins here. The serum proteins showed a markedly higher concentration, at between 35 and 53 mg/g d.w., as compared

Advances in Neurosurgery, Vol. 13
Edited by H. Dietz, M. Brock, and M. Klinger

with the tumor tissue. The CBV of the tumor tissue was calculated as 2.32 ± 0.53 ml/100 g w.w. In the meningiomas, the water content levels were widely scattered between 78% and 84% and showed no correlation with the serum protein concentration, which was between 1 and 16 mg/g d.w. In the peritumoral tissue, a correlation could be suspected between a serum protein concentration of 25-40 mg/g d.w. and a water content of 79%-82.5%. The CBV of the tumor tissue was calculated as 2.86 ± 0.63 ml/100 g w.w.

In the glioblastomas, an inverse proportionality was found between the dexamethasone concentration and the serum protein content both in the tumor and in the peritumoral tissue (Fig. 3). The dexamethasone concentrations were between 0.48 and 2.6 μg/g d.w. In the meningiomas, the dexamethasone concentration was relatively homogeneous both in the tumor and in myaloid tissue, in a range between 0.9 and 2.6 μg/g d.w. (Fig. 4). With almost identical dexamethasone concentrations in the peritumoral tissue, the serum protein concentrations differed, being between 24.7 and 39.6 mg/g d.w. A similar relationship was found between dexamethasone concentration and water content. In tumor tissue of glioblastomas dexamethasone concentrations were 0.0209-0.451 μg/g w.w., while water content ranged from 82.04% to 86.2%. Corresponding values for peritumoral tissue of glioblastomas were 0.072 to 0.3622 μg/g w.w. at water contents of 80.1%-82.0%. Dexamethasone concentrations in meningiomas correlated with water content neither in the tumor tissue (0.2136-0.4040 μg/g w.w. at 77.8%-84.1%) nor in peritumoral tissue (0.1901-0.2324 μg/g w.w. at 79.2%-82.6% water content).

The sodium concentration in glioblastomas was 11.6-20.4 μg/mg P. In the peritumoral tissue, concentrations were found between 11.8 and 15.8 μg/mg P. Both for the tumor and the peritumoral tissue, there were proportional correlations with the water content, which was higher in the tumor than in the peritumoral tissue. A proportional relationship between the sodium concentration and the water content was also found in the meningiomas. In the tumor tissue the sodium concentration were 8-15.8 μg/mg P and in the peritumoral tissue 11.3-16.0 μg/mg P at water concentrations of 79.5%-82.6%.

Discussion

The results in the glioblastomas confirm the correlation between water content and serum protein concentration already reported in experimental studies. This correlation also applied to the peritumoral tissue (7). Such a correlation can at best be suspected for the peritumoral tissue in meningeal tumors, since the material available so far does not permit a representative evaluation. The higher serum protein concentrations throughout the peritumoral tissue in glioblastomas are striking, although here the water content was markedly less than that of the tumor tissue; there is thus a dissociation between a relatively high protein and a markedly lower water content. It must be critically noted that the values obtained were not necessarily representative for the entire tumor. In addition, corresponding control values were lacking. Nevertheless, the results appear to be relevant, since various typical components of vasogenic brain edema were correlated and one can also assume known values, e.g., for the normal water content of the brain (2, 6, 13, 15). The effect of dexamethasone on the extravasation of serum proteins is evident in glial tumors. This correlation may have been masked by the differences of dexamethasone contents per gram wet weight. However, when wet weight contents of dexamethasone are correlated with water contents, the relationship is reconfirmed. The dissociation of a relatively high protein concentration and a markedly lower water content in the peritumoral tissue can likewise only be understood as an effect of dexamethasone, although the water content in reabsorption of the edema has evidently diminished more rapidly than the tissue protein content.

Conclusions

Only consideration of the correlations between the three major components of the tumor edema, namely the water content, the serum proteins, and the electrolytes, permits a differentiated quantitative analysis. The value of immunohistochemical determinations of serum proteins in the tumor and in the peritumoral tissue is evident, even though the material available so far in tumors not speficic to the brain does not permit a representative appraisal.

References

1. Aarabi, B., Long, D.M.: Dynamics of cerebral edema. The role of an intact vascular bed in the production and propagation of vasogenic brain edema. J. Neurosurg. 51, 779-784 (1979)
2. Adachi, M., Feigin, I.: Cerebral oedema and the water content of normal white matter. J. Neuro. Neurosurg. Psychiat. 29, 446-450 (1966)
3. Baithmann, A., Öttinger, W., Fleischer, B., Moritake, K., Jesch, F.: Corticosteroids stimulate cerebral energy metabolism; support for a metabolic action of steroids on brain edema. Adv. Neurosurg. 6, 187-192 (1978)
4. Bodsch, W., Hürter, T., Hossmann, K.-A.: Immunochemical method for quantitative evaluation of vasogenic brain edema following cold injury of rat brain. Brain Res. 249, 111-121 (1982)
5. Brock, M., Wiegand, H., Zillig, C., Zywietz, C., Mock, P., Dietz, H.: The effect of desamenthasone on intracranial pressure in patients with supratentorial tumors. In: Pappius, H.M., Feindel, W. (eds.) Dynamics of brain edema, pp. 330-336. Springer, Berlin Heidelberg New York 1976
6. Hadjidimos, A.A., Reulen, H.J., Brock, M., Deruaz, J.P., Brost, F., Fischer, F., Samii, M., Schürmann, D.: rCBF, tissue water content and tissue lactate in brain tumours. in: Ross Russel, R.W. (ed.) Brain and blood flow, pp. 378-385. Pitman, London 1971
7. Hossmann, K.-A., Hürter, T., Oschlies, U.: The effect of dexamethasone on serum protein extravasation and edema development in experimental brain tumors of cats. Acta Neuropathol. 60, 223-231 (1983)
8. Hossmann, K.-A., Wechsler, W., Wilmes, F.: Experimental peritumorous edema. Morphological and pathophysiological observations. Acta Neuropathol. 45, 195-203 (1979)
9. Klatzo, I., Chui, E., Fujiwara, K., Spatz, M.: Resolution of vasogenic brain edema. Adv. Neurol. 28, 359-373 (1980)
10. Klatzo, I., Wisniewski, H., Steinwall, O., Streicher, E.: Dynamics of cold injury edema. In: Klatzo, I., Seitelberger, F. (eds.) Brain edema, pp. 554-563. Springer, Berlin Heidelberg New York 1962
11. Meinig, G., Aulich, A., Wende, S., Reulen, H.J.: Resolution of peritumoral brain edema following a combination therapy with dexamethasone and furosemide. Acta Neurochir. 36, 278-279 (1977)

12. Meinig, G., Reulen, H.J., Wende, S., Schürmann, K.: Use of dexamethasone and furosemide in brain edema. In: Hartmann, A., Brock, M. (eds.) Treatment of cerebral edema, pp. 139-155. Springer, Berlin Heidelberg New York 1982

13. Pach, M.P., Tweed, W.A.: Tissue albumin and water content in the early stages of vasogenic brain edema formation. Canad. J. Neurol. Sci. 6, 423-426 (1979)

14. Reulen, H.J., Jadjidimos, A.A., Schürmann, K.: The effect of dexamethasone on water and electrolyte content and on rCBF on perifocal brain edema in man. In: Reulen, H.J., Schürmann, K. (eds.) Steroids and brain edema, pp. 239-252. Springer, Berlin Heidelberg New York 1972

15. Yates, A.J., Thelmo, W., Pappins, H.M.: Postmortem changes in the chemistry and histology of normal and edematous brains. Am. J. Pathol. 79, 555-564 (1975)

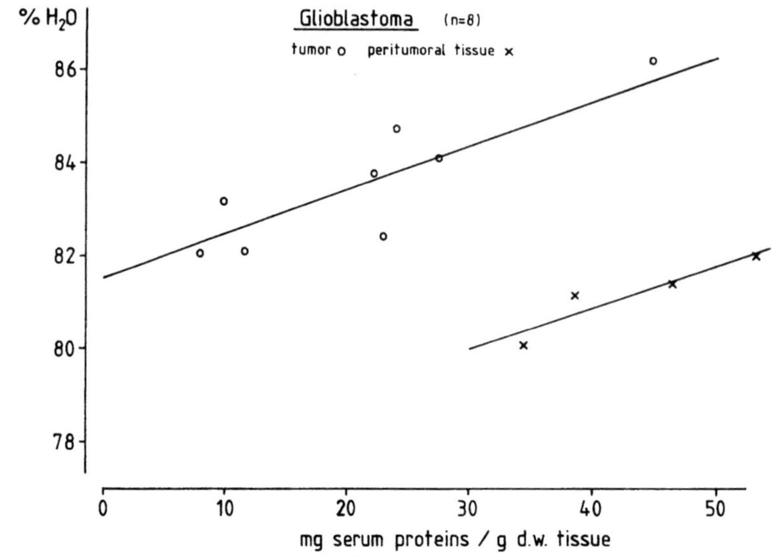

Fig. 1. Relationship between serum proteins and water content in glioblastomas and the peritumoral tissue. Venous hematocrit (Htk_V): 38.2 ± 1.41 vol%. Cerebral blood volume (CBV) of tumor tissue: 2.32 ± 0.53 ml/100 g.w.w. Values represent measured parameters; curves were obtained by linear regression

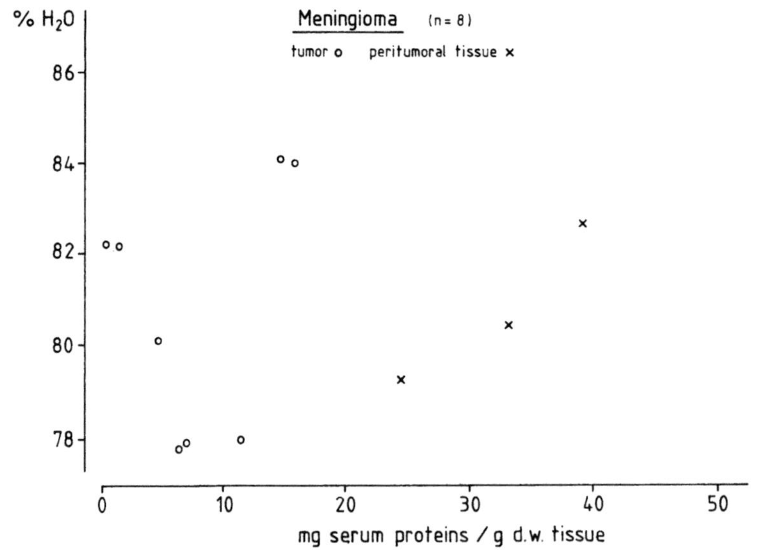

Fig. 2. Relationship between serum proteins and water content in meningiomas and the peritumoral tissue. Htk_V 38.85 ± 2.98 vol%. CBV of tumor tissue: 2.86 ± 0.63 ml/100 g.w.w.

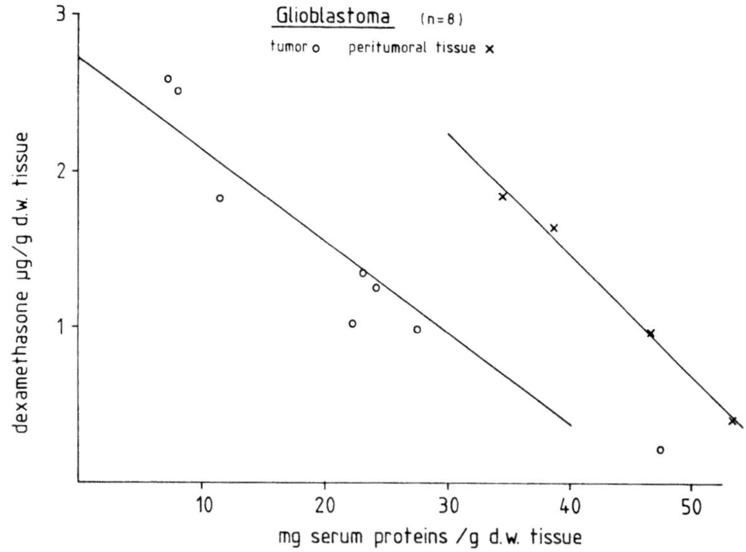

Fig. 3. Relationship between dexamethasone and serum proteins in glioblastomas and the peritumoral tissue. CBV and Htk_V: see Fig. 1

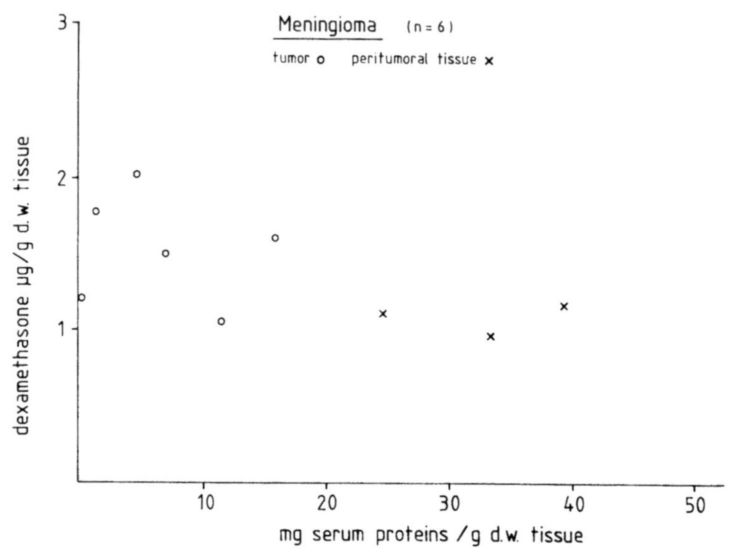

Fig. 4. Relationship between dexamethasone and serum proteins in meningiomas and the peritumoral tissue. CBV and Htk_V: see Fig. 2

Melatonin: A Marker for Tumors of the Pineal Region

H.-E. Clar[1], L. Tharandt[2], C. Schrenk[2], F. Rosanowski[2], G. Benker[2], and D. Reinwein[2]

[1]Abteilung für Neurochirurgie, [2]Medizinische Abteilung, Universitätsklinikum der Gesamthochschule Essen, Hufelandstraße 55, D-4300 Essen 1

Introduction

In patients with tumors of the pineal region, endocrine abnormalities appear to be more frequent than was previously assumed. It has been suggested that these abnormalities originate in the hypothalamus (1, 3). Melatonin is secreted by the pineal gland and may thus serve as a tumor marker in patients with tumors in this area. Recently, a sensitive radioimmunoassay of melatonin was developed which enabled us to study serum levels of the hormone in patients with pineal tumors. Surprisingly, up to now there have been only single reports on melatonin in neoplastic pineal disease.

Patients

Serum levels of melatonin were studied in 11 patients with tumors in the pineal region during daytime nadir (11 a.m. to 3 p.m.) and in 11 normal controls (6, 7). Diagnosis was by CT scan and histological examination and by cytological examination of cerebrospinal fluid in three cases.

Method

Melatonin was analyzed by the method of ROLLAG and NISWENDER (5), using NISWENDER's highly specific antimelatonin serum. The profile of melatonin in normal controls (Fig. 1) showed a typical nyctohemeral rhythm. Daytime nadir was low [12.3-42.5 pg melatonin/ml (2 s range)] with little variation between 11 a.m. and 3 p.m. At night, we observed high melatonin levels (58.2-94.5 pg/ml serum) with more variability in the normal control group.

Results

Serum levels of melatonin in patients with verified tumors in the pineal region taken at the daytime nadir were increased above normal levels (Fig. 2). Two groups were differentiated:

Group 1: Extremely high melatonin levels (patients 1-4) which were more than double the normal range (87.8-230 pg/ml serum). All these patients showed signs of tumor progression at the time of clinical examination and on CT scan (Figs. 2, 3).

Group 2: Modestly elevated melatonin levels (47.4-72.6 pg/ml serum). In these patients (5-11) the tumor was treated successfully by irra-

 Advances in Neurosurgery, Vol. 13
Edited by H. Dietz, M. Brock, and M. Klinger

diation. CT scan and clinical examination showed no signs of tumor activity. In six of these cases (patients 5-10) the existence of residual, nonprogressive tumors has been known for years. Patient no. 10 had a normal CT scan five years after pineal tumor irradiation, with an only slightly elevated melatonin level (65 pg/ml) (Figs. 2, 4).

Discussion

Endocrine abnormalities are quite common in patients with tumors of the pineal region, as in patients with craniopharyngiomas. However, the endocrine activity of the pineal region in these patients could not previously be studied, as methods for the determination of melatonin did not become available until recently. Our study of 11 patients with pineal tumors shows that the disease was always associated with increased serum melatonin levels during daytime nadir. Melatonin levels remained elevated even in a patient in whom the tumor was no longer detectable on CT scan after successful irradiation. Similar results were obtained in patients with nonprogressive tumors. Progressive disease – as shown by CT scan – was always associated with high levels of serum melatonin. Similarly, BARBER et al. (2) and NEUWELT and LEWY (4) have described elevated melatonin in patients with progressive tumors of the pineal region.

The increased melatonin secretion may result either from hormone production by the tumor itself or from the effects of the tumor on the normal pineal tissue (stimulation or loss of inhibition). The exact mechanism is not yet understood.

Conclusion

These data obtained from 11 patients indicate that:

1. Tumors in the pineal region are associated with increased serum melatonin levels.
2. High levels of melatonin are associated with marked tumor progression as shown by CT scans.
3. Melatonin can be considered a marker for tumors in the pineal region in general.

References

1. Andler, W., Clar, H.E.: Hypothalamic function in patients with tumors of the pineal area. Helv. paediatr. Acta 37, 323-329 (1982)
2. Barber, S.G., Smith, J.A., Hughes, R.C.: Melatonin as a tumor marker in a patient with pineal tumor. Brit. Med. J. 2, 328 (1978)
3. Clar, H.E., Andler, W.: Diencephale hormonelle Funktionsstörungen bei Tumoren der Pinealisregion. Verh. Dtsch. Ges. Neurol. I, pp. 447-450. Springer, Berlin Heidelberg New York 1980
4. Neuwelt, E.A., Lewy, A.: Disappearance of plasma melatonin after removal of neoplastic pineal gland. New Engl. J. med. 308, 1132-1135 (1983)
5. Rollag, M.D., Niswender, G.D.: Endocrinology 98, 482 (1976)
6. Tharandt, L., Reinwein, D.: Melatonin, ein klinisch bedeutsames Hormon? Dtsch. med. Wschr. 10, 470-474 (1983)
7. Tharandt, L., Schrenk, C., Rosanowski, F., Kirsch, W., Reinwein, D.: Aufgehobene Melatoninrhythmik bei Akromegalie. Vortrag Dtsch. Ges. Endokrinologie, Heidelberg 1984

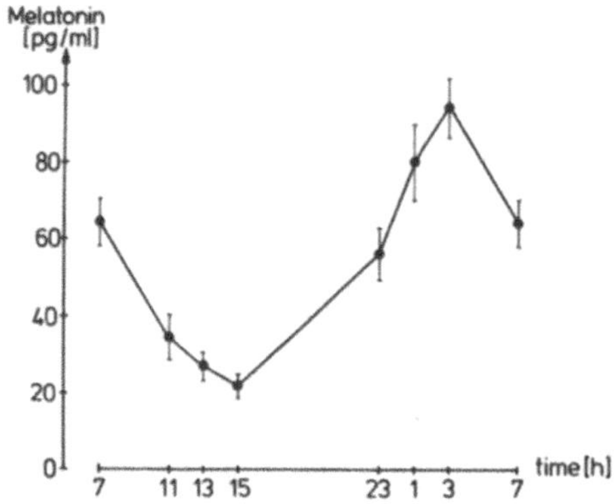

Fig. 1. Melatonin serum levels in 11 normal controls over a 24-h period. Levels were constantly low between 11 a.m. and 3 p.m.

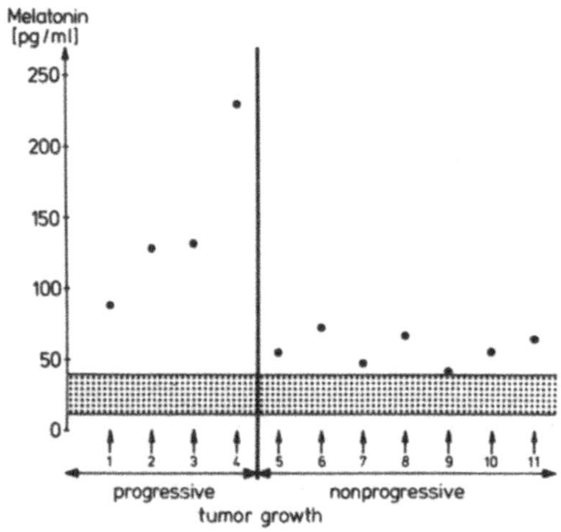

Fig. 2. Melatonin levels in 11 patients with treated pineal tumors at the daytime nadir (11 a.m. to 3 p.m.)

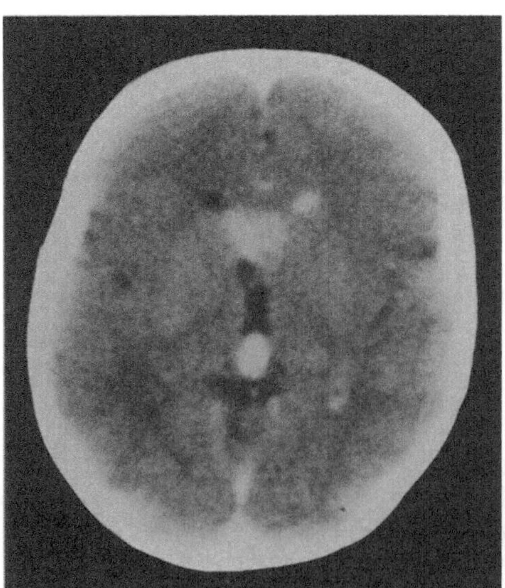

Fig. 3. CT scan of a 20-year-old man with metastatic pineal tumor growth (case No. 3)

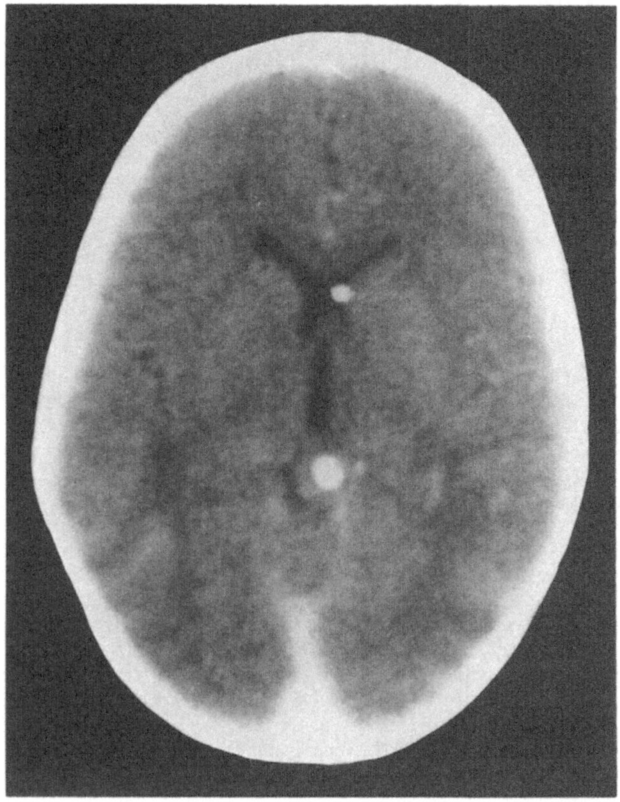

Fig. 4. CT scan of a 10-year-old boy five years after radiation of a pineal tumor with no signs of tumor recurrence

Optical Properties of Brain Tissue and Brain Tumors at the Wavelength of the Nd-YAG Laser ($\lambda = 1060$ nm)

H. R. Eggert

Neurochirurgische Universitätsklinik, Klinikum der Albert-Ludwigs-Universität, Hugstetter Straße 55, D-7800 Freiburg

According to the increasing number of reports on clinical (2, 4, 6, 8, 10, 13, 16) and experimental (1, 7, 15) observations of the effect of Nd-YAG laser irradiation on intracranial tumors and vascular lesions, the Nd-YAG laser provides a useful tool for shrinking brain tumors and coagulating vessels. However, there is a lack of information about the optical properties of normal brain tissue and brain tumors at a wavelength of 1060 nm, which influence the effects of laser irradiation. These optical properties are the reflection, extinction, and transmission capabilities. Extinction consists of absorption and scattering. The biological effect of surgical laser irradiation is determined by the amount of energy absorbed by the tissue. Up to now, optical properties of human brain tissue in comparison to brain tumors have not been made the subject of experimental studies. With regard to the methodological difficulties, the present study attempts to evaluate the relative levels of absorbance and transmittance of normal human brain tissue in comparison with brain tumors based on experiments performed in vitro.

Material and Methods

Tissue samples were derived from five cadaver brains and from brain tumors removed surgically. Five samples of frontal gray matter, frontal white matter, and basal ganglia and two specimens of pons and medulla oblongata were obtained from each brain. Tumor samples included 23 meningiomas, 14 astrocytomas, and 14 glioblastomas. To obtain information on the absorption capability of tissue, tissue samples of 1 mm thickness filled into quartz cuvettes were irradiated with the focussed beam (calculated focus diameter 2.9 mm, output power 30 and 50 W, power density with regard to 4% loss of power due to 1 mm of quartz glass 443 and 737 W/cm^2) of an Nd-YAG laser (medilas, Fa. MBB, Munich, Germany). The power transmitted by the tissue samples was measured with the power meter (LMG-01, Fa. MBB, Munich, Germany) fitted so closely to the back side of the cuvette that the entire measuring opening of the instrument was covered. The measured power was plotted against time. Using this experimental design, it was observed that after a variable period of irradiation, in which the transmitted power remained nearly unchanged, the transmitted power increased steeply, with visible vaporization of the tissue sample (Fig. 1). Since absorption of energy is a precondition for vaporization, this time (penetration time, PT) corresponds mainly to the energy absorbed by the tissue. In tumor samples pale and more or less reddish colored portions could be distinguished. The penetration time of these parts was determined separately. In each specimen, penetration time was determined four to

 Advances in Neurosurgery, Vol. 13
Edited by H. Dietz, M. Brock, and M. Klinger

six times, depending on the diameter of the pale halo occurring around the focus.

The relative level of transmission was measured in tissue homogenates filled in plastic cuvettes of 1 mm thickness. The cuvettes were irradiated with the focussed beam of the Nd-YAG laser using an output power of 20 W with regard to a normal saline blank. The power transmitted by the tissue homogenates was measured with a power meter, the measuring opening of which rested closely behind the cuvette. Tissue homogenates were obtained by homogenizing 1 g of tissue in 10 ml of normal saline at 1000 rpm for 3 min and diluting 1 ml of this homogenate with 4 ml of normal saline. The transmission capability of tissue homogenates was expressed in the percentage of output power in relation to a normal saline blank. The concentration of hemoglobin in tissue homogenates was determined photometrically using the hemoglobin-cyanide method (9). A modification of the method so that the samples were centrifuged at 3000 rpm before reading seemed necessary due to a delicate white precipitation which was observed after mixing brain tissue homogenates mainly containing myelin with the potassium cyanide solution.

Results

Penetration Time (Table 1)

Significant differences were observed between cortical gray matter and white matter, on the one hand, and basal ganglia and medulla oblongata on the other (Fig. 2). In tumor samples, the penetration time was significantly shorter in reddish colored parts compared with pale parts. It was significantly longer in meningiomas than in astrocytomas or glioblastomas. The most striking differences were observed when comparing normal brain tissue with brain tumors. In every case, the penetration time of brain tissue was evidently longer than in brain tumors. While in brain tumors the penetration time corresponded quite strongly with the concentration of the hemoglobin in normal brain tissue, no statistical correlation could be found (Fig. 3).

Transmission (Table 1)

The transmittance of cortex and basal ganglia was significantly higher than that of the other brain regions. Homogenates of meningiomas and astrocytomas transmitted more power than homogenates of glioblastomas. The transmittance of brain tumors in general was significantly higher than that of brain tissue. In normal brain tissue as well as in brain tumors the transmittance depended strongly on the hemoglobin concentration (Fig. 4).

Discussion

According to the law of energy conservation, the total amount of optical tissue properties adds up to one. Therefore, given the relative levels of absorption determined by the penetration time and the relative levels of transmission measured in tissue homogenates, the relative levels of reflection can be estimated. Measurements of tissue absorption coefficients are methodologically difficult and seem of little value, especially if output powers are applied, which are known to alter physical and chemical properties of the tissue (11, 15). Since it has been shown by theoretical considerations (14) as well as by experimental investigations (5) that the tissue blood flow does not sig-

Table 1. Experimental results, mean values ± SD. PT 30 = penetration time using an output power of 30 W; PT 50 = penetration time using an output power of 50 W

		n	Hb (g%)	Transmission (%)	PT 30 (s)	PT 50 (s)
Cortex		25	0.28 ± 0.10	25.0 ± 5.0	11.3 ± 2.6	3.4 ± 1.0
White matter		25	1.23 ± 0.48	7.4 ± 0.5	12.1 ± 4.0	2.9 ± 1.0
Basal ganglia		25	0.45 ± 0.17	16.0 ± 6.0	8.5 ± 3.3	2.1 ± 0.9
Pons		10	0.91 ± 0.30	9.0 ± 1.0	11.1 ± 4.1	3.8 ± 1.5
Medulla oblongata		10	0.90 ± 0.37	9.0 ± 1.0	8.0 ± 2.3	3.1 ± 1.8
Meningiomas	Pale	23	0.69 ± 0.5	67.0 ± 15.0	5.5 ± 2.2	2.4 ± 1.3
	Red				2.4 ± 1.6	0.8 ± 0.6
Astrocytomas	Pale	14	0.74 ± 0.5	57.0 ± 18.0	3.1 ± 2.0	0.9 ± 0.6
	Red				1.0 ± 0.7	0.3 ± 0.2
Glioblastomas	Pale	14	1.57 ± 0.7	47.0 ± 11.0	2.7 ± 1.8	1.4 ± 1.1
	Red				1.5 ± 0.7	0.8 ± 1.0

nificantly influence the thermal and optical (3) response of tissue to laser irradiation, in vitro studies of optical properties of tissue are not only of theoretical interest but also – at least to a certain degree – of practical significance. As our results indicate, the interactions of Nd-YAG laser light and brain tissue are predominantly ruled by the high reflectance of brain tissue (comparatively long penetration time, low transmittance). Also at $\lambda = 633$ nm a rather high reflection coefficient of 0.6 was measured in cow brain (3). The rather high standard deviation in measurements of the penetration time may be due to the rather rough experimental design. However, they may also indicate different absorption coefficients due to a different hemoglobin content of closely neighboring areas of tissue, since the concentration of hemoglobin was measured in tissue homogenates and could not be determined in every tissue area in which the penetration time was measured. The observation that in the brain tissue no statistical correlation could be found between penetration time and hemoglobin concentration may be caused by the same reason. On the other hand, with regard to absorption, hemoglobin and myelin act against each other, since the scattering coefficient is increased by the content of myelin (12). This may also explain the fact that in spite of a comparatively high hemoglobin concentration, the longest penetration time and the lowest transmittance were found in cerebral white matter. Both values indicate that white matter reflects most of the incident Nd-YAG laser light.

In contrast to normal brain tissue, the interactions of Nd-YAG laser light and cerebral tumors are dominated by the absorption of the light due to the hemoglobin content of tumor tissue. In general, the light of the Nd-YAG laser is absorbed by tumor tissue to a far higher degree than by brain tissue. On the basis of these observations, the Nd-YAG laser may be somewhat safer in microsurgical operations on brain tumors than the commonly used CO_2 laser if tumor coagulation is intended before dissection is completed.

Conclusions

From the results obtained the following conclusions may be drawn:

1. At the wavelength of the Nd-YAG laser ($\lambda = 1060$ nm) quite pronounced differences in optical properties exist between different brain regions as well as between different brain tumors and between normal brain tissue and brain tumors.
2. Tissue derived from basal ganglia and medulla oblongata seems to be more sensitive to the radiation than cortical gray matter, white matter, and pons, probably due to a different content of myelin.
3. Cerebral tissue reflects the incident light of the Nd-YAG laser to a far higher degree than does tumor tissue.
4. The absorption of the Nd-YAG laser light by brain tumors depends strongly on their content of hemoglobin.

Acknowledgments. The author is indebted to Prof. Dr. Kracht, Department of Pathology, University of Gießen, for his willingness to provide the cadaver brains. This study was supported by the Deutsche Forschungsgemeinschaft (SFB 70).

References

1. Beck, O.J., Wilske, J., Schönberger, J.L., Gorisch, W.: Tissue changes following application of lasers to the rabbit brain. Neurosurg. Rev. 1, 31-36 (1979)
2. Beck, O.J.: The use of the ND:YAG and the CO_2 laser in neurosurgery. Neurosurg. Rev. 3, 261-266 (1980)
3. Doiron, D.R., Svaasand, L.O., Profio, A.E.: Light dosimetry in tissue: application to photoradiation therapy. In: Kessel, D., Dougherty, T.J. (eds.) Porphyrin photosensibilisation. Plenum Press, New York London 1982
4. Edwards, M.S.B., Boggan, J.E., Fuller, T.A.: The laser in neurological surgery. J. Neurosurg. 59, 555-566 (1983)
5. Eichler, J., Knof, J., Lenz, H., Salk, J., Schäfer, G.: Temperature distribution in tissue during laser irradiation. Radiat. Environ. Biophys. 15, 277-287 (1978)
6. Fasano, V.A., Urciuoli, R., Ponzio, R.M.: Photocoagulation of cerebral arteriovenous malformations and arterial aneurysms with the neodymium-aluminium-garnet or argon laser: preliminary results in twelve patients. Neurosurgery 11, 754-760 (1982)
7. Jain, K.K., Gorisch, W.: Repair of small blood vessels with the neodymium-YAG laser: A preliminary report. Surgery 85, 684-688 (1979)
8. Jain, K.K.: Lasers in neurosurgery: a review. Lasers in Surgery and Medicine 2, 217-230 (1983)
9. Vankampen, E.J., Zijlistra, W.G.: Standardization of hemoglobinometry. II. The hemoglobin-cyanide method. Clin. Chim. Acta 6, 538-544 (1961)
10. Leheta, F., Wilske, J., McCord, R.C.: Erste klinische Erfahrungen mit dem Nd:YAG-Laser in der Neurochirurgie. Lasers in Medicine and Biology, GSF-Bericht BPT 5, Proc. of the Sympos., Neuherberg, 22-25 June, 1977, pp. 4-1/4-7
11. Polanyi, T.G.: Physics of surgery with the CO_2 laser. In: Adrews, A.M., Polanyi, T.G. (eds.) Microscopic and endoscopic surgery with the CO_2 laser. John Wright PSG, Boston Bristol London 1982

12. Swaasand, L.O., Ellingsen, R.: Optical properties of human brain. Photochem. Photobiol. 38, 293-299 (1983)

13. Takeuchi, J., Handa, H., Taki, W., et al.: The Nd:YAG laser in neurological surgery. Surg. Neurol. 18, 140-142 (1982)

14. Welch, A.J., Wissler, E.H., Priebe, L.A.: Significance of blood flow in calculation of temperature in laser irradiated tissue. IEEE Trans. Bio-medical Engng. 27, 164-166 (1980)

15. Wharen, R.E., Anderson, R.E., Scheithauer, B., Sundt, T.M.: The Nd:YAG laser in neurosurgery. Part 1. Laboratory investigations: close-related biological response of neural tissue. J. Neurosurg. 60, 531-539 (1984)

16. Wharen, R.E., Anderson, R.E., Sudt, T.M.: The Nd-YAG laser in neurosurgery. Part 2. Clinical studies: an adjunctive measure for hemostasis in resection of arteriovenous malformations. J. Neurosurg. 60, 540-547 (1984)

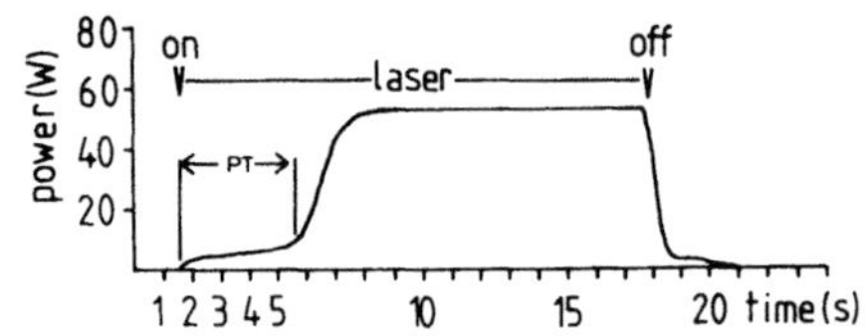

Fig. 1. Irradiation of a tissue sample of a meningioma (thickness 1 mm) with a power of 50 W; laser beam focussed on the surface of the sample (focus diameter 2.9 mm). Transmitted power plotted against irradiation time. During the penetration time *(PT)* the transmitted power remains nearly unchanged

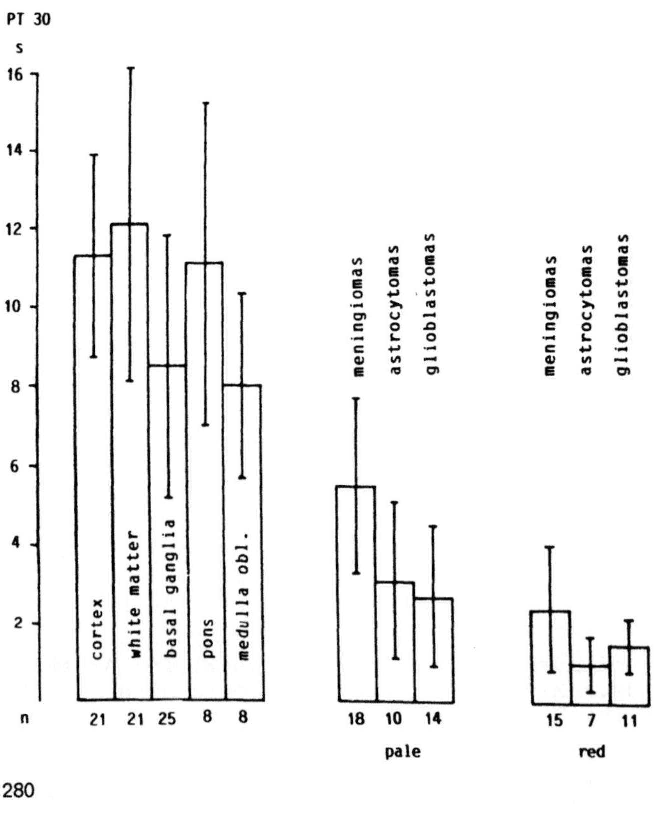

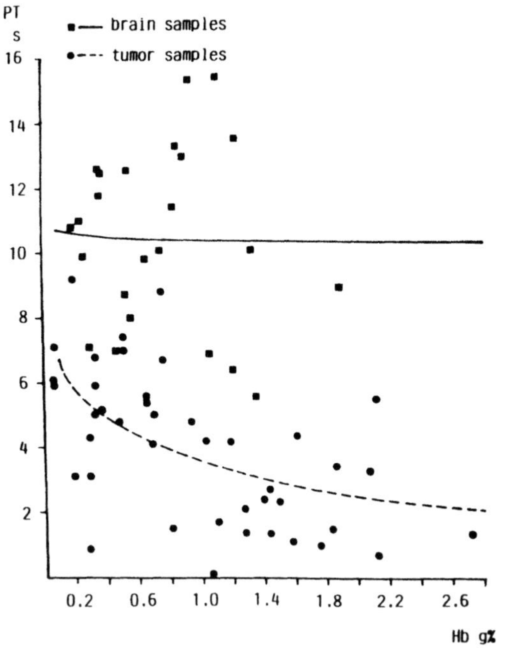

Fig. 3. Penetration time obtained with an output power of 30 W in brain tissue and pale parts of tumor samples plotted against hemoglobin concentration measured in tissue homogenates. In tumor tissue a statistically significant correlation ($r = -0.560$, $0.001 > P$) is evident

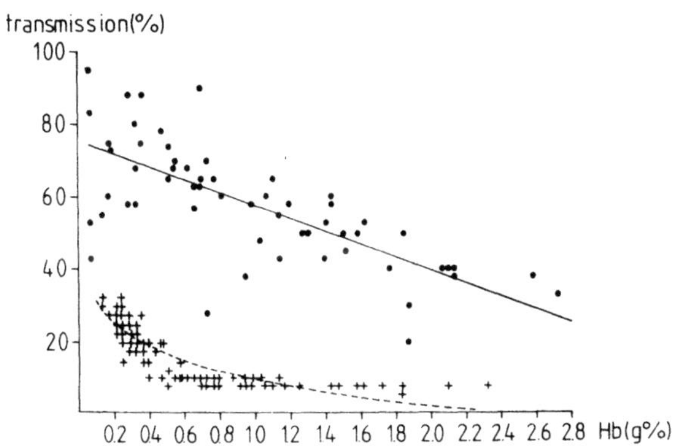

Fig. 4. Transmission of homogenates from normal brain tissue *(crosses, interrupted line)* and brain tumors *(points, solid line)* plotted against hemoglobin concentration. In homogenates of normal brain tissue ($r = -0.881$) as well as in homogenates of brain tumors ($r = -0.445$), there is a statistically significant ($0.01 > P > 0.001$) correlation between transmission and hemoglobin concentration

Fig. 2. Penetration time of brain tissue and tumor samples using an output power of 30 W. Differences between cortex and white matter on the one hand and basal ganglia and medulla oblongata on the other are statistically significant ($0.005 > P > 0.001$, t-test) as well as the difference between pale and red parts of tumors ($0.001 > P$, t-test) and differences between meningiomas and astrocytomas ($0.01 > P > 0.005$, t-test). Differences between brain tissue and tumor tissue are statistically significant in every case ($0.001 > P$, t-test)

Clinical Differential Diagnosis of Cerebral Manifestations of Lymphoma

L. Gerhard[1], H. C. Nahser[2], and V. Reinhardt[1]
[1] Institut für Neuropathologie, [2] Neurochirurgische Universitätsklinik, Universitätsklinikum der Gesamthochschule Essen, Hufelandstraße 55, D-4300 Essen

Introduction

Among primary brain tumors and their metastatic secondary manifestations, increasing attention is being given to lymphomas, which have also been termed reticulum cell sarcomas (3-7). Since advances in treatment have already been achieved for extracerebral lymphomas based on their appropriate classification, the recognition and proper diagnosis of cerebral lymphoma seems very urgent.

Material and Approach

Between 1977 and 1984, 51 cases of lymphoma of the CNS have been recognized among our patients and the patients of various other hospitals[1]. According to Figs. 1 and 2, there are distinct differences in terms of age between the group of patients with spinal lymphomas and secondary manifestations of extracerebral lymphomas and the group with primary cerebral lymphomas. The histological patterns of the tumors, their clinical course, and autopsy findings have been compared. Eight patients underwent treatment with radiation and cytostatic drugs (1). The clinical courses of all 51 cases, including these with radiation and cytostatic treatment, have been followed up to the present.

Results

Comparison of the clinical course, clinical symptoms, and morphology, including topography (Table 1), led us to differentiate four major types (Table 2) of distribution pattern, which correspond to the clinical symptoms (2). Although there may be overlapping developments, especially with the tumorous type, in most patients the disease is confined to one of the four different patterns: (1) tumorous type,

[1] We are indebted to the Departments of Neurosurgery in Duisburg (Prof. Bettag), Recklinghausen (Prof. Kretschmar), Bochum (Prof. Lausberg), and Essen Krupp Krankenhaus (Prof. Mücke); the Neurological Departments in the University of Essen (Prof. Lehmann), Oberhausen (Dr. Lang), Essen Krupp Krankenhaus (Prof. Brandt), Duisburg (Dr. Beneicke), (Prof. Leven); and the Radiological Department of the University of Essen (Prof. Scherer, Prof. Löhr, Dr. Bamberg)

 Advances in Neurosurgery, Vol. 13
Edited by H. Dietz, M. Brock, and M. Klinger

Table 1. Localization of tumorous type of cerebral lymphoma

	Left	Right
Frontal	3	4
Parietal	-	2
Temporal	1	-
Occipital	2	3
Cerebellum	2	4
Brainstem	3	
Suprasellar	1	
Multifocal	7	
Supratentorial	2	
Infratentorial	1	

Table 2. Patterns of distribution of cerebral lymphoma

A TUMOROUS TYPE	**C PSEUDOENCEPHALITIC TYPE**
B PSEUDOMENINGITIC TYPE	**D EMBOLIC TYPE** (angioendotheliomatosis neoplastica)
mainly primary cerebral lymphomas	mainly secondary cerebral involvement in generalized lymphomas

(2) pseudomeningitic type, (3) pseudoencephalitic type, and (4) embolic type ("endotheliomatosis neoplastica"). This explains the very different clinical symptoms, including the CT results. CT is only reliable in the tumorous type, although even in these cases symmetric tumors occasionally cause serious problems. In the pseudomeningitic type CT is negative but the diagnosis can be made by CSF controls. The pseudoencephalitic and embolic types may be silent on CT or demonstrate diffuse spread of hemorrhagic or demyelinating lesions, including true colliquation necrosis. This may cause suspicion of circulatory or inflammatory diseases.

In the early stages all lymphomas react promptly to steroid therapy and some lesions disappear definitively.

Discussion

Manifestations of lymphoma in the central nervous system account for about 2% of the malignant brain tumors in our patients, and we would therefore not consider it to be a rare tumor. Since three of our cases have had a depressed immune response, we may consider that, in accordance with the literature, in all patients with depressed immune response there is a higher risk of developing a cerebral lymphoma than exists among the general population. This means that one can expect an increase in such cases as the use of immunosuppressive therapy continues to grow. The different types of distribution of lymphomas in the CNS and their different diagnostic consequences, especially in respect of the results of CT scans, have to be known in order to establish a preoperative diagnosis of lymphoma of the CNS. This has only occasionally been achieved, but it alone would make possible the immediate use of those special tissue preparations in the operating room which are already used for extracerebral lymphomas.

References

1. Bamberg, M., et al.: Radiotherapy of primary cerebral lymphomas (in preparation)
2. Gerhard, L., Nahser, H.C., Bamberg, M., Reinhardt, V., Wu, K.: Histology, distribution pattern and clinical symptoms and approaches to treatment in cerebral lymphomas. Acta Neurochirurgica (to be published)
3. Henry, J.M., Heffner, R.R., Dillard, S.H., Earle, K.M.: Primary malignant lymphomas of the central nervous system. Cancer 34, 1293-1302 (1974)
4. Jellinger, K., Radiaszkewitz, T.: Involvement of the central nervous system in malignant lymphomas. Virchows Arch. Abt. A (Path. Anat.) 370, 345 (1976)
5. Kazner, E., Wilske, J., Steinhoff, H., Stochdorph, O.: Computer assisted tomography in primary malignant lymphomas of the brain. J. Comp. Assist. Tomogr. 2, 125-134 (1978)
6. Mendenhall, N.P., et al.: Primary lymphomas of the central nervous system. Cancer 52, 1993-2000 (1983)
7. Russell, D.S., Marshall, A.H.E., Smith, F.B.: Microgliomatosis. Brain 521, 1-15 (1948)

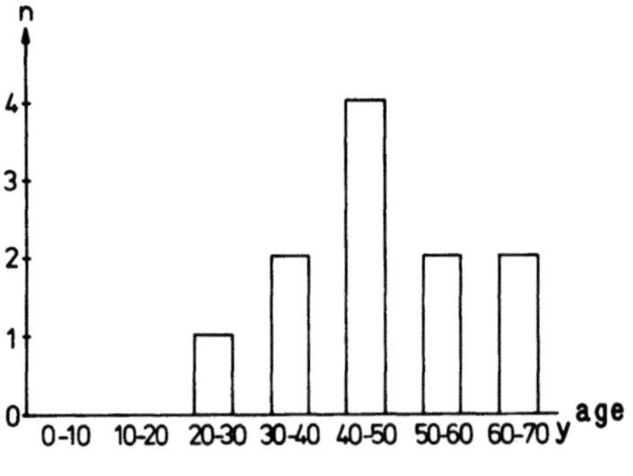

Fig. 1. Spinal and secondary cerebral manifestations, age distribution

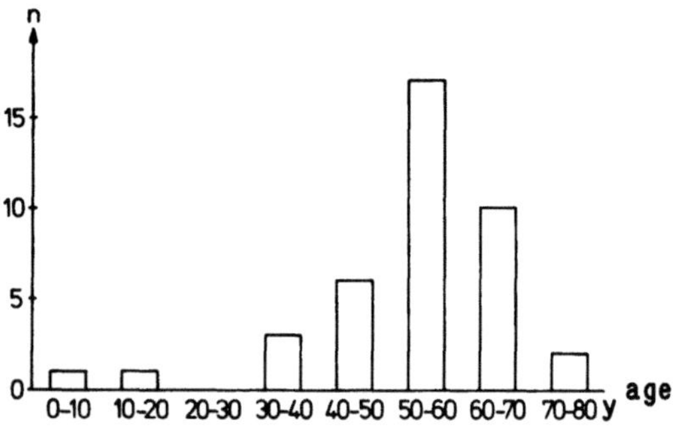

Fig. 2. Primary cerebral manifestations, age distribution

A Computerized Analysis of ICP for the Determination of Intracranial Tightness: Experimental Results and Clinical Significance*

A. Brawanski, M. R. Gaab, and H. E. Heißler
Neurochirurgische Universitätsklinik, Josef-Schneider-Straße 11, D-8700 Würzburg

Introduction

During recent years various groups (3, 4, 6) have studied the possibility of direct evaluation of intracranial tightness by analyzing the height of the ICP pulse amplitude (Amp) without further invasive procedures. The mathematical model (4, 6) underlying this type of assessment requires either the elastance (E) or the cerebral pulse volume (ΔV) to be constant. As recent reports have shown (3, 4, 6), however, these a priori conditions are only partly fulfilled, implying that a *general quantitative* relationship between Amp and E cannot be firmly established. Similar results were obtained by a separate group (8) who performed an analysis of the *ICP modulations*.

Using the PA/ICP relationship and a Fourier analysis on the ICP modulations, we studied the clinical yield of these two mathematical approaches, both in animals and in a selected patient population.

Animal Experiments and Clinical Study

Animal Experiments

An infusion test at different rates in the cisterna magna was performed in ten adult cats (four normal, six hydrocephalic). ICP course and amplitudes of cardiac (PA) as well as respiration (RA) induced ICP modulations were simultaneously recorded, using digital filter techniques for the latter two measurements. The correlation between systolic ICP (ICP_S) and unfiltered pulse amplitude (Amp) was calculated by means of a regression and correlation analysis for the complete infusion test. Furthermore, a Fourier analysis was performed on the two main ICP oscillations (PA, RA).

Clinical Evaluation

The ICP course of 40 head injured patients was recorded using an epidural pressure transducer (5). All patients had diffuse brain swelling and underwent barbiturate coma and hyperventilation (pCO_2 30-32 mmHg). In addition to the standard on-line ICP registration, the PA and RA components of ICP were also recorded. As in the animal experiments, a Fourier analysis of the ICP modulations was performed in addition to the Amp/ICP_S correlation calculation. No additional external volume load via lumbar puncture or ventricular catheter was attempted. As op-

*Supported by grants from DFG (Br 843/1-1)

Edited by H. Dietz, M. Brock, and M. Klinger

posed to the animal preparations, only *short time* intervals were evaluated in this group of patients. The collected data were compared to the clinical status as determined by a modified Glasgow coma scale (2).

Results

Animal Experiments

ICP and PA increased simultaneously with rising intracisternal volume (Fig. 1a). The reverse phenomenon was observed at the end of the infusion test. In nearly all instances of intracranial volume changes, PA reacted earlier than ICP. The respiration-induced modulations (RA) either increased or decreased at different ICP levels. However, no general trend could be established. A significant regression and correlation between ICP_s and Amp was found for the complete infusion test. In addition, a significant correlation between intracranial elastance (E) and the regression slopes (k) was found in the *hydrocephalic* cats.

Clinical Study

Figures 1b and 2 show the clinical application of our models. A significant positive regression and correlation between ICP and Amp was found in over 80% of all evaluated time intervals. With rising ICP, the steepness of the regression slope k also increased. The most significant results were found for the regression line of ICP_s and Amp. It was frequently observed that before an actual ICP increase could be determined, an increasing k-slope concomitant with a still low mean ICP predicted the subsequent intracranial hypertension. At very high pressure levels (ICP > 50 mmHg) a decrease in cerebral perfusion pressure (CPP) was accompanied by decreasing Amp and negative k-slopes. A therapeutic lowering of ICP also resulted in flattening of the k-slope.

The Fourier analysis yielded two prominent modulations, one induced by cardiac action (PA), the other by respiration (RA) (Fig. 2b). At low ICP levels we found RA to be higher than PA, giving a low PA/RA quotient. The opposite occurs when ICP rises: then, PA continuously decreases whereas PA increases in amplitude, resulting in a high PA/RA quotient.

Discussion

Our animal data were found to be in good agreement with the results of other authors (3, 4, 6). In the present study we also found a significant linear regression between Amp and mean ICP (Fig. 1a), adducing evidence that ΔV is constant within a certain pressure range (ICP < 40 mmHg) while E increases. This finding, however, was not conclusively supported by our clinical evaluation of the head-injured patient group (Fig. 1b). A significant linear fit was found for the complete ICP/Amp data set of most patients, whereby an exponential curve could often be approximated as well, thus indicating that two different regression lines have to be assumed. This was specifically observed when high ICP levels (ICP > 40 mmHg) were recorded. These results consequently imply that neither ΔV nor E is constant at high ICP levels (4, 6, 7).

In comparison to all other published reports pertaining to this subject, we additionally studied *short time intervals* in respect of Amp and ICP regression. Usually no major changes of ΔV should occur within these time intervals and the results could thus be explained in terms of changing E (however, respecting the level of the mean ICP; see above). Our clinical results confirm these assumptions (Fig. 2a). The steepness of the regression slope k increases concomitantly with rising ICP, and vice versa, indicating an increase in E. The obtained results were statistically significant in more than 80% of the investigated time intervals. Furthermore, using this method, therapeutic procedures could be verified, decreasing CPP monitored, and imminent ICP increases predicted by a steep k-slope while ICP levels were evidently still low (1). The Fourier analysis of ICP modulation during short time intervals yielded additional data. PA was found to increase together with ICP, whereas RA decreased. The former indicated an arterialization of the ICP modulations whereas the respiratory changes RA, which are transferred by the venous system, were increasingly reduced. Moreover, the Fourier components were apparently not as variable as the k-slope. In fact, a good correlation between the PA/RA quotient and the clinical status was found (Fig. 2b).

Conclusions

The present study shows that ICP evaluations during short time intervals using a regression model and Fourier analysis yields valuable clinical information regarding head-injured patients. While the results obtained with both mathematical models were in good agreement with the underlying pathophysiological changes, we could find no quantitative interdependences between the calculated parameters and intracranial elastance.

References

1. Brawanski, A., Gaab, M.R., Heissler, H.E.: Computer analysis of ICP modulations: Clinical significance and prediction of ICP dynamics. In: Intracranial Pressure V, 186-190 (1983)
2. Brihaye, J., Frowein, R.A., Loew, F.: Coma scaling. Report on the meeting of the W.F.N.S. Neuro-traumatology committee. J. Neurol. Sci. 10, 215-239 (1970)
3. Castel, J.P., Cohadon, F.: The pattern of cerebral pulse: Automatic analysis. In: Intracranial Pressure III, 303-307 (1976)
4. Eijndhoven, J.H.M., Cees, J., Avezaat, J.: Cerebrospinal fluid pulse pressure as parameter of intracranial elastance. In: Wood, J.H. (ed.) Neurobiology of cerebrospinal fluid 2, 643-660. Plenum Publishing Corporation 1983
5. Gaab, M.R., Knoblich, O.E., Dietrich, K.: Miniaturisierte Methoden zur Überwachung des intrakraniellen Druckes. Techniken und klinische Ergebnisse. Langenbecks Arch. Chir. 350, 13-31 (1979)
6. Gaab, M.R., Haubitz, I., Brawanski, A., Faulstich, F., Heissler, H.E.: Pressure-volume (P/V)-test and pulse wave (PA)-analysis of ICP. Methods and clinical significance. In: Advances in neurosurgery, Vol. 10, pp. 367-377. Springer, Berlin Heidelberg New York 1981
7. Guinane, J.E.: Cerebrospinal fluid pulse pressure and brain compliance in adult cats. J. Neurol. 25, 559-564 (1975)
8. Szewszykowski, J., Sliwka, S., Kunicki, A., Dytko, P.W., Korsak-Sliwka, J.: A fast method of estimating the elastance of the intracranial system. J. Neurosurg. 47, 19-26 (1977)

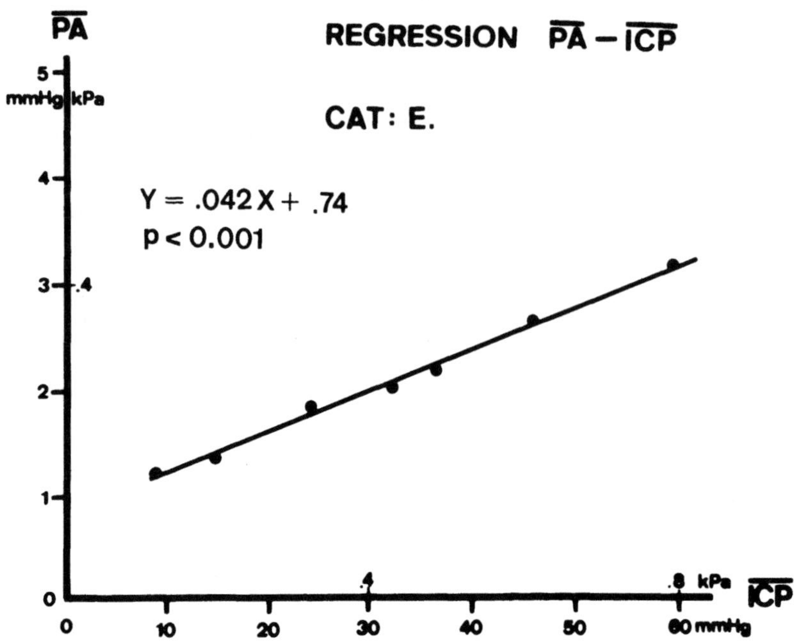

a

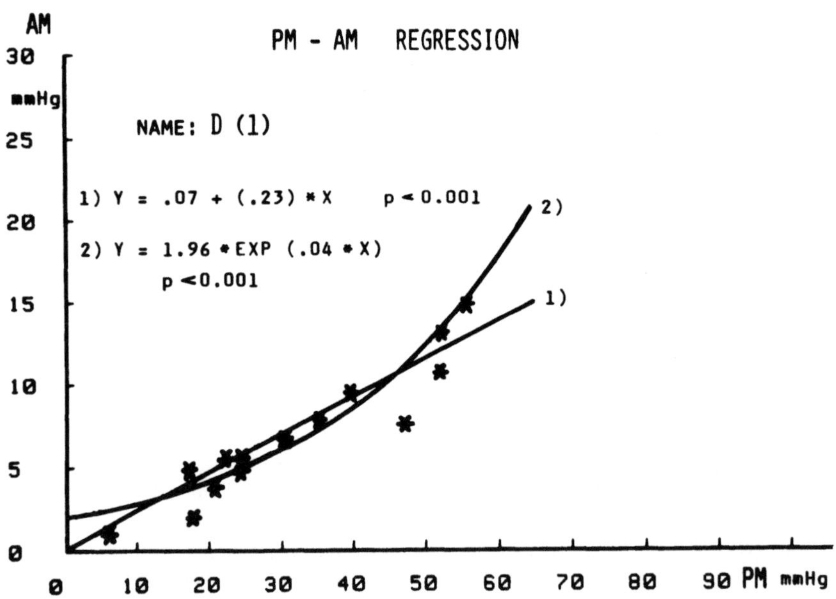

b

Fig. 1. Amp-ICP regression in a an animal experiment and b a clinical study (head injury). A significant exponential regression can be approximated to clinical data as well, indicating an inconstant E or ΔV at higher ICP levels (ICP > 40 mmHg)

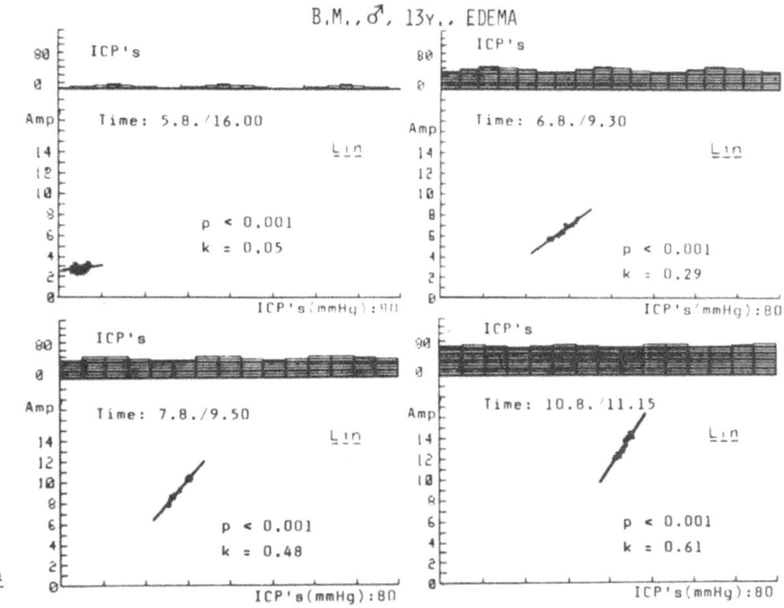

a

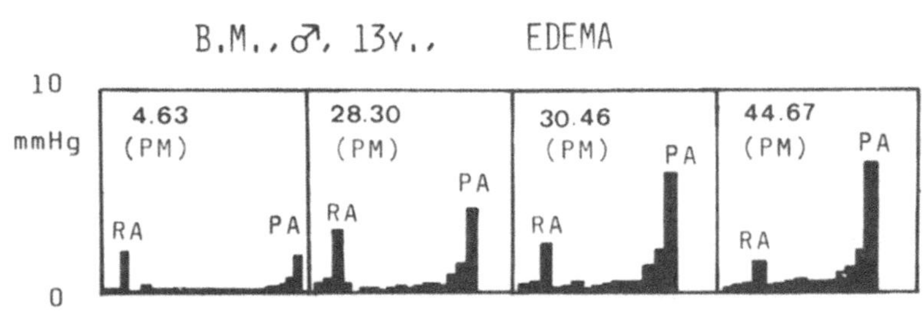

TIME	5.8./16.00	6.8./9.30	7.8./9.50	10.8./11.15
ΔF	0.08	0.11	0.11	0.15
PA/RA	0.91	1.35	2.41	4.29
CLINICS	Coma I	Coma II	Coma III	Coma III

b

Fig. 2. a Amp-ICP regression and b Fourier analysis of a head-injured patient within short time intervals. The regression slope k (a) as well as the cardiac amplitude PA of the Fourier spectrum (b) increase with rising mean ICP (*PM*). However, the respiratory component RA (b) decreases when PM is high. In addition, the time factor ΔF of the frequency spectrum, the quotient PA/RA, and the clinical condition are given

Motor Activity, Intracranial Pressure, and Vegetative Signs During Decerebration

N. Klug, O. Hoffmann, and J. Zierski

Neurochirurgische Abteilung, Universität Göttingen, Klinikstraße 29, D-6300 Gießen

Introduction

Factor analysis was performed to study the relationship between muscle activity, intracranial pressure, and vegetative parameters during paroxysms of decerebration. Factor analysis is a multivariate statistical method assuming the correlations between the observed variables to be the result of variations of few factors. Usually these factors cannot be measured directly. The complex pattern of interrelations is reduced to a more simple structure. Twenty-five patients were investigated during the state of decerebrate rigidity (DR). Change in intracranial pressure (ICP), integrated electromyogram (IEMG), arterial blood pressure (ABP), central venous pressure (CVP), respiration rate (RR), and heart rate (HR) were calculated at 22 intervals immediately before a DR episode and after the onset of DR.

Patients and Method

Patients

Twenty-five patients aged between 11 and 68 years (mean ± SD: 35 ± 15 years) have been investigated. There were 15 cases of severe head injury and 10 cases of acute vascular brain lesions. The patients were investigated within the first week after the onset of DR, during the phase of clinically evident DR paroxysms occurring spontaneously or upon application of noxious stimuli.

Method

In each patient CT scan (2-mm sections) was performed within 24 hours before or after the investigation. According to the width of the perimesencephalic cisterns, the patients were divided into three groups: group I, patent cisterns; group II, partially occluded cisterns; group III, complete obstruction of cisterns.

In each group a subdivision into spontaneous and induced DR episodes was made. In total, 356 DR episodes were analyzed, including 246 spontaneous and 110 induced ones. Details of monitoring, equipment, data recording, and computing have been reported earlier (3, 4, 7, 10). In addition to the already statistically analyzed changes in the variables, factor analysis was performed to obtain further information on the relationship between muscle activity, intracranial pressure, and vegetative parameters during paroxysms of decerebration.

Advances in Neurosurgery, Vol. 13
Edited by H. Dietz, M. Brock, and M. Klinger

Results

Frequency of DR Episodes

With increasing occlusion of the perimesencephalic cisterns there was a remarkable decrease in spontaneous DR episodes related to each patient and recording (I: 15, II: 10, III: 3).

During DR episodes similar simultaneous and synchronous increases in motoricity and other variables were observed clinically but scrutiny of isolated episodes revealed marked differences (Fig. 1).

Parameters Directly Recorded

The arithmetic means and standard deviations of the variables investigated during spontaneous DR episodes are summarized in Table 1.

Table 1. Arithmetic means and standard deviations of examined and derived parameters (spontaneous DR episodes)

	DR-epis.	ΔEMG (J)	MICP (mmHg)	ΔICP (mmHg)	MABP (mmHg)	ΔABP (mmHg)	ΔCPP (mmHg)
I	106	0.22 ±0.12	15 ±9	2.0 ±6.1	117 ±42	9.8 ±19.2	9.1 ±14.2
II	104	0.18 ±0.07	21 ±6	4.0 ±6.8	93 ±22	14.8 ±15.9	10.7 ±12.9
III	36	0.14 ±0.09	45 ±14	11.9 ±7.3	124 ±27	22.5 ±11.4	10.6 ±8.5

With an increasing degree of occlusion of the perimesencephalic cisterns, motor activity decreased during DR episodes. In group III the mean ICP was found to be significantly increased ($P < 0.01$) in comparison to group I, whereas only a slight increase was observed in group II. The same relationship was found for the change in ICP (ΔICP): The greatest changes in ICP and ABP were observed in group III, whereas in group II the reactions were less pronounced and in group I they were smallest.

In all groups during spontaneous as well as during induced DR episodes MABP rose on average by more than MICP, resulting in a net increase in the cerebral perfusion pressure (CPP = MABP-MICP). Since MABP remained high when MICP began to fall (Fig. 2), the increase in CPP outlasted the DR episode. This effect was observed in 87% of the analyzed DR episodes.

Partial Correlation Analysis

Linear correlations between the variables do not lead to logically explicable conclusions because all parameters are interrelated. To avoid spurious correlations the method of partial correlation was used, the results of which are summarized in Fig. 3.

During spontaneous DR episodes in group I, a high number of significant correlations was observed. With progressive obstruction of the cisterns the number of correlations diminished. Several interrelationships were observed during spontaneous and induced episodes. During induced episodes in patients with patent cisterns there was a negative correlation between MICP and ΔICP, whereas in patients with occluded cisterns a positive relationship existed.

Factor Analysis

Factor analysis was performed only in spontaneous DR episodes. Four factors were extracted to explain the 55 correlations between the 11 variables (Fig. 4):

1. Intracranial state before onset of DR episode (cisternal obstruction, intracranial pressure, intracranial compliance)
2. CSF and hemodynamic interaction (autoregulation, venous compensation of ICP changes)
3. Reaction of the cardiorespiratory center
4. State of the cardiorespiratory center before onset of DR.

Discussion

The causative factors that lead to decerebrate rigidity in acute midbrain syndrome are still unknown. Clinical and experimental findings revealed that DR may occur with and without compression of the midbrain at the tentorial hiatus (2, 5, 6, 9). Not very much is known so far about the relationship between ICP and DR. It has been demonstrated that DR may be accompanied by increased as well as by normal ICP (1, 2, 4, 8). In our patients the ICP was always at least moderately increased in those with free and partially occluded cisterns and markedly increased in patients with obstructed cisterns. Our investigations show that cisternal obstruction at the incisural level with subsequent loss of the possibility to compensate acute ICP influences the pattern of reaction during decerebration. Partial correlation analysis leads to two findings: Firstly, there is a remarkable network of relations during spontaneous DR episodes in group I; this network is less in group II and small in group III. Secondly, the complexity measured by the number of interrelations diminishes when comparing spontaneous and induced episodes in each group. There is a loss of complexity of reactions with increasing obstruction of the perimesencephalic cisterns. However, the causative factors leading to DR and determining the reaction during a DR episode are still unknown. The application of factor analysis may help to clarify their nature. Factors 1 and 4 are essentially related to the situation before the onset of DR and seem to be connected with the initiation of DR. Factors 2 and 3 define the pattern of the DR episode.

References

1. Fleischer, A.S., Payne, N.S., Tindall, G.T.: Continuous monitoring of intracranial pressure in severe close injury without mass lesion. Surg. Neurol. 5, 31-34 (1976)

2. George, B.: Neurophysiological effects of experimental intracranial hypertension on three different structures of the brain stem in the cat. Rostrocaudal deterioration. Acta Neurochir. (Wien) 55, 71-83 (1980)

3. Klug, N., Hoffmann, O., Zierski, J., Buss, K.: Intracranial pressure and muscle activity in patients with decerebrate rigidity. Acta Neurochir. (Wien) 60, 155-167 (1982)

4. Klug, N., Hoffmann, O., Zierski, J., Buss, K., Laun, A., Agnoli, A.L.: Decerebrate rigidity and vegetative signs in the acute midbrain syndrome with special regard to motoricity and intracranial pressure. Acta Neurochir. (Wien) (1984) (to be published)

5. Pia. H.W.: Die Schädigung des Hirnstammes bei raumfordernden Prozessen des Gehirns. Springer, Wien 1957

6. Pia, H.W.: Central dysregulation. Z. Neurol. (Berlin) 204, 1-21 (1973)

7. Schepelmann, F.: Human motor activity in decerebrate states and their sequelae. Acta Neurochir. (Wien) 46, 185-217 (1979)

8. Tsementzis, S.A., Gillingham, F.J., Gordon, A., Hitchcock, E.R.: The effect of decerebrate rigidity on ICP as modified by brain elastance. In: Shulman, K., et al. (eds.) Intracranial Pressure IV. Springer, Berlin Heidelberg New York 1980

9. Weinstein, J.D., Langfitt, T.W., Bruno, L., Zaren, H.A., Jackson, J.L.F.: Experimental study of patterns of brain distortion and ischemia produced by an intracranial mass. Surg. Forum 18, 430-432 (1967)

10. Zierski, J.: Extradural, ventricular and subdural pressure recording. Comparative clinical study. In: Shulman, K., et al. (eds.) Intracranial Pressure IV. Springer, Berlin Heidelberg New York 1980

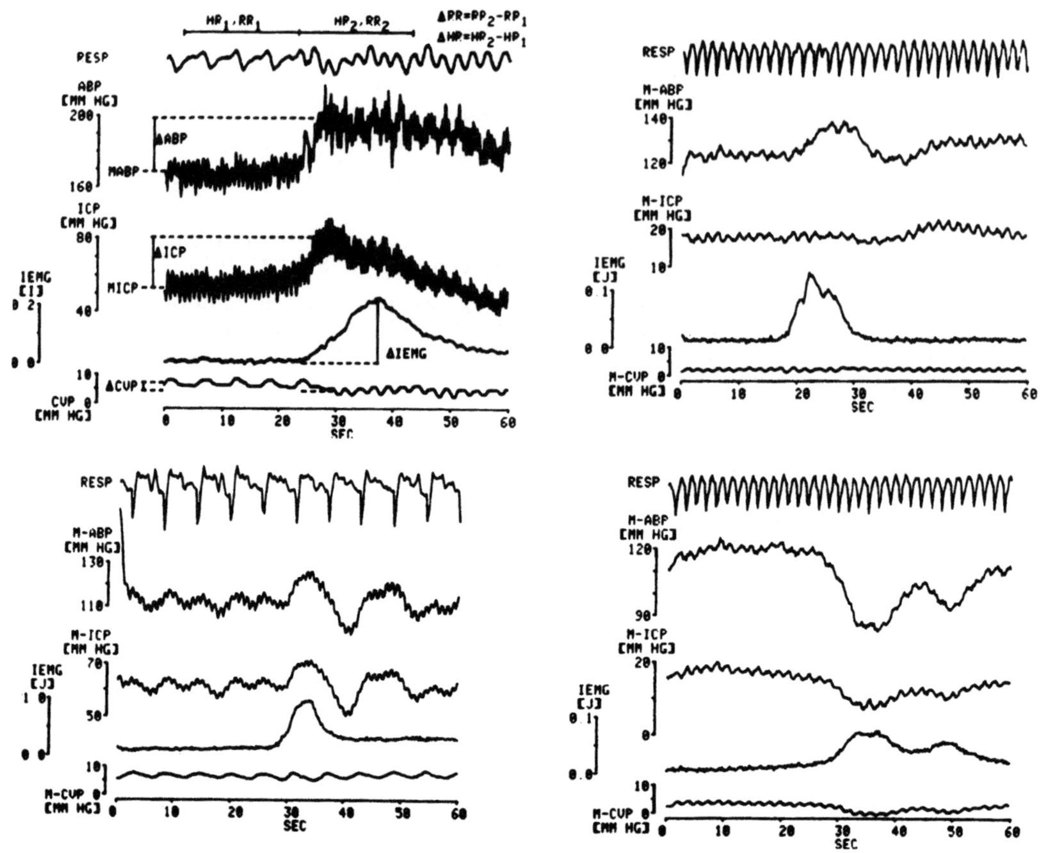

Fig. 1. Different types of spontaneous DR episode

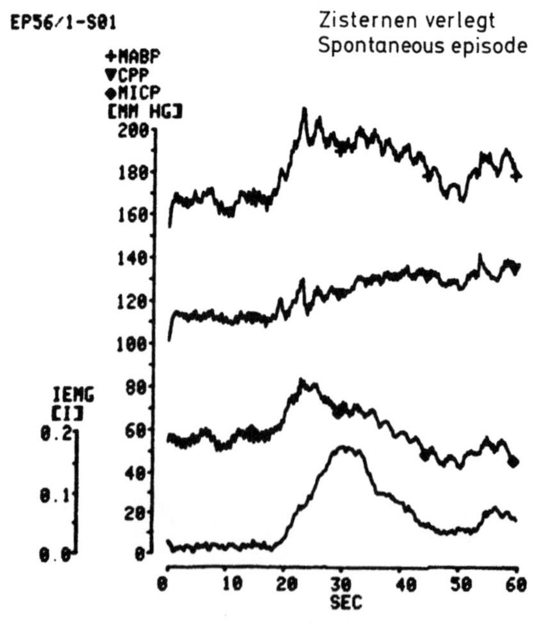

Fig. 2. Spontaneous DR episode (group III). Increase of cerebral perfusion pressure outlasting the DR episode

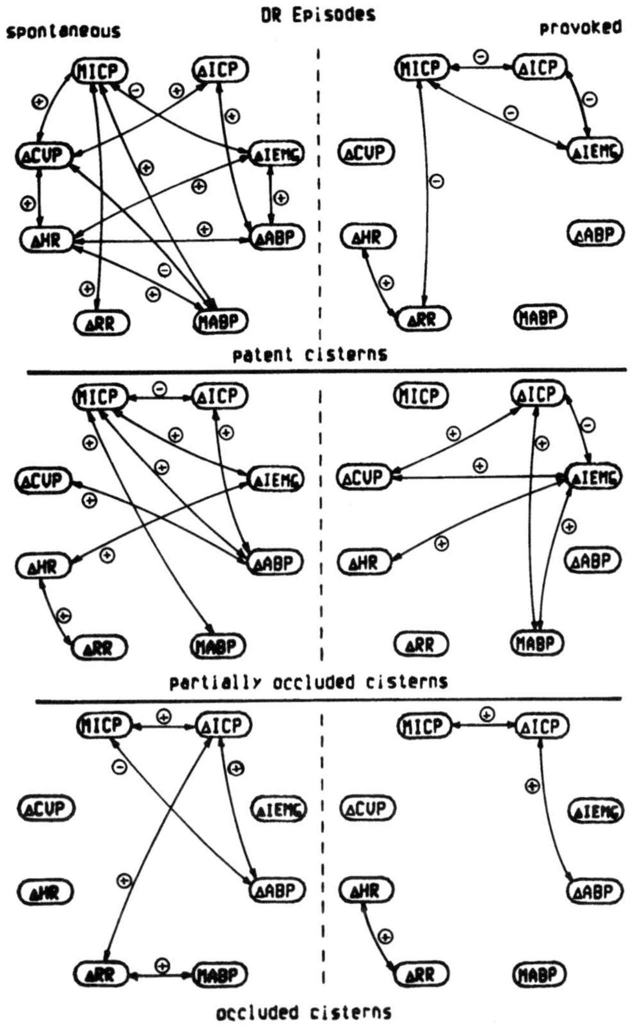

Fig. 3. Results of partial correlation analysis. Each line represents a significant relation at the 99% confidence level. +, positive correlation; -, negative correlation

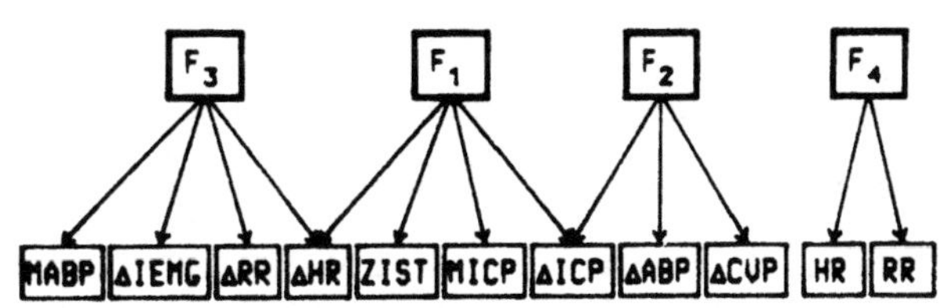

Fig. 4. Factor analysis of spontaneous DR episodes

Pre- and Postoperative Studies of Sleep Levels in Patients with Normal Pressure Hydrocephalus for an Indication of Operative Treatment

H. Kuchiwaki[1], N. Misu[1], N. Hirai[1], S. Inao[1], A. Ikeda[1], S. Takada[1], H. Ishiguri[1], N. Kageyama[2], and M. Terashima[1]

[1] Department of Neurosurgery, Nagoyo University School of Medicine, [2] Division of Neurophysiology, Clinical Laboratory, Nagoya University Hospital, 65 Tsurumai-Cho, Showa-Ku, Nagoya, 466 Japan

Introduction

Among patients who show abnormal ventricular dilatation, those with normal pressure hydrocephalus (NPH) should be discriminated because they have a neurosurgically treatable disease (1). However, NPH is not so easily diagnosed because similar symptoms are presented by dementia caused by brain atrophy within the same age distribution. From the analysis of the pathophysiological mechanism of NPH, the authors have reported previously that the so-called sleep stage of NPH patients is frequently interrupted by arousal responses accompanied by pressure waves (8).

The aim of this study is to clarify the pathologic factors in the progressive deterioration of patients with NPH by means of comparative examinations of pre- and postoperative polygraphic findings on sleep level, including associated phenomena.

Clinical Material and Methods

Case Summary and Neurological Examination

During the period 1980-1983, 19 patients were examined for NPH suspected because of ventricular dilatation identified by CT scan. Case summaries are shown in Table 1. The duration between onset and operative treatment ranged from three to twelve months. However, these differences hardly appeared to be related to operative results in this series.

Other Preoperative Evaluations

Radioisotope (RI) cisternography was performed by intrathecal injection of 1 mCi ^{111}In DTPA. Results of the examinations showed ventricular reflux in all of the cases, including delayed patterns of RI disappearance. Electroencephalography (EEG) generally showed slow waves as the basic rhythm and no pattern of epileptic discharges. Cerebral blood flow also showed abnormally diffuse low flow states (mean 32.9 ml/100 g/min; normal mean value for adult, 49.7 ml/100 g/min) which correlated well with EEG findings. WAIS score was under 60 points except in two patients who were unable to perform the test.

 Advances in Neurosurgery, Vol. 13
Edited by H. Dietz, M. Brock, and M. Klinger

Table 1. Summary of clinical and postoperative follow-up data for 19 patients (+, positive neurological state)

Group	Case no.	Age (yrs)	Sex	Etiology	Symptoms D	G	I	Follow-up
Op. group	1	63	M	Unknown	+	+	+	T.R. → died
	2	59	M	Unknown	+	+		F.R.
	3	68	M	Unknown		+	+	G.R.
	4	66	M	Unknown	+	+	+	F.R.
	5	57	M	SAH	+	+	+	F.R.
	6	43	F	SAH	+	+	+	Died
	7	53	M	Trauma	+	+	+	G.R.
	9	69	M	Unknown	+	+	+	F.R.
	11	66	M	Meningitis	+	+	+	G.R.
	13	63	M	Meningitis	+	+	+	F.R.
	15	71	M	Unknown	+	+	+	F.R.
	16	66	M	Unknown	+	+	+	S.H.
	17	72	M	Unknown	+	+	+	F.R.
	18	69	M	Unknown	+	+	+	F.R.
	19	63	F	Unknown	+	+	+	G.R.
Mean		63.2						
Nonop. group	8	71	M	Unknown	+	+	+	Unchanged
	10	43	M	Unknown	+	+	+	F.R.
	12	53	M	Trauma	+	+	+	Unchanged
	14	68	M	Unknown	+	+	+	Unchanged
Mean		58 (61.2)						

Abbreviations: D, dementia; G, gait disturbance; I, incontinence; SAH, subarachnoid hemorrhage; G.R., good recovery; F.R., fair recovery; T.R., transient fair recovery; S.H., subdural hematoma

Analysis of Sleep Levels, Apneas, and Their Relationship to Pressure Waves

On the third day of 3-day ICP measurements patients were examined using polygraphic methods. Polygraphic monitorings consisted of EEG, electro-oculography (EOG), electromyography (EMG), and electrocardiography (ECG), and respiratory movements were evaluated from nasal and oral airflow, including simultaneous recordings of the movement at both the chest and abdomen. By these procedures apneas caused by obstruction of the upper respiratory tract (peripheral type) or by the stopping of all the respiratory movements (mixed or central type) can be distinguished. Sleep levels were classified according to the standards of the American Sleep Association for the Physiological Study of Sleep.

Operative Indications

A monitored level of ICP (intracranial pressure) above 15 mmHg was evaluated as an operative indication. Almost all cases of NPH showed less than 15 mmHg ICP during the day, in contrast to high pressure at night, including continuous appearance of pressure waves and apneas. Delayed disappearance and ventricular reflux by RI cisternography were also thought to be operative indications. However, patients with psychosis were not considered for surgery, even if the criteria mentioned above were sufficiently demonstrated.

Clinical Materials for Postoperative Examinations

Postoperative follow-up studies were conducted 4-15 months after the last operation. Symptoms of NPH were improved and recovery was rated as fair to good. It is interesting that patients' families reported that the patients' sleep was without snoring and was better than in the preoperative state. Among these patients, six who improved postoperatively were evaluated by polygraphic methods without the monitoring of ICP.

Results

Preoperative ICP Monitoring

Pressure waves appeared in all of the cases. ICP levels oscillated during the day within the normal levels; however, most were raised over 15 mmHg at night and early in the morning. Table 2 shows in detail the levels of ICP and B waves. No A waves were observed. Figure 1 demonstrates the characteristic long-term correlation between apnea and B waves. There are two types of increase in ICP in patients with NPH. In one type, ICP increases during repeated appearances of pressure waves. In the other type, peaks of pressure waves become abnormally high in spite of the normal basal level of ICP.

Table 2. Results of ICP monitoring. ICP level at which B waves occurred with maximal peak and amplitude. A waves did not appear (-)

Case no.	ICP 15 mmHg	B waves (mmHg)			A waves
		Amplitude	Level	Peak	
3	Yes	11.0	6.0	27.0	(-)
4	Yes	8.0	3.0	25.0	(-)
7	Yes	10.0	8.0	30.0	(-)
15	Yes	7.4	22.1	29.4	(-)
17	Yes	10.2	10.2	22.8	(-)
18	Yes	18.3	18.3	25.0	(-)

Correlation of Changes in EEG and Respiratory Movements at Preoperative Study (Fig.2)

Spectral analysis of EEG and respiratory movements is shown in Fig. 2 for case 4. Apnea with slow waves and respiratory movements with fast waves appear alternately. As shown by the power array of EEG, the periodic appearance of fast waves correlated well with the resumption of respiration. The coincidence of fast waves and EMG was recorded for a short period. These polygraphic findings show arousal responses near the peak of the pressure waves. In another words, so-called sleep in these patients was interrupted many times at night and during the early morning.

Analysis of Apnea

Table 3 shows the total time of the data recordings, the number of apnea, their maximal spells, and types of apnea presented by percentage of total number of apneas. In each column values to the left of the slash show preoperative data and those to the right show postoperative data.

As shown in Table 3, a remarkable decrease occurred in the occurrence of apnea and its duration. These findings correlated well with decreases in snoring during patients' sleep as detected by their families. Peripheral type apnea decreased in four cases, while central and mixed types decreased in two cases. In case 17 the sleep time of the patient was less than half of the total recording time, resulting in a remarkable decrease of apnea.

Table 3. Pre- and postoperative results by polygraphic evaluation in patients with NPH (preop./postop.). Maximum duration of apnea is shown. Under REM, + indicates appearance of REM sleep

Case no.	Recording time (min)	REM	Apnea		Type of apnea (%)	
			No.	Duration (s)	Central + mixed	Peripheral
3	480/550	(+)/(+)	79/33	70/42	6 /79.5	94.0/20.5
4	556/480	(+)/(+)	221/36	108/48	48.0/83.3	52.0/16.7
7	473/470	(+)/(+)	37/ 7	24/20	22.6/42.9	77.4/57.1
15	500/500	(+)/(+)	67/42	25/25	65.7/38	34.3/62
17	500/480	(-)/(-)	126/ 3	40/20	54 /100	46 / 0
18	482/480	(+)/(+)	45/34	60/50	44.4/20.5	55.6/79.5

Comparison of Pre- and Postoperative Sleep Levels

Representative illustrations in case 3 by analysis of sleep are shown in Fig. 3. In the preoperative state, the sleep level alternated frequently between stage W and 1, including an abnormally short period of REM, while rarely going into stages 2, 3, or 4. However, in the postoperative condition of the same patient, stage 2 sleep level increased and the number of apnea was reduced. But no stage 3 and 4 sleep was observed even during this follow-up study.

Discussion

The level of intracranial pressure (ICP) is an important factor in the treatment of hydrocephalus. Pressure dynamics in NPH become transiently abnormal, especially during sleep. Pressure waves in patients with NPH appeared characteristically as well as frequently during sleep. The mechanism promoting the transient abnormal increased level of ICP (pressure waves) is not well understood and should be studied further.

The authors reported previously that simultaneous occurrence of pressure waves and periodic respirations are due to dysregulation of the brainstem (7). Our polygraphic studies revealed that each pressure wave is accompanied by arousal responses, resulting in frequent interruption of sleep. The sleep of NPH patients hardly ever enters into stage 3 or 4.

KRIEGER et al. (6) studied the changes in EEG before and after an apnea and speculated that apnea in stage 2 causes disappearance of deeper sleep than stage 2.

There are in fact many complicated opinions about the diagnostic value of the appearance of pressure waves (9, 11). The occurrence of various types of pressure waves is well known in REM stage (2). Judging by our experience in this series, however, patients with NPH do not have enough REM stage for pressure waves to appear. To understand the background of the appearance of pressure waves, an analysis of sleep level is important. The diagnostic value of pressure waves in non-REM sleep should be appreciated in patients with NPH.

In the age range most suspectable to NPH an apnea may originate from many causes. SUZUKI (10) reported that sleep in mentally deteriorated patients contained a remarkably decreased period of stage 3 and 4 sleep. Patients with sleep apnea syndrome (4) as well as NPH exhibited very similar symptoms. Apneas in NPH decreased after the shunt operation. However, treatment of apnea by cerebrospinal fluid (CSF) bypass operation has never been reported.

As shown by ROCCO et al. (3), repeated and pulsating pressure for a long time impairs the ependyma. In moderately advanced hydrocephalus with marked ventricular dilatation even a minimum increase in pressure level has some influence on the regulation of the biological rhythm center.

INOUE et al. (5) reported from their animal experiments that the biological timer in the suprachiasmatic nucleus (SCN) acts as a pacemaker of the sleep-awake state in the hypothalamus. SCN also has a great influence on the whole brain via amplification of the reticular activating system. From these basic observations, the rhythm in the sleep-awake state seems to bear some relation to the SCN and hypothalamus. In patients with NPH, progressive ventricular dilatation and periventricular edema indicating abnormal CSF absorption are intimately correlated with progressive symptoms of NPH.

Conclusion

The prominent finding in our follow-up studies was decreased apnea. We think that the evaluation of sleep level in patients with NPH is a sensitive and precise procedure for the diagnosis of normal pressure hydrocephalus.

References

1. Adams, R.D., Fischer, C.M., Hakims, S., et al.: Symptomatic occult hydrocephalus with "normal" cerebrospinal fluid pressure. A treatable syndrome. New Engl. J. Med. 273, 117-126 (1965)
2. Cooper, R., Hulme, A.: Intracranial pressure and related phenomena during sleep. J. Neurol. Neurosurg. Psychiatry 29, 564-570 (1966)
3. Di Rocco, C., Di Trapani, G., Pettorossi, V.E., et al.: On the pathology of experimental hydrocephalus induced by artificial increase in endoventricular CSF pulse pressure. Child's Brain 5, 81-95 (1979)
4. Guillemault, C., Eldrige, F.L., Dement, W.C.: Insomnia with sleep apnea: A new syndrome. Science 181, 856-858 (1973)

5. Inoue, S.T., Kawamura, H.: Persistence of circadian rhythmicity in a mammalian hypothalamic "island" containing the suprachiasmatic nucleus. Proc. Natl. Acad. Sci. USA 76, 5962-5966 (1979)

6. Krieger, J., Kurtz, D.: EEG changes before and after an apnea. In: Guillemault, C., Dement, W.C. (eds.) Sleep apnea syndromes, pp. 161-176. Alan R. Liss, New York 1978

7. Kuchiwaki, H., Furuse, M., Nakaya, T., et al.: Intracranial dynamics associated with experimentally induced pressure waves. In: Schulman, K., Marmarou, A., Miller, J.D., et al. (eds.) Intracranial pressure IV, pp. 147-149. Springer, Berlin Heidelberg New York 1980

8. Kuchiwaki, H., Kageyama, N., Hirai, N., et al.: Sleep levels and oscillations of intracranial pressure in patients with normal pressure hydrocephalus (NPH). In: Annual Report of the Ministry of Health and Welfare "NPH" Research Committee, pp. 81-86 (Jpn) 1982

9. Nornes, H., Rootwelt, K., Spastad, O.: Normal pressure hydrocephalus. Eur. Neurol. 9, 261-274 (1973)

10. Suzuki, Y.: Sleep encephalography of presenile and senile psychosis. Psychiatr. Neurol. 68, 512-525 (1968) (Jpn)

11. Symon, L., Dorsch, N.W.C. Stephens, R.J.: Pressure waves in so-called low pressure hydrocephalus. Lancet II, 1291-1292 (1972)

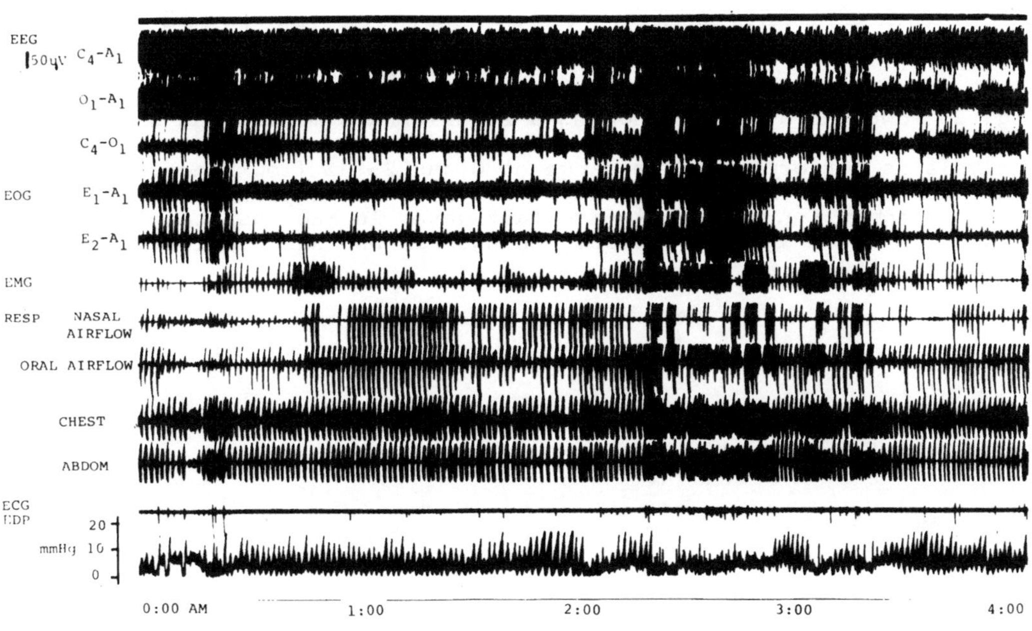

Fig. 1. A representative polygraphy for case 4 is shown for a period from 0:00 to 4:00 a.m. *EEG*, electroencephalography; *EOG*, electrooculography; *EMG*, electromyography; *RESP*, respiration; *ECG*, electrocardiography; *EDP*, intracranial pressure measured with epidural pressure transducer. Time (hours) at the bottom. With the exception of 2:30 to 3:00 a.m., B waves are well defined throughout the recording, with apnea followed by arousal responses in EMG and EOG

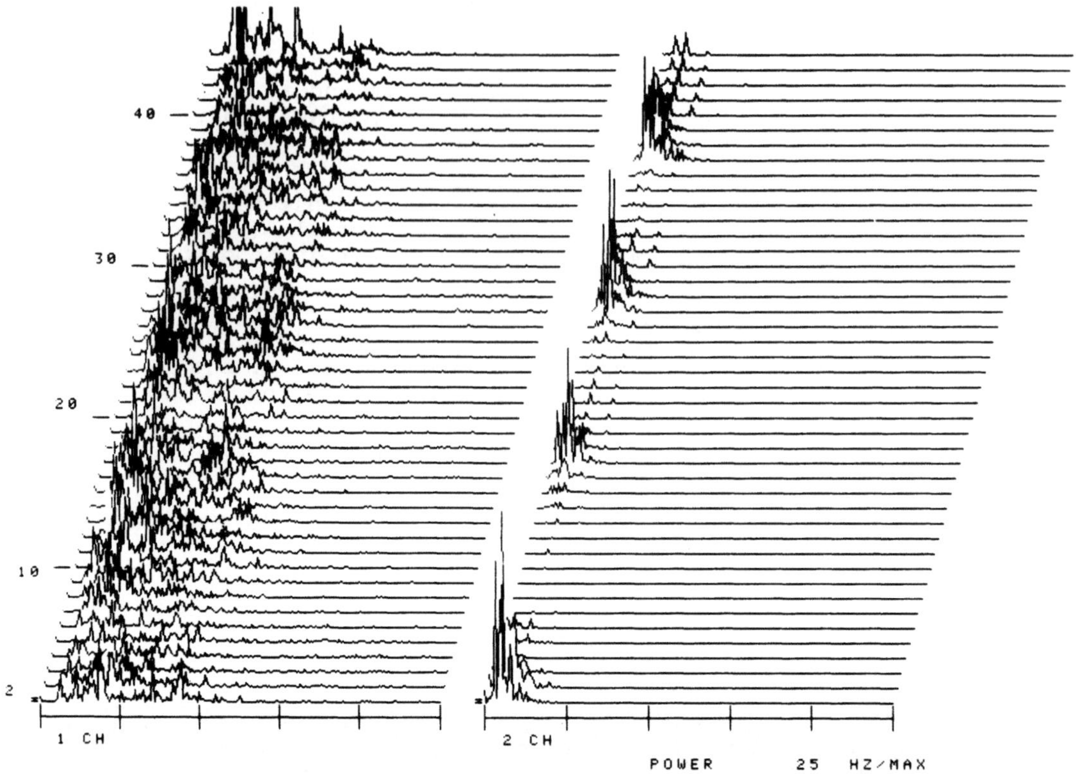

Fig. 2. Power array graph showing a serial and simultaneous analysis of EEG (*1 CH*) and respiratory movement (*2 CH*) in case 3. Frequency analysis is performed over a range of 0 and 25 Hz (low frequency cut less than 1 Hz in EEG) on a line of 8.0 s. Time-elapsed increase from *bottom* to *upper line*. Note relative fast waves in EEG just before the resumption of breathing. Periodic changes in EEG and respiration are characteristic

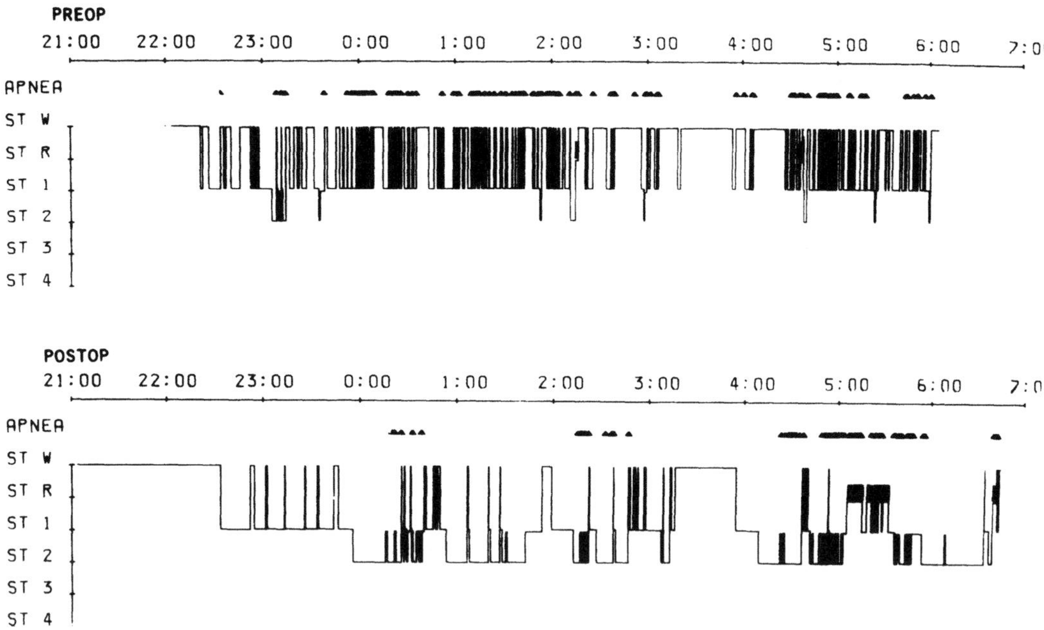

Fig. 3. Pre- (*Preop*) and postoperative (*Postop*) evaluation of sleep levels in case 3. *Closed triangles* show apnea. The *upper trace* shows the preoperative conditions and the *lower trace* demonstrates the postoperative condition. Note reducing frequency in apnea and rich appearance of stage 2 level and REM sleep after operation. However, no stage 3 and 4 levels are observed

Influence of Age, Hypertension, Vasospasm, and Other Factors on the Results of Aneurysm Surgery

E. Kraus[1], F. Scheil[1], J. Hedderich[2], and H. Bünning[2]

[1] Neurochirurgische Universitätsklinik, Weimarer Straße 8, D-2300 Kiel
[2] Abteilung Medizinische Statistik und Dokumentation der Christian-Albrechts-Universität Kiel, Brunswicker Straße 2a, D-2300 Kiel

Introduction

The success of an aneurysm operation depends not only on the technical outcome of the operation. We know of numerous other factors which influence the result; however, we know too little, or even nothing, of the weight of their influence and their significance. Therefore, we investigated the following 22 factors: age, sex, the interval between bleeding and admission to hospital, the neurological status on admission, high blood pressure in the case history, blood in the subarachnoid space, intracerebral hematoma, ventricular hemorrhage, mass lesion, local and generalized spasm, mild and severe arteriosclerosis, recurrent hemorrhage, the preoperative neurological condition, the postoperative local and generalized spasm, arterial occlusion, postoperative hemorrhage, brain edema, ischemic lesion, aneurysm localization and size, and the interval between bleeding and operation.

Material and Approach

We used the data of the Cooperative Study, whose results we presented two years ago (3, 6, 9), while in a position to proceed from 1045 cases of ruptured intracranial aneurysms. Those found intraoperatively or as late as during an autopsy were excluded for the purpose of homogenization of the case material. The remaining 851 cases all had an angiographically identified single aneurysm subjected to the same operative technique, i.e., elimination by clip.

The graduation of the neurological status was carried out on the basis of the International Cooperative Study:

Grade I	No symptoms
Grade II	Minor symptoms (headache, meningism, diplopia)
Grade III	Neurological focal symptoms with consciousness fully maintained
Grade IV	Impaired consciousness with defensive reactions maintained
Grade V	Weak defensive reactions with vital signs stable
Grade VI	No reaction to address or shaking, no response to pain stimuli, and increasing instability of vital signs

The check of contingency tables for independence was performed by means of the chi-square test. The 1% and 5% stages were chosen as significance levels. The strength of the relationship between two variables can be directly read from the calculated corrected contingency coefficient (CC_C) according to Pawlik, whose value always ranges between 0 and 1. The value of 1 would mean a 100% relationship or complete dependence, while 0 would denote no relationship at all.

Edited by H. Dietz, M. Brock, and M. Klinger

Results

First we considered the statistical relationship between the single factors and the result after the aneurysm operation. Out of the 22 investigated factors, 18 were found to exercise a significant influence on the operative result. The computed magnitude of their influence is represented graphically in Fig. 1. It appears that the neurological status at surgery and on admission as well as the postoperative complications exert the strongest influence on the result. These conclusions are based on the univariate method of analysis, where each and every factor is investigated separately. The factors, however, also influence one another mutually. This we investigated with regard to the neurological condition, the most important preoperative factor. Figure 2 shows the close statistical correlation between most factors and the preoperative neurological status. No correlation, however, resulted in respect of age, sex, hypertension, arteriosclerosis, local postoperative spasm, and postoperative hemorrhage.

The influence of the factors on the result, taking into account the preoperative neurological grade, was investigated in the next step because of the importance of the preoperative neurological status. In this way, the sometimes statistically highly significant correlation between a factor and the preoperative condition is eliminated, with only the effect of each factor on the result being determined. This effect was statistically significant for age at grades I and II, the neurological status on admission at grades II and III, arteriosclerosis at grades I, II, and III, blood in the subarachnoid space at grades V and VI, brain edema at all grades, the ischemic lesion at grades I-IV, postoperative local spasm at grade I, postoperative generalized spasm at grades II and III, arterial occlusion at grade II, and postoperative hemorrhage at grades I and II (Fig. 3).

Discussion

Numerous publications have dealt with the factors that influence the result of aneurysm operations (1, 2, 4, 7, 8, 10, 11). Many of these papers, however, have proceeded from relatively small case numbers, thus preventing their statements from being universally accepted. Frequently, the interdependence of the factors is not considered. Very often one is quite mistaken in applying inadmissible statistical procedures if – regardless of the scale analysis and distribution of the characteristics – a multivariate regression analysis is calculated and the computed multiple correlation coefficient is called upon for an evaluation and weighting of the variables.

Owing to the fact that our data were chiefly scaled nominally, the check of contingency tables for independence was carried out by means of the chi-square test. It stands to reason that our results are only conditionally comparable with those of other publications because of the different case groups and the statistical treatment of the data. We have amply discussed the pertinent literature for each factor elsewhere (5).

It is remarkable that both at grade IV and at grades V and VI solely two factors influenced the result in a statistically significant way. In respect of preoperative grades V and VI, the reason for this resides in the fact that bad surgical results exclusively rest on the bad neurological status, so that it makes almost no difference which additional factors are present. In grade IV the relatively heterogeneous composition of the group explains the findings.

The results of our investigation can be summed up as follows:

1. The outcome of aneurysm surgery is decisively determined by the preoperative neurological status.
2. Additionally, it is – statistically speaking – significantly influenced by the patient's age, the neurological status on admission to hospital, and the possible occurrence of arteriosclerosis.
3. Of great importance is the influence of postoperative complications, especially brain edema and ischemic lesion.
4. Angiographic and computer tomographic findings prior to the operation – such as aneurysm size, aneurysm localization, vasospasm, recurrent hemorrhage, intracerebral hematoma, ventricular hemorrhage, and mass lesion – chiefly influence the preoperative neurological condition and are effective through the latter. A statistically significant influence of these factors on the operative result cannot be recognized.
5. Of particular interest in respect of the discussion on timing of surgery is the fact that we were unable to demonstrate statistically any dependence of the results upon the timing of the operation, taking into account the preoperative grade.

Conclusion

The preoperative condition represented by the neurological grade determines the result of aneurysm surgery to a very great extent. In future, we intend to investigate more closely the neurological grade or what it stands for: the disturbance of the brain function. Perhaps it will be possible to identify clinical or other parameters which will define it more precisely and permit better management and treatment of ruptured intracranial aneurysms.

References

1. Andrews, R.J., Spiegel, P.K.: Intracranial aneurysms. Age, sex, blood-pressure and multiplicity in an unselected series of patients. J. Neurosurg. 51, 27-32 (1979)

2. Artiola i Fortuny, L., Prieto-Valiente, L.: Long-term prognosis in surgically treated intracranial aneurysms. Part 1: Mortality. J. Neurosurg. 54, 26-34 (1981)

3. Jensen, H.-P.: Acute, non-traumatic intracranial hemorrhage – Critical remarks on the results of the Cooperative Study. In: Jensen, H.-P., Brock, M., Klinger, M. (eds.) Advances in neurosurgery, vol. 11, pp. 32-37. Springer, Berlin Heidelberg New York 1983

4. Jomin, M., Lesoin, F., Lozes, G.: Prognosis with 500 ruptured and operated intracranial arterial aneurysms. Surg. Neurol. 21, 13-18 (1984)

5. Kraus, E.: Inauguraldissertation der Christian-Albrechts-Universität Kiel 1984 (in preparation)

6. Kraus, E., Hedderich, J.: Acute, non-traumatic intracranial hemorrhage – Treatment and prognosis. In: Jensen, H.-P., Brock, M., Klinger, M. (eds.) Advances in neurosurgery, vol. 11, pp. 23-31. Springer, Berlin Heidelberg New York 1983

7. Paul, R.L., Arnold, J.G.: Operative factors influencing mortality in intracranial aneurysm surgery. Analysis of 186 consecutive cases. J. Neurosurg. 32, 289-294 (1970)

8. Post, K.D., Flamm, E.S., Goodgold, A., Ransohoff, J.: Ruptured intracranial aneurysms. Case morbidity and mortality. J. Neurosurg. 46, 290-295 (1977)

9. Scheil, F., Hedderich, H.: Acute, non-traumatic intracranial hemorrhage - diagnosis and timing. In: Jensen, H.-P., Brock, M., Klinger, M. (eds.) Advances in neurosurgery, vol. 11, pp. 11-22. Springer, Berlin Heidelberg New York 1983

10. Wheelock, B., Weir, B., Watts, R., et al.: Timing of surgery for intracerebral hematomas due to aneurysm rupture. J. Neurosurg. 58, 476-481 (1983)

11. Yoshimoto, T., Uchida, K., Kaneko, U., Kayama, T., Suzuki, J.: An analysis of follow-up results of 1000 intracranial saccular aneurysms with definitive surgical treatment. J. Neurosurg. 50, 152-157 (1979)

FACTOR	CC_C (Corrected contingency coefficient)
Brain edema	0,73
Ischemic lesion	0,69
Neurological grade preoperativly	0,64
Postoperative spasm generalized	0,53
Neurological grade on admission	0,50
Arterial occlusion	0,49
Time hemorrhage to operation	0,38
Blood in subarachnoid space (CT)	0,36
Ventricular hemorrhage	0,34
Mass lesion	0,33
Intracerebral hematoma	0,31
Age	0,30
Postoperative hemorrhage	0,29
Arteriosclerosis minor/major	0,28
Recurrent hemorrhage	0,27
Preoperative spasm local/generalized	0,26
Hypertension	0,24
Size of aneurysm	0,23

Fig. 1. Importance of various factors for surgical results (statistical significance: $P < 0.01$)

FACTOR	CC_C (Corrected contingency coefficient)
Neurological grade on admission	0,79
Time hemorrhage to operation	0,56
Mass lesion	0,53
Arterial occlusion	0,51
Intracerebral hematoma	0,50
Brain edema	0,43
Postoperative spasm generalized	0,41
Ventricular hemorrhage	0,40
Recurrent hemorrhage	0,39
Blood in subarachnoid space (CT)	0,34
Preoperative spasm local/generalized	0,33
Ischemic lesion	0,33
Time hemorrhage to admission	0,26
Location of aneurysm	0,26
Size of aneurysm	0,24

Fig. 2. Relation of factors to preoperative neurological status (statistical significance: $P < 0.01$)

FACTOR	GRADE	CCc (Corrected contingency coefficient)
Age	I	0,39
	II	0,35
	III	n.s.s.
	IV	n.s.s.
	V+VI	n.s.s.
Neurological grade on admission	I	n.s.s.
	II	0,39
	III	0,45
	IV	n.s.s.
	V+VI	n.s.s.
Arteriosclerosis minor/major	I	0,39
	II	0,32
	III	0,40
	IV	n.s.s.
	V+VI	n.s.s.
Blood in subarachnoid space (CT)	I	n.s.s.
	II	n.s.s.
	III	n.s.s.
	IV	n.s.s.
	V+VI	0,57
Brain edema	I	0,77
	II	0,69
	III	0,72
	IV	0,64
	V+VI	0,71
Ischemic lesion	I	0,82
	II	0,77
	III	0,57
	IV	0,57
	V+VI	n.s.s.
Postoperative spasm local	I	0,69
	II	n.s.s.
	III	n.s.s.
	IV	n.s.s.
	V+VI	n.s.s.
Postoperative spasm generalized	I	n.s.s.
	II	0,64
	III	0,62
	IV	n.s.s.
	V+VI	n.s.s.
Arterial occlusion	I	n.s.s.
	II	0,47
	III	n.s.s.
	IV	n.s.s.
	V+VI	n.s.s.
Postoperative hemorrhage	I	0,45
	II	0,27
	III	n.s.s.
	IV	n.s.s.
	V+VI	n.s.s.

Fig. 3. Importance of various factors for surgical results with regard to the preoperative neurological status; statistical significance: $P < 0.05$; *n.s.s.*, not statistically significant

Endarterectomy and Angioplasty in Long-Segment or High Located Carotid Stenoses

L. Solymosi and H. Wassmann

Neuroradiologische Abteilung, Neurochirurgische Universitätsklinik, Sigmund-Freud-Straße 25, D-3500 Bonn-Venusberg

Introduction

The modified balloon dilatation technique, i.e., percutaneous transluminal angioplasty, developed by DOTTER (1) and GRÜNTZIG (3), is a relatively new method of treating vascular stenoses and obstructions. The results achieved with this method, which has already become a routine procedure in angiology and vascular surgery, are very good (7). It has, however, rarely been applied to the cervical vessels. One of the principal indications is nonarteriosclerotic angiostenoses such as fibromuscular dysplasia (5). Although the use of percutaneous transluminal angioplasty on arteriosclerotic cerebral vessels is problematic since it can easily embolize plaques into the cerebral circulation and subsequently produce a cerebral infarct, complication-free courses have been reported in the literature (2, 6, 8).

The surgical treatment of narrowing and obstruction of arteries supplying the brain has made considerable progress in the last 20 years. Endarterectomy of the carotid bifurcation and extracranial-intracranial bypass operations have developed into reliable methods for treatment of cerebrovascular occlusions. One unsolved problem is the treatment of high located or long-segment stenoses of the internal carotid artery. On the one hand, these stenoses cannot be reached via the direct approach and, on the other, bypass surgery, as we know from the literature, can result in secondary occlusion of the stenosed artery with additional neurologic deficits due to hemodynamic changes (4).

Method

For more than one year we have used a combined surgical and neuroradiological method for the treatment of this sort of obliterating process in our hospital. After establishment of the diagnosis by angiography and exposure of the carotid bifurcation, all visible material deposited on the wall and plaques are removed. Inaccessible segments are dilated through the incision in the carotid artery by "open angioplasty" and concurrently disobliterated. A balloon catheter is passed through the incised carotid, advanced as far as the basis cranii, inflated several times, and then withdrawn somewhat. This procedure is repeated until the catheter reaches the incision in the carotid. The balloon is then reinserted as far as the siphon and withdrawn in the inflated state. If the effect is still unsatisfactory, the entire procedure is repeated. With this technique, dislodged plaque is not flushed into the cerebal circulation, since retrograde blood flow washes it out of the distal carotid segment.

Advances in Neurosurgery, Vol. 13
Edited by H. Dietz, M. Brock, and M. Klinger

Results

We would like to demonstrate the results which can be achieved by way of two typical cases. The first is a 65-year-old woman who was referred to us for bypass surgery with the angiographic diagnosis of internal carotid artery occlusion. The referral angiogram (Fig. 1) showed filiform filling along the course of the internal carotid artery. Repeat angiography with an extended series at our hospital showed filiform carotid segments extending as far as the siphon. We therefore elected to perform the technique described above. No flow through the internal carotid artery could be demonstrated on intraoperative Doppler examination. Retrograde flow of the internal carotid artery was still not achieved after a conventional endarterectomy in the carotid bifurcation. A sudden flow of blood upon withdrawal of the balloon catheter, however, washed out a pea-sized thrombus. Blood flow measurement after closure of the arteriotomy showed a flow rate of 250 ml/min. The postoperative course was uneventful. Control angiography (Fig. 2) demonstrated adequate filling of the internal carotid artery and the associated hemisphere. No further ischemic attacks were detectable in the interval from nine months after surgery.

The second case illustrates that recanalization is also possible with this method. The 46-year-old man in question had suffered from transitory ischemic attacks for approximately one year. Angiography showed obstruction of the right common and internal carotid artery (Fig. 3). "Cross filling" had already resulted in anastomosis formation in the internal carotid artery as well as from the vertebral artery and out of the deep cervical artery into the external carotid artery. After removal of atheromatous material from the bifurcation, patency of the common and internal carotid artery could not be achieved during surgery. The common carotid artery was then dilatated with a catheter passed from the femoral artery. A 3 cm long thrombus was removed with a second balloon catheter advanced proximally through the carotid incision. The internal carotid artery obstruction was located in the intracavernous segment, which was removed by a balloon catheter advanced distally. Control angiography showed good orthograde filling of the common carotid artery as well as the internal carotid artery and its intracranial branches (Fig. 4). The postoperative course was also uneventful.

All in all we treated ten patients with such a procedure and were able to achieve a distinct additional increase of blood flow through the internal carotid artery in nine of them.

Conclusion

In suitable cases, a pronounced increase of flow in the internal carotid artery can be achieved with combined carotid endarterectomy and angioplasty; no neurological complications have been observed thus far. The method appears to be particularly well suited for patients with almost total obstruction of the carotid and those patients with extended or high located stenoses of the internal carotid artery for whom extracranial-intracranial anastomosis would previously have been indicated. On the basis of our experience, we feel that long-term controls of this combined procedure in additional cases would definitely be valuable.

References

1. Dotter, C.T., Judkins, M.P.: Transluminal treatment of arteriosclerotic obstruction: description of a new technique and a preliminary report of its application. Circulation 30, 654-670 (1964)
2. Freitag, G., Freitag, J., Koch, R.D.: Perkutane transluminale Angioplastik von Karotisstenosen. Fortschr. Röntgenstr. 140, 209-212 (1984)
3. Grüntzig, A., Hopf, H.: Perkutane Rekanalisation chronischer arterieller Verschlüsse mit einem neuen Dilatationskatheter. Dtsch. Med. Wschr. 99, 2502-2505 (1974)
4. Gumerlock, M.K., Ono, H., Neuwelt, E.A.: Can a patent extracranial-intracranial bypass provoke the conversion of an intracranial stenosis to a symptomatic occlusion? Neurosurgery 12, 391-399 (1983)
5. Hasso, A.N., Bird, C.R., Zinke, D.E., Thompson, J.R.: Fibromuscular dysplasia of the internal carotid artery: Percutaneous transluminal angioplasty. AJR 136, 955-960 (1981)
6. Mathias, K.: Perkutane transluminale Katheterbehandlung supraaortaler Arterienobstruktionen. Angio 3, 47-50 (1981)
7. Zeitler, E., Grüntzig, A., Schoop, W. (eds.) Percutaneous vascular recanalization. Technique, application, clinical results. Springer, Berlin Heidelberg New York 1978
8. Ritter, H., Grossmann, K., Basche, S. Heerklotz, I., Schiffmann, R., Schumann, E.: Die perkutane transluminale Angioplastik (PTA) von Aortenbogenästen. Fortschr. Röntgenstr. 136, 365-370 (1982)

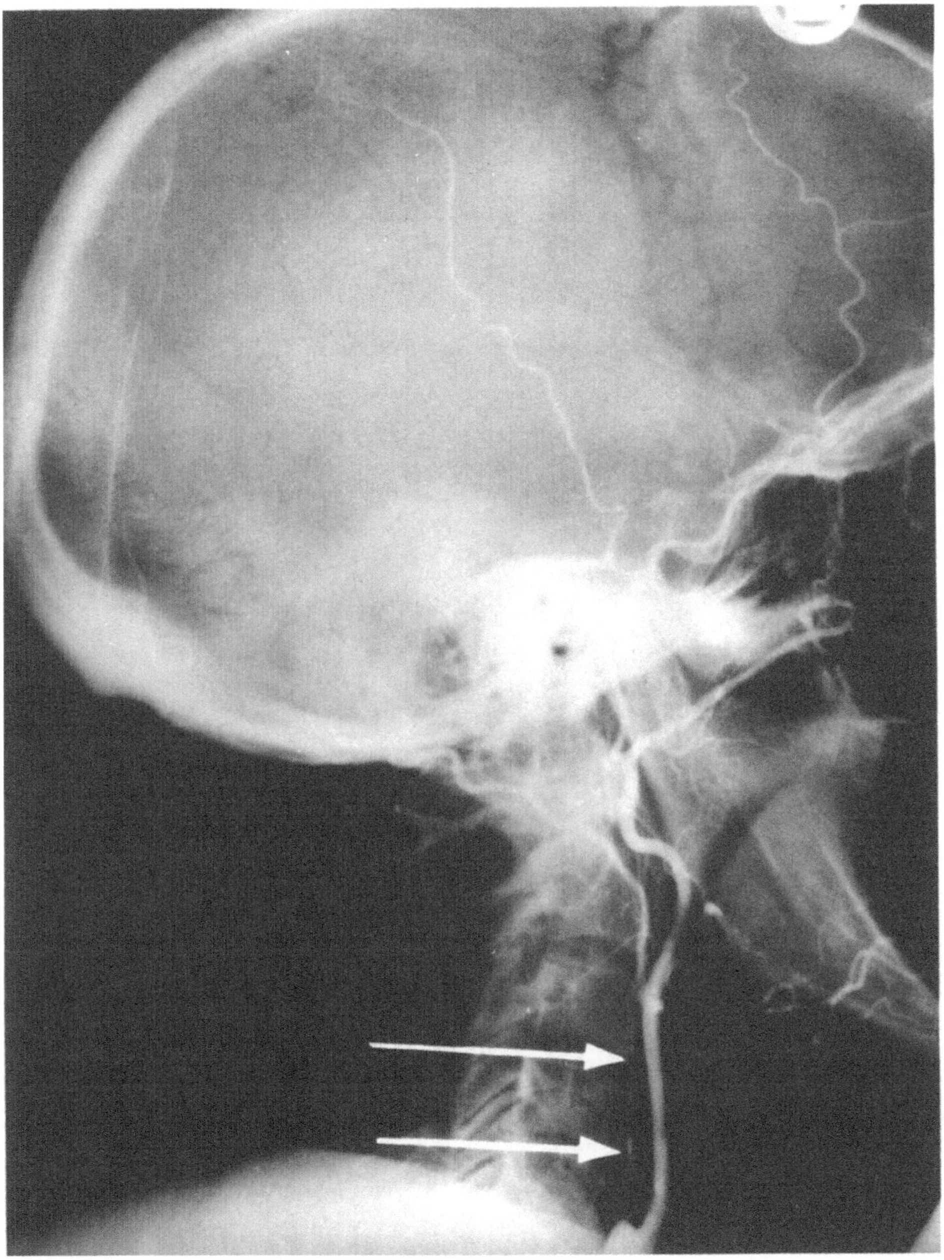

Fig. 1. Carotid angiogram of the first patient. Diagnosis at admission was occlusion of the internal carotid artery. A filiform column of contrast medium can be seen in the cervical segment (*arrows*)

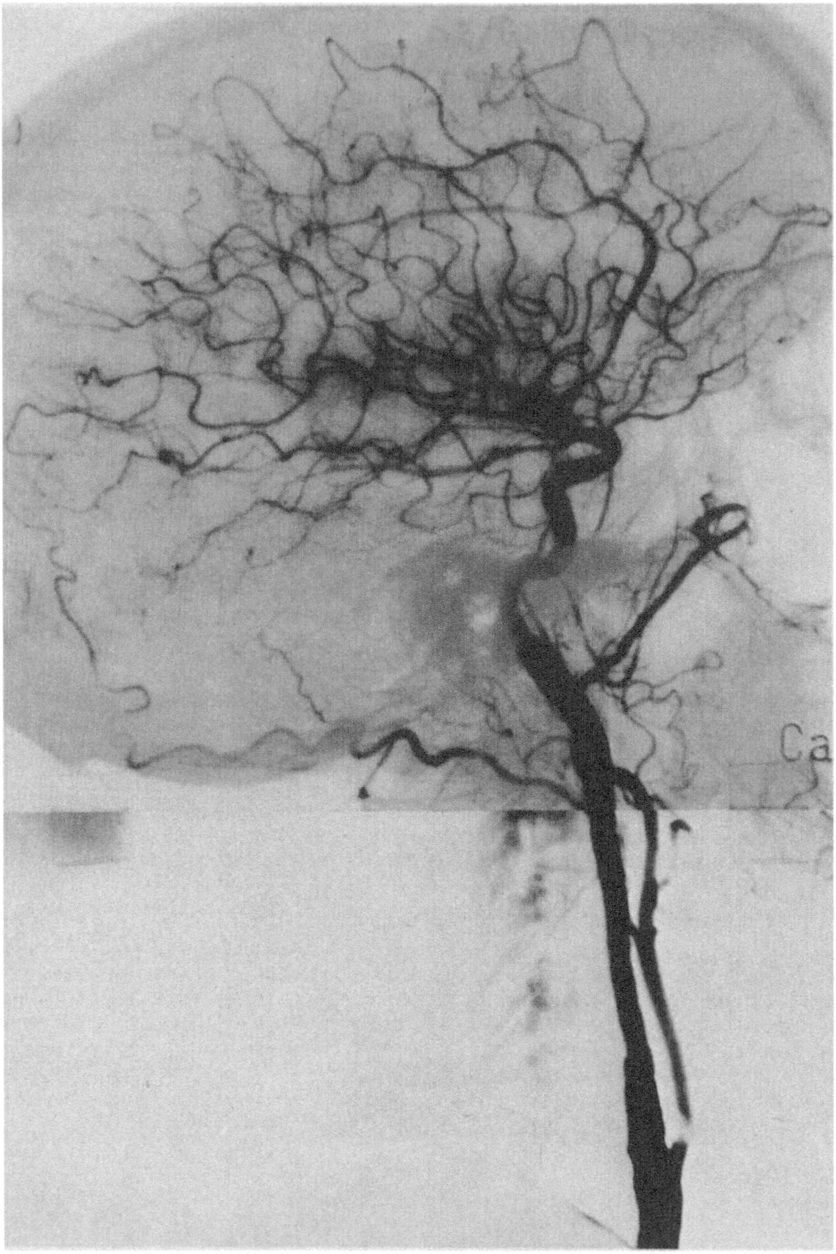

Fig. 2. Control angiogram showing the internal carotid artery with adequate caliber and good orthograde filling of the associated hemisphere

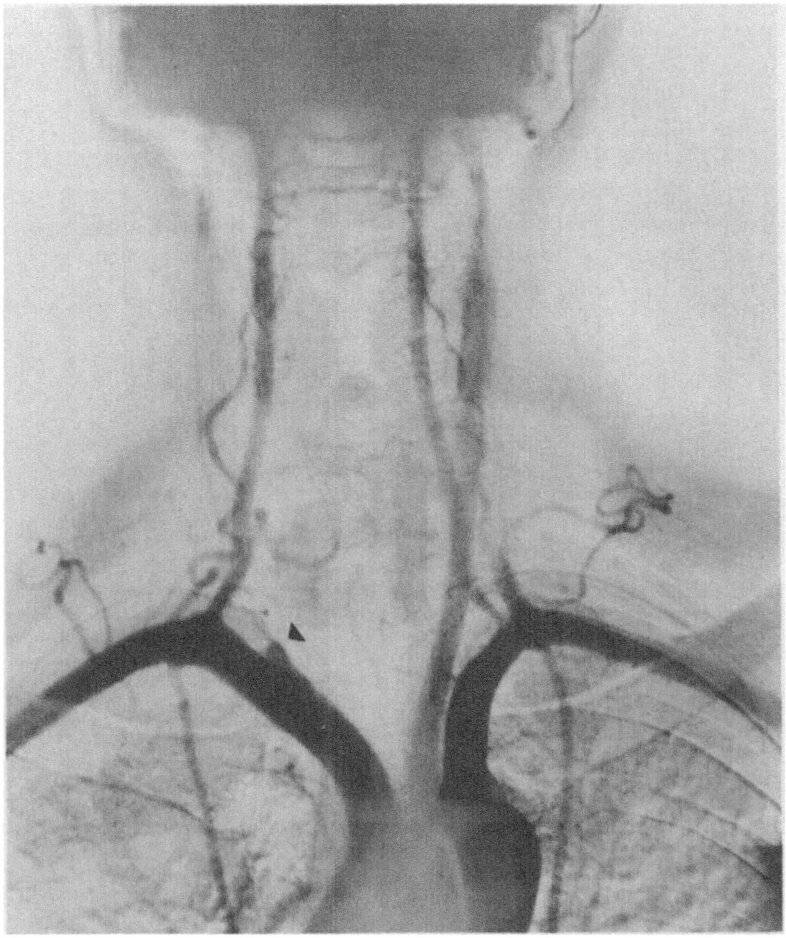

Fig. 3. Visualization of the aortic arch of the second patient. The common carotid artery is totally occluded (*arrow*). The internal carotid artery was not filled even by collateral arteries

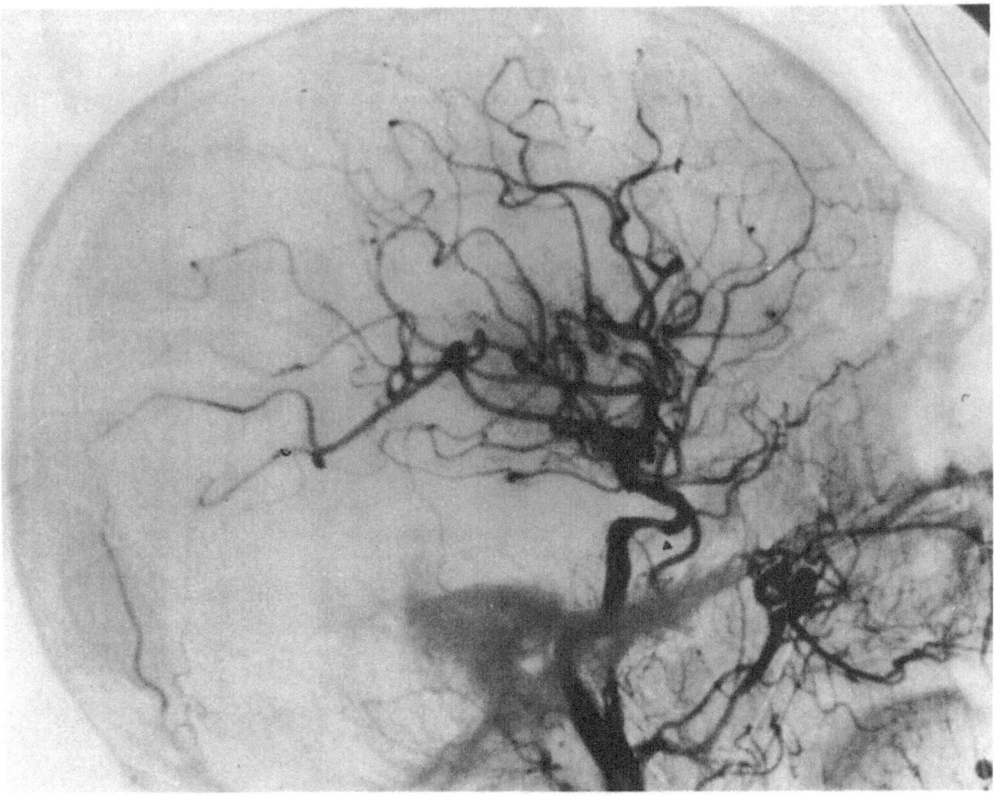

Fig. 4. Control angiography showing good orthograde filling of the internal carotid artery and its intracranial branches

nrCBF and EEG Monitoring During Probatory Balloon Occlusion of the Internal Carotid Artery

P. Ulrich[1], B. Ludwig[2], W. Süss[3], and G. Meinig[1]

[1] Abteilung für Neurochirurgie, [2] Abteilung für Radiologie, [3] Abteilung für Neurologie, Klinikum der Johannes Gutenberg-Universität Mainz, Langenbeckstraße 1, D-6500 Mainz 1

Introduction

Surgical treatment of tumors in the neck and throat rounding the carotid artery or of giant aneurysms originating from this vessel often makes ligation or resection of the internal carotid artery necessary. This procedure carries a 15%-30% morbidity from cerebral ischemia according to the literature (2, 7).

Common methods of avoiding ischemic complications, like the MATAS test (3) and gradual occlusion of the carotid by adjustable clamps, have proved unreliable (6) and may sometimes be hazardous because of thromboembolic events. Therefore a procedure was developed (1, 2, 4) in order to increase the reliability and safety of patient selection for permanent carotid artery occlusion.

Material and Methods

We investigated 31 patients (25 male; mean age 47; range 18-62 years). Twenty patients suffered from tumors of the throat or neck rounding the carotid artery, five from tumors of the skull base, and six from giant aneurysms originating from the internal carotid artery.

In local anesthesia a double line 5 or 7 French balloon catheter was inserted transfemorally into the proximal part of the internal carotid artery and blocked. Angiography of the contralateral side was performed using a second catheter. The motor functions of the corresponding side of the body and the state of consciousness were observed continuously. EEG was registered in all patients and interpreted by additional computerized frequency analysis in 50%. In ten patients regional cerebral blood flow was measured by the ^{133}Xe-inhalation technique (nrCBF).

Results

In most cases we found cross-flow from the opposite side to be greater when the carotid artery was occluded by balloon than when it was occluded by hand. In the case of a 52-year-old man with lymph node metastases from an epiglottic carcinoma, the left carotid artery was probatorily occluded. Angiography revealed poor cross-filling from the right side (Fig. 1). EEG showed a parietal alpha-reduction on both sides (and especially the left) prior to occlusion, and a further alpha-reduction and increase of theta-activity under transitory occlusion (Fig. 2).

Edited by H. Dietz, M. Brock, and M. Klinger

nrCBF measurement showed a flow decrease in the left hemisphere of 30% and falls in the initial slope index (ISI) (9) and in flow in the fast clearing compartment (F_1) to below a level of 30 or 40 ml/100 g/min (Figs. 3, 4). Therefore permanent ligation had to be regarded as dangerous (5) and was avoided in the neck dissection performed later.

In our group of 31 patients (Fig. 5), 17 (group A) showed neither ischemic neurological symptoms nor any EEG changes during 30 min of occlusion. Nevertheless, in two of six patients with CBF measurement, ISI fell below the critical level mentioned above. However, permanent occlusion was performed and no ischemic deficit occurred. In nine patients (group B) there was only EEG slowing. Three of these patients had CBF measurements and only one showed a significant deterioration of flow and therefore did not undergo ligation.

The remaining five patients (group C) developed ischemic neurological signs and EEG deterioration after about 6 min of occlusion. One of these patient's CBF revealed no major reduction, and ligation was therefore performed; there were no complications.

Discussion

Summarizing our results, in 16% of trial occlusions ischemic symptoms occurred after a short period of time, i.e., less than the figure reported in the literature (7). There were no late ischemic complications in the 14 patients who underwent permanent carotid artery ligation. In 45% EEG slowing occurred. In those cases in which we registered EEG and CBF in parallel ($n = 10$), we found a positive correlation between the two parameters in only 50%. This means that EEG changes were seen in cases where neither neurological deficit nor significant CBF reduction could be registered.

Conclusion

Probatory balloon occlusion of one carotid artery has been proved to be an efficient technique with a low complication rate. Observation of the neurological status and EEG and nrCBF registration in the awake patient under occlusion provide, in combination, useful hints on imminent cerebral ischemia, even if no close correlation exists between EEG and CBF and no clearcut threshold for ischemic risk can be defined by this study.

References

1. Günther, R., Süss, W., Kuffner, H.D., Meinig, G.: Ballonokklusionstest vor Karotisligatur. Fortschr. Röntgenstr. 135/5, 532-534 (1981)
2. Hacke, W., Zeumer, H., Ringelstein, E.: EEG controlled occlusion of the internal carotid artery during angiography. Neuroradiology 22, 19-22 (1981)
3. Matas, R.: Testing the efficiency of the collateral circulation as a preliminary to the occlusion of the great surgical arteries. Ann. Surg. 53, 1-43 (1911)
4. Meinig, G., Günther, R., Ulrich, P., et al.: Reduced risk of ICA ligation after balloon occlusion test. Neurosurg. Rev. 5, 95-98 (1982)

5. Miller, J.D., Jawad, K., Jennett, B.: Safety of carotid ligation and its role in the management of intracranial aneurysms. J. Neurol. Neurosurg. Psychiat. 40, 64-72 (1977)

6. Mount, L.A.: Results of treatment of intracranial aneurysms using the Selverstone clamp. J. Neurosurg. 16, 611-618 (1959)

7. Nishioka, H.: Results of treatment of intracranial aneurysms by occlusion of the carotid artery in the neck. J. Neurosurg. 25, 660-682 (1966)

8. Odom, G.L., Tindall, G.T.: Carotid ligation in the treatment of certain intracranial aneurysms. Clin. Neurosurg. 15, 101-116 (1968)

9. Risberg, J., Ali, Z., Wilson, E.M., et al.: rCBF by 133 xenon-inhalation. Preliminary evaluation of an initial slope index in patients with unstable flow compartments. Stroke 6, 142-148 (1975)

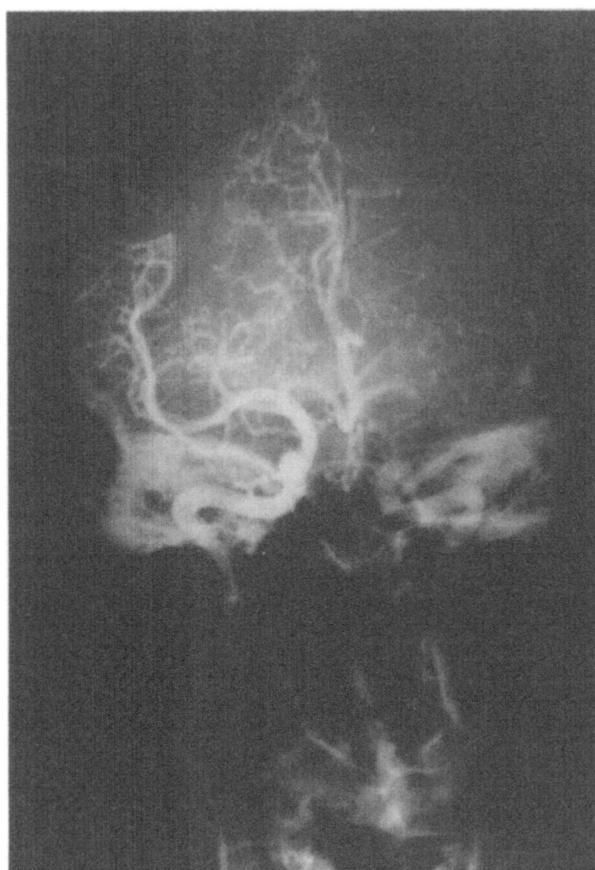

Fig. 1. Anteroposterior carotid angiography from the right during balloon occlusion of the left side

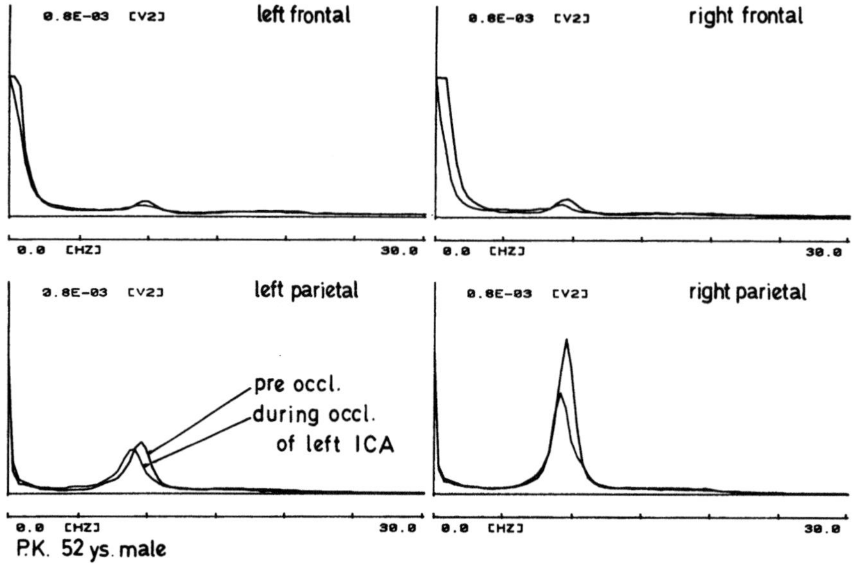

Fig. 2. Computerized EEG frequency analysis

Fig. 3. nrCBF under standard conditions (resting flow); slight tumor stenosis of the left internal carotid artery in the neck

Fig. 4. nrCBF under balloon occlusion of the left internal carotid artery

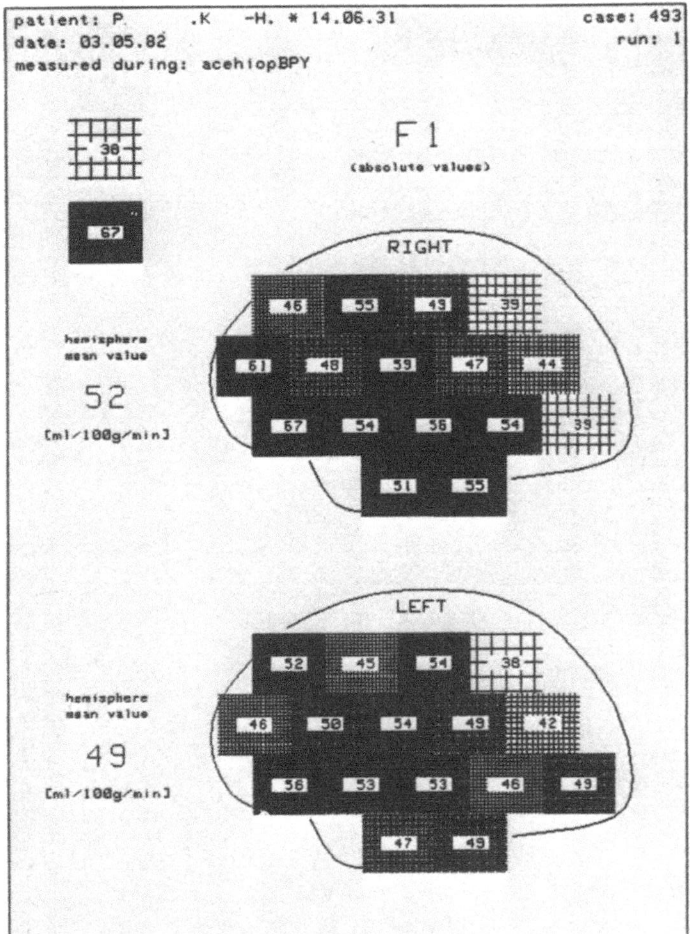
patient: P. .K -H. * 14.06.31
case: 493
date: 03.05.82
run: 1
measured during: acehiopBPY
F1
(absolute values)
RIGHT
LEFT
hemisphere mean value
52
[ml/100g/min]
hemisphere mean value
49
[ml/100g/min]

Fig. 3

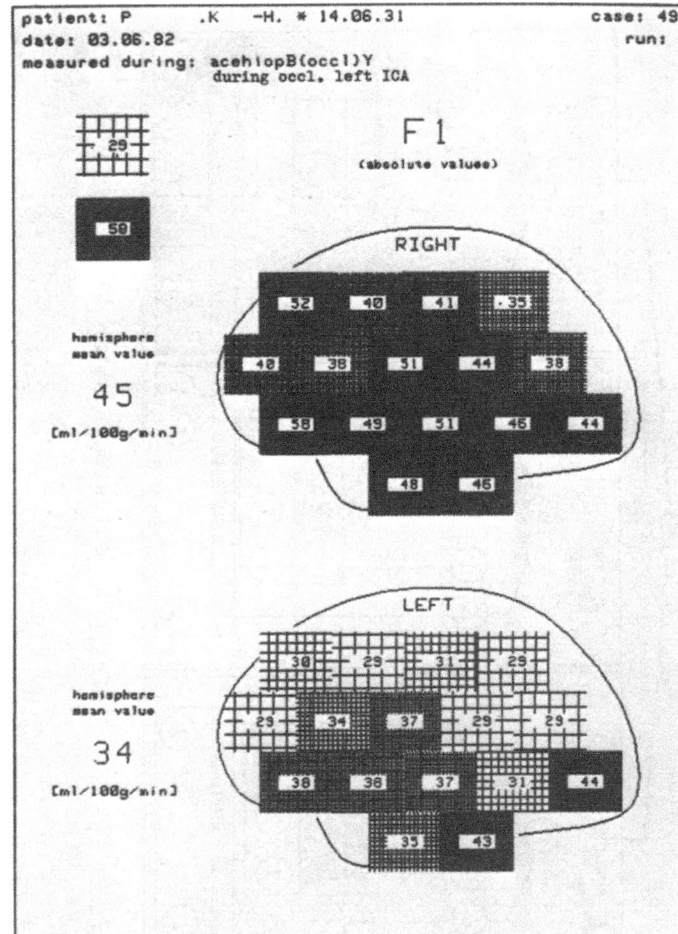
patient: P .K -H. * 14.06.31
case: 493
date: 03.06.82
run: 2
measured during: acehiopB(occl)Y
during occl. left ICA
F1
(absolute values)
RIGHT
LEFT
hemisphere mean value
45
[ml/100g/min]
hemisphere mean value
34
[ml/100g/min]

Fig. 4

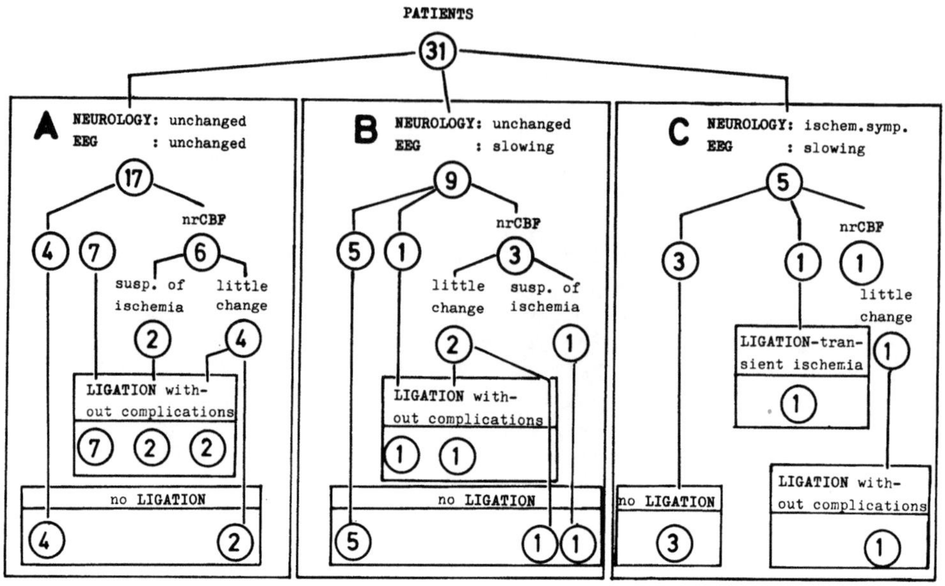

Fig. 5. Results of balloon occlusion test in 31 patients

Effects of Arachidonic Acid on Blood-Brain Barrier Function*

M. Wahl[1], A. Unterberg[2], and A. Baethmann[2]

[1]Abteilung Physiologie, Pettenkoferstraße 12, D-8000 München 2

[2]Institut für Chirurgische Forschung, Klinikum Großhadern, Universität München, Marchioninistraße 15, D-8000 München 70

Introduction

Increased concentrations of free fatty acids, especially arachidonic acid (AA), have been found in brain tissue under several conditions, such as ischemia (9), severe hypoxia (5) or hypoglycemia (1), cold injury (4), and seizures (8). In addition, release of AA into edema fluid sampled from perifocal brain areas surrounding a cold lesion has been detected (7). AA or its products obviously influence membrane function of parenchymal cells since they may induce cytotoxic edema (3). Electron microscopic investigations have shown lesions of endothelial cells of cerebral vessels exposed to AA (6). Therefore, AA and its metabolites may act as mediators of secondary brain damage, i.e., vasogenic edema. It was the aim of the present study to investigate the effects of AA on the blood-brain barrier (BBB) and the caliber of extraparenchymal cerebral arteries and veins when superfusing the cortical surface.

Methods

The experiments were performed in cats anesthetized with α-chloralose (50 mg/kg i.v.) and immobilized during artificial ventilation. Arterial pH, PCO_2, and PO_2 were controlled. End-tidal CO_2, arterial blood pressure and body temperature were continuously measured. After opening of the skull in the parietal region, a fluid reservoir was made around the trephined area using rapid polymerizing dental cement. Thereafter, the dura was covered with paraffin oil and slit. Then, the cortical surface was superfused (10 ml/30 min) with inert, artificial cerebrospinal fluid (mock CSF) via plastic tubes perforating the wall of the reservoir. Subsequently, ascending concentrations (3×10^{-5} to 3×10^{-3} M) of sodium arachidonate (Sigma) dissolved in mock CSF were superfused.

Na^+-fluorescein (MW 376) or fluorescein-labeled dextran (FITC-dextran, MW 19 400 or 62 000) were administered as BBB indicators into a femoral vein. The response of the diameter of pial arteries, arterioles, veins, and venules as well as extravasation of the tracers were documented microphotographically using a Wild Photomacroscope M400 combined with a Wild MPS 55/51 photoautomat. Photographs were taken after 1 and 30 min of each exposure period.

---

*Supported by the Deutsche Forschungsgemeinschaft

Advances in Neurosurgery, Vol. 13
Edited by H. Dietz, M. Brock, and M. Klinger

Table 1. Change of vascular diameter (% of control) of pial arterioles and arteries (60-190 μm) after 1 and 30 min of cortical superfusion with Na^+-arachidonate in ascending concentrations

		Na^+-arachidonate (M)		
		3×10^{-5}	3×10^{-4}	3×10^{-3}
	$\bar{x}$	- 8.05	-10.12	+ 1.05
1 min	SEM	± 1.65	± 1.79	± 3.88
	n	12	14	13
	$\bar{x}$	-12.22	- 9.31	+ 9.42
30 min	SEM	± 3.10	± 2.24	± 4.24
	n	9	14	13

Table 2. Change of vascular diameter (% of control) of pial venules and veins (70-190 μm) after 1 and 30 min of cortical superfusion with Na^+-arachidonate in ascending concentrations

		Na^+-arachidonate (M)		
		3×10^{-5}	3×10^{-4}	3×10^{-3}
	$\bar{x}$	+ 2.18	- 0.35	- 1.62
1 min	SEM	± 1.72	± 1.76	± 3.41
	n	14	15	11
	$\bar{x}$	- 2.34	- 3.77	- 2.82
30 min	SEM	± 2.22	± 2.89	± 2.92
	n	10	16	9

Results and Discussion

Table 1 summarizes the effect of AA on the diameter of pial arteries and arterioles with a resting diameter of 60-190 μm. At concentrations of 3×10^{-5} and 3×10^{-4} M AA induced a reduction of diameter by about 10% after 1 and 30 min of cortical superfusion. This is in disagreement with the findings of others (2, 10) who reported dilatation of feline pial arteries at 3.3 to 6.6×10^{-4} M AA. In the present study an increase of arterial diameter by about 10% was only found after 30 min superfusion with 3×10^{-3} M AA.

As shown in Table 2, the diameter of cerebral veins with a resting diameter of 70-190 μm was not changed by administration of AA, either after 1 or after 30 min.

During the control periods (superfusion with mock CSF), no leakage of any BBB indicators was observed. AA, however, caused extravasation of the tracers used. Fluorescent spots were first detected adjacent to small veins, but later a diffuse fluorescence was observed within the parenchyma. Penetration of Na^+-fluorescein into the parenchyma was induced by AA in 28.5% of the experiments at 3×10^{-5} M, in 43% at 3×10^{-4} M, and in 28.5% at 3×10^{-3} M. Leakage of FITC-dextran was only detected at 3×10^{-3} M AA.

Conclusions

Superfusion of the parietal cortex with mock CSF containing AA induced extravasation of intravascularly applied fluorescent tracers without markedly changing vessel diameter. Therefore, we conclude that leakage of the markers is caused by an increase of BBB permeability. We suggest that large functional pores are opened since penetration of tracers with an MW up to 62 000 was found. These results support the hypothesis that AA released in damaged brain is involved in the formation of BBB dysfunction.

References

1. Agardh, C.D., Siesjö, B.K.: Hypoglycemic brain injury: phospholipids, free fatty acids and cyclic nucleotides in the cerebellum of the rat after 30 and 60 minutes of severe insulin-induced hypoglycemia. J. Cereb. Blood Flow Metabol. 1, 267-275 (1981)
2. Busija, D.W., Heistad, D.: Effects of indomethacin on cerebral blood flow during hypercapnia in cats. Am. J. Physiol. 244, H519-H524 (1983)
3. Chan, P.H., Fishman, R.A.: Brain edema: induction in cortical slices by polyunsaturated fatty acids. Science 201, 358-360 (1978)
4. Chan, P.H., Fishman, R.A.: Phospholipid degradation and the early release of polyunsaturated fatty acids in the evolution of brain edema. In: Go, K.G., Baethmann, A. (eds.) Recent progress in the study and therapy of brain edema, pp. 193-202. Plenum Press, New York 1984
5. Gardiner, M., Nilsson, B., Rehncrona, S., Siesjö, B.K.: Free fatty acids in the rat brain in moderate and severe hypoxia. J. Neurochem. 36, 1500-1505 (1981)
6. Kontos, H.A., Wei, E.P., Povlishock, J.T., Dietrich, W.D., Magiera, C.J., Ellis, E.F.: Cerebral arteriolar damage by arachidonic acid and prostaglandin G_2. Science 209, 1242-1245 (1980)
7. Maier-Hauff, K., Lange, M., Schürer, L., Guggenbichler, C., Vogt, W., Jacob, K., Baethmann, A.: Glutamate and free fatty acid concentrations in extracellular vasogenic edema fluid. In: Go, K.G., Baethmann, A. (eds.) Recent progress in the study and therapy of brain edema, pp. 183-192. Plenum Press, New York 1984
8. Siesjö, B.K., Ingvar, M., Westerberg, E.: The influence of bicuculline-induced seizures on free fatty acid concentrations in cerebral cortex, hippocampus, and cerebellum. J. Neurochem. 39, 796-802 (1982)
9. Shiu, K.G., Nemmer, J.P., Nemoto, E.M.: Reassessment of brain free fatty acid liberation during global ischemia and its attenuation by barbiturate anesthesia. J. Neurochem. 40, 880-884 (1983)
10. Wei, E.P., Ellis, E.F., Kontos, H.A.: Role of prostaglandins in pial arteriolar response to CO_2 and hypoxia. Am. J. Physiol. 238, H226-H230 (1980)

Blood Flow, Metabolism, and Function of the Brain During Cerebral Administration of Bradykinin*

A. Unterberg, U. Hack, and A. Baethmann

Institut für Chirurgische Forschung, Klinikum Großhadern, Universität München, Marchioninistraße 15, D-8000 München 70

Introduction

The kallikrein-kinin system is considered a mediator of secondary brain damage, e.g., evolving from traumatic lesions or cerebral ischemia (1). The kinin peptides are powerful dilatory substances of the peripheral vasculature and they increase its permeability (3, 6). Activation of the system and release of kinins occur in tissue injury associated with coagulation and inflammation (3, 6). Evidence of pathophysiological effects in the CNS induced by kinins has been provided. Superfusion of cerebral cortex with bradykinin opens the blood-brain barrier to small molecules and dilates cerebral arteries (8, 10). Moreover, ventricle perfusion with bradykinin was found to cause cerebral edema, and focal injury of the brain to result in cerebral uptake of plasma kininogens and formation of kinins (5, 7).

In the current experiments, cerebral blood flow and metabolism were assessed together with the electrical activity of the brain during cerebral administration of bradykinin by ventriculocisternal perfusion. The electrical impedance of brain tissue was determined in addition as a measure of the extra-intracellular fluid distribution.

Methods

The experiments were conducted in mongrel cats (3-3.5 kg b.w.) under chloralose anesthesia (50 mg/kg b.w.). Ventriculocisternal perfusion of the brain commenced with artificial cerebrospinal fluid at a flow rate of 0.4 ml/min. After a control period of 1 h, perfusion continued with either mock CSF (controls) or with bradykinin (3 μM) dissolved in experimental animals for 3 h.

Cerebral blood flow was measured as clearance of ^{133}Xe injected into the lingual artery. CBF measurements, including a test of the CO_2 reactivity, were made during the control period. CBF was then measured at 5, 30, and 180 min after the start of perfusion with bradykinin. The flow studies were combined with determinations of the cerebral O_2 and glucose uptake. For that purpose, O_2 and glucose were analyzed in arterial and cerebrovenous blood. EEG was carried out at 30-min intervals as 1-min samples by two frontal and occipital electrodes placed on the dura. Tissue impedance was measured every 5 min using an R-C

---

*Supported by Deutsche Forschungsgemeinschaft (Ba 452/6-3)

Edited by H. Dietz, M. Brock, and M. Klinger

bridge. Blood pressure, intracranial pressure, temperature, and blood gases were continuously monitored throughout the experiment.

Results and Discussion

Cerebral Blood Flow and Metabolism

Five minutes after the start of ventricle perfusion with mock CSF or bradykinin, CBF fell somewhat in both groups for no obvious reasons. Then, however, CBF increased significantly in experimental animals, exceeding the initial control value at 3 h (Table 1). Control animals also had a tendency to normalization of blood flow, which, however, was less pronounced than in experimental animals.

Both the control and the experimental preparations had a tendency to increase oxygen uptake with recovery from anesthesia, whereas the cerebral glucose consumption was clearly different between the two groups. Cerebral administration of bradykinin led to a marked stimulation of cerebral glucose uptake, to 217% of what was found during the initial control period (Table 2). In controls, the glucose uptake remained largely unchanged throughout the experiment. Stimulation of glucose uptake into brain tisse by bradykinin is in agreement with findings on glucose consumption by muscle tissue in man (2).

Electrical Function

Contrary to the findings on cerebral uptake of glucose secondary to ventriculocisternal perfusion with bradykinin, the peptide was found to depress the EEG activity as demonstrated by power spectrographic analysis. Depression of the EEG was particularly prominent 30 min and 1 h after the start of perfusion with bradykinin; it became attenuated with the further experimental course (9). Depression of nervous activity by kinins was also found in other studies, where it was attributed to kinin metabolites rather than to the peptide itself (4).

Electrical Tissue Impedance

Figure 1 gives the electrical conductivity of brain tissue (i.e., the reciprocal of impedance) in a control and an experimental animal during bradykinin perfusion. After impalement of the electrodes into the brain tissue, the electrical conductivity rose initially until a constant level was reached. In the control animal (Fig. 1, top) conductivity remained largely stable during the remaining experimental observation period. On the other hand, ventriculocisternal perfusion with bradykinin was observed to induce a further rise in conductivity until the end of the experiment. It is considered that this response, i.e., a decrease of impedance secondary to bradykinin, probably results from an expansion of the extracellular fluid space indicative of interstitial brain edema.

Summary and Conclusions

Cerebral administration of bradykinin by ventriculocisternal perfusion led to a marked increase of the cerebral glucose uptake, whereas blood flow and oxygen consumption were only marginally affected. Bradykinin was found to depress transiently the cerebral electrical activity as concluded from a delay in recovery of the EEG power during anesthesia.

Table 1. Cerebral blood flow (ml/100 g per minute; mean ± SEM) during ventriculocisternal perfusion with bradykinin or mock CSF (controls)

	Control phase	5 min	30 min	180 min
Mock CSF	28.6 ±1.0 (n = 10)	25.2[a] ±1.6 (n = 6)	25.5 ±1.3 (n = 10)	27.3 ±1.0 (n = 9)
Bradykinin	27.1 ±1.3 (n = 9)	25.2 ±1.8 (n = 9)	26.1 ±1.1 (n = 8)	30.2[a] ±1.7 (n = 9)

[a]$P < 0.05$ (compared to control phase)

Table 2. Cerebral glucose consumption (mean ± SEM) in percent of the initial value obtained in the control phase during ventriculocisternal perfusion with bradykinin or mock CSF (controls)

	5 min	30 min	180 min
Mock CSF	109.0 ±17.1 (n = 6)	96.9 ±16.2 (n = 10)	100.1[a] ±19.2 (n = 9)
Bradykinin	120.4 ±21.8 (n = 9)	201.3[b] ±40.9 (n = 8)	217.2[a,c] ±46.9 (n = 9)

[a]$P < 0.05$ (comparison between control and bradykinin-perfused experiments)

[b]$P < 0.05$ (compared to the initial control value)

[c]$P < 0.02$ (compared to the initial control value)

The electrical tissue impedance was found to decrease specifically in experimental animals, this being indicative of interstitial fluid accumulation. The latter finding provides further support for edema-inducing properties of kinins in central nervous tissue, increasing the probability that the kallikrein-kinin system has a mediator function in an acute cerebral process. Moreover, enhancement of the cerebral glucose uptake by kinins may result in an energy failure of the brain when the cerebral blood flow is liable to become decreased.

Acknowledgments. The excellent technical and secretarial assistance of Ruth Demmer, Ulrike Goerke, and Angelika Konrad is greatly appreciated.

References

1. Baethmann, A., Kempski, O., Unterberg, A., Maier-Hauff, K., Lange, M., Schürer, L.: Entstehung und Therapie zerebraler Sekundärschäden. Münchn. Med. Wschr. 124, 941-944 (1982)

2. Dietze, G., Wicklmayr, M.: Effekt von Bradykinin auf die Glukoseaufnahme durch die Muskulatur beim Menschen. Klin. Wschr. 55, 357-358 (1977)

3. Frey, E.K., Kraut, H., Werle, E., Vogel, R., Zickgraf, G., Trautschold, I. (eds.): Das Kallikrein-Kinin-System und seine Inhibitoren. Enke, Stuttgart 1968

4. Kariya, K., Iwaki, H., Ihda, M., Maruta, E., Morase, M.: Central action of bradykinin. I. Electroencephalogram of bradykinin and its degradation system in rat brain. Japn. J. Pharmacol. 31, 261-267 (1981)

5. Maier-Hauff, K., Baethmann, A., Lange, M., Schürer, L., Unterberg, A.: The kallikrein-kinin system as mediator in vasogenic brain edema. II. Studies on kinin-formation in focal and perifocal brain tissue. J. Neurosurg. 61 (1983)

6. Svensjö, E., Arfors, K.-E., Raymond, R.M., Grega, G.J.: Morphological and physiological correlation of bradykinin-induced macromolecular efflux. Am. J. Physiol. 236, H600-H606 (1979)

7. Unterberg, A., Baethmann, A.: The kallikrein-kinin system as mediator in vasogenic brain edema. I. Cerebral exposure to bradykinin, or plasma. J. Neurosurg. 61 (1983)

8. Unterberg, A., Wahl, M., Baethmann, A.: Effects of bradykinin on cerebrovascular permeability and resistance. J. Cereb. Blood Flow Metabol. 3 (Suppl. 1), S234-S235 (1983)

9. Unterberg, A., Baethmann, A., Hack. U.: Cerebral blood flow and metabolism during bradykinin exposure. In: Baldy-Moulinier, M., Ingvar, D.H., Meldrum, W.S. (eds.) Cerebral blood flow, metabolism and epilepsy, pp. 174-179. John Libbey Eurotext, London Paris 1983

10. Wahl, M., Young, A.R., Edvinsson, L., Wagner, F.: Effects of bradykinin on pial arteries and arterioles in vitro and in situ. J. Cereb. Blood Flow Metabol. 3, 231-237 (1983)

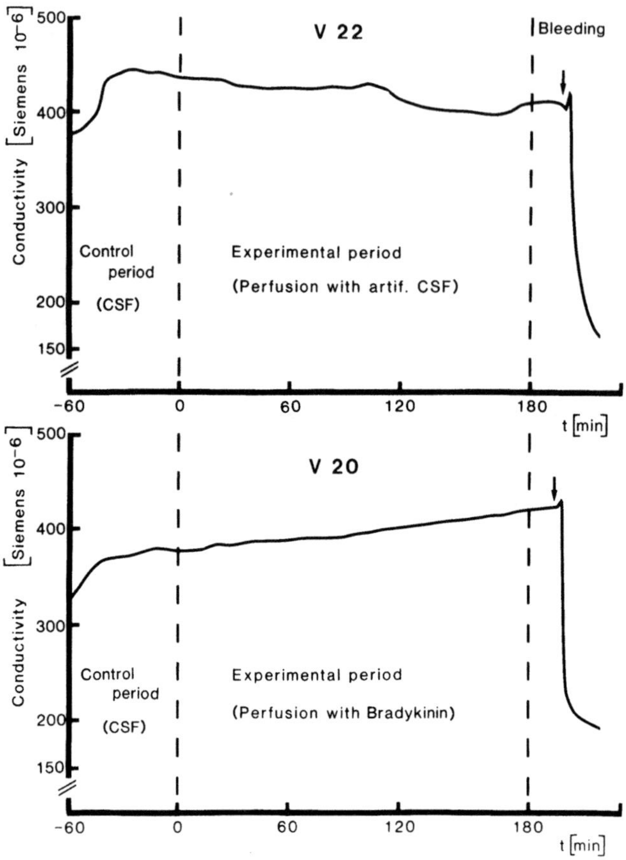

Fig. 1. Electrical tissue conductivity (reciprocal of impedance) of a control and an experimental animal. In the control animal the cerebral ventricles were perfused with artificial CSF *(V 22)*; in the experimental animal bradykinin (3 μM) dissolved in artificial CSF was used instead *(V 20)*. The experiments were terminated by exsanguination for measurement of the ischemic impedance response of the brain. As seen, this led to a marked drop in the electrical conductivity to approximately 50%

The Course of Intracranial Pressure During Experimental Long-Time Perfusion with Prostacyclin

V. Seifert, D. Stolke, and H. Dietz

Neurochirurgische Klinik der Medizinischen Hochschule Hannover, Konstanty-Gutschow-Straße 8, D-3000 Hannover 61

Introduction

Although many treatments for cerebral vasospasm following subarachnoid hemorrhage (SAH) have been proposed, the ideal medical approach remains controversial. However, in recent research it has been demonstrated that certain metabolites of arachidonic acid may be involved in the genesis of cerebral vasospasm (2, 4, 11, 13-15, 18, 19, 23, 24). Under physiological conditions a precise balance is thought to exist between two short-lived prostaglandins, i.e., thromboxane A2 (TXA_2, a powerful vasoconstrictor with platelet aggregating properties which is synthesized in the platelets itself) and prostacyclin (PGI_2, which is generated in the endothelium of the vessel wall and is a potent vasodilator and inhibitor of platelet aggregation). During the course of SAH, there is diminished synthesis of prostacyclin due to an inhibition of prostacyclin synthetase. On the other hand, it has been shown that the endothelial cell which is the major site of PGI_2 synthesis in the blood vessel undergoes ultrastructural changes during the course of experimental SAH (8, 12, 25). It is suggested that these two events proceed in parallel and lead to an imbalance in the TXA_2 - PGI_2 homeostasis. Because of the decreased synthesis of PGI_2, the relationship between these two prostaglandins is shifted towards a disproportionate concentration of TXA which is followed by cerebral vasospasm and platelet aggregation (7, 16, 17, 20, 23, 24, 26).

It is expected that correction of the disturbed homeostasis between TXA_2 and PGI_2 by exogenously administered prostacyclin may be a useful therapeutic model for the release or even prevention of cerebral vasospasm. In recent investigations this model has proved to be effective in releasing experimentally induced vasospasm in vitro and in animals (1, 3-6, 21, 22). An essential prerequisite for a possible therapeutic use of a strong vasodilator like PGI_2 is the fact that no adverse side-effects concerning the intracranial pressure are allowed to occur during intravenous infusion of the drug. It was the aim of our study to investigate the course of intracranial pressure during continuous infusion with different dosages of prostacyclin.

Material and Methods

Twenty adult cats of both sexes, weighing between 2.1 and 3.7 kg, were used for the experiments. After induction of general anesthesia, the left femoral vein was cannulated for continuous infusion of the anesthetic drugs, and the left femoral artery for recording of the systemic arterial blood pressure and for withdrawal of arterial blood samples. The right femoral vein was used for continuous infusion of pro-

Advances in Neurosurgery, Vol. 13
Edited by H. Dietz, M. Brock, and M. Klinger

stacyclin. A tracheostomy was performed and the animals were mechanically ventilated with a small animal respirator. Arterial blood gases were frequently checked and maintained within physiological limits by adjusting the rate and tidal volume of the respirator. After a midline incision in the scalp, a burr hole 1 cm in diameter was made in the right temporoparietal region and an epidural pressure device implanted.

Continuous recording of systemic blood pressure and epidural pressure was made on a multichannel recorder.

The animals were assigned to four trial groups using a different prostacyclin (Deutsche Wellcome, FRG) dosage (ng/kg per minute) for each group:

Group 1: 20 ng/kg per minute
Group 2: 100 ng/kg per minute
Group 3: 500 ng/kg per minute
Group 4: 1000 ng/kg per minute

A control group was infused with the diluent of the drug which consists of a glycin buffer (pH 10.5).

For statistical evaluations of ICP and SBP after 1, 2, and 3 h of prostacyclin infusion, Student's *t*-test was employed.

Results

During continuous infusion with the two lower dosages (20 and 100 ng/kg per minute), the courses of systemic blood pressure (SBP) and intracranial pressure (ICP) were almost identical to those in the control group. In Fig. 1 original recordings of the first 30 min of SBP and ICP during administration of prostacyclin are shown. This is underlined by the graphic presentations in Fig. 2, which demonstrate nearly parallel courses of ICP in the 20 ng and 100 ng groups and in the control group. The SBP seemed to show a slightly elevated course in the treated group, but the differences were not statistically significant.

However, in the two groups with intravenous administration of 500 and 1000 ng/kg per minute, the course of ICP was somewhat different (Fig. 3). Immediately after commencement of treatment, there was a sharp rise in the ICP which was paralleled by a fall in the SBP. While these changes were already obvious in the 500 ng group, they were even more pronounced at the highest dosage of 1000 ng. After 1-3 min, the ICP and SBP returned to the starting levels. After this there was a continuous increase in ICP which was only partially paralleled by a slight fall in SBP. In the 500 ng group the ICP was elevated for about 90 min, the differences in the ICP between the treated and the untreated group being statistically significant after 1 h of infusion.

In the 1000 ng group the increase in ICP was maintained throughout the entire experiment, the differences in ICP between the treated and nontreated group being statistically significant after 1, 2, and 3 h (Fig. 4).

Discussion

In recent investigations the possible therapeutic use of intravenous or intra-arterial prostacyclin (PGI_2) has been demonstrated during experimental and clinical treatment of different states of impaired brain perfusion following SAH or cerebral ischemic infarction. QUINTANA et al. (22) demonstrated release of experimentally induced vasospasm in cats using a dosage of 50 ng/kg per minute during a continuous intravenous infusion for 5 h. AWAD et al. (1), using a model of focal cerebral ischemia after middle cerebral occlusion in cats, suggested a possible protective effect of PGI_2 on the blood-brain barrier while using a dosage of 100 ng/kg per minute intra-arterially for 6 h. GRYGLEWSKI et al. (9), in a non-double-blind clinical trial, reported dramatic regression of neurological deficits in ten patients with ischemic stroke treated with 2.5-5.0 ng/kg prostacyclin per minute in four to ten courses of continuous infusion for 6 h. However, a strong vasodilating substance of the cerebral vessels like prostacyclin increases the cerebral blood flow and its therapeutic application would thus carry the risk of a dangerous rise in ICP, especially under pathological conditions like SAH and ischemic events. As already stated, it is therefore an essential prerequisite for the therapeutic use of prostacyclin, like any other potent vasodilator, that no adverse side-effects in respect of the ICP were allowed to occur.

From our experimental studies it can be concluded that during continuous infusion of up to 100 ng/kg prostacyclin per minute, which is already within the spasmolytic therapeutic range, no increase in ICP has to be expected. However, there is a significant rise in ICP following continuous application of 500 and 1000 ng/kg per minute, which is beyond the probable threshold of 100 ng/kg per minute for an adverse effect on the ICP. Despite the fact that we cannot yet explain the brief rise in ICP and fall in SBP at the beginning of the infusion (which seem to be direct pharmacodynamic effects of the drug), the dose-dependent increase in ICP when administering high dosages of prostacyclin during experimental or clinical trials should be taken into consideration.

Acknowledgment. The excellent technical assistance of Mrs. U. Strewe is gratefully acknowledged.

References

1. Awad, I., Little, J.R., Lucas, F., et al.: Treatment of acute cerebral ischemia with prostacyclin. Stroke 14, 203-209 (1983)
2. Boullin, D.J., Bunting, S., Blaso, W.P., et al.: Responses of human and baboon arteries to prostaglandin endoperoxides and biologically generated and synthetic prostacyclin: their relevance to cerebral arterial spasm in man. Brit. J. Clin. Pharmacol. 7, 139-147 (1979)
3. Boullin, D.J.: Potential use of prostacyclin in the treatment of vasospasm. In: Wilkins, R.H. (ed.) Cerebral arterial spasm, pp. 533-539. Williams and Wilkins, Baltimore London 1980
4. Brandt, L., Ljunggren, B., Andersson, K.E., et al.: Effects of indomethacin and prostacyclin on isolated human pial arteries contracted by CSF from patients with aneurysmal SAH. J. Neurosurg. 55, 877-883 (1981)
5. Chapleau, C.E., White, R.P.: Effects of prostacyclin on the canine isolated basilar artery. Prostaglandins 17, 573-580 (1979)
6. Chapleau, C.E., White, R.P., Robertson, J.T.: Cerebral vasodilation and prostacyclin. J. Neurosurg. 53, 188-192 (1980)
7. Ellis, E.F., Nies, A.S., Oates, J.A.: Cerebral arterial smooth muscle contraction by thromboxane A_2. Stroke 8, 480-483 (1977)

8. Fein, J.M., Flor, W.J., Cohan, S.L., et al.: Sequential changes of vascular ultrastructure in experimental cerebral vasospasm. Myonecrosis of subarachnoid arteries. J. Neurosurg. 41, 49-58 (1974)

9. Gryglewski, R.J., Nowak, S., Kostka-Trabka, E., et al.: Treatment of ischaemic stroke with prostacyclin. Stroke 14, 179-183 (1983)

10. Hallenbach, J.M., Furlow, T.W.: Prostaglandin I_2 and indomethacin prevent impairment of post-ischemic brain reperfusion in the dog. Stroke 10, 629-637 (1979)

11. Holst von, H., Granström, E., Hammarström, S., et al.: Effect of leucotrines C4, D4, prostacyclin and thromboxane A_2 on isolated human cerebral arteries. Acta Neurochir. 62, 177-185 (1982)

12. Hughes, J.T., Schianchi, P.M.: Cerebral artery spasm. A histological study at necropsy of the blood vessels in cases of subarachnoid hemorrhage. J. Neurosurg. 48, 515-525 (1978)

13. Jarmann, D.A., Du Boulay, G.H., Kendall, B., et al.: Responses of baboon cerebral and extracerebral arteries to prostacyclin and prostaglandin endoperoxide in vitro and vivo. J. Neurol. Neurosurg. Psychiatry 42, 677-686 (1979)

14. Maeda, Y., Tani, E., Miyamoto, T.: Prostaglandin metabolism in experimental cerebral vasospasm. J. Neurosurg. 55, 779-785 (1981)

15. Moncada, S., Herman, A.G., Higgs, E.A., et al.: Differential formation of prostacyclin (PGX or PGI_2) by layers of the arterial wall. An explanation for the antithrombotic properties of vascular endothelium. Thromb. Res. 11, 323-344 (1977)

16. Moncada, S.: Biological importance of prostacyclin. Brit. J. Pharmacol. 76, 3-31 (1982)

17. Moncada, S.: Biology and therapeutic potential of prostacyclin. Stroke 14, 157-168 (1983)

18. Moskowitz, M.A., Coughlin, S.R.: Basic properties of the prostaglandins. Stroke 12, 696-701 (1981)

19. Okamoto, S., Handa, H., Toda, N.: Role of intrinsic arachidonate metabolites in the vascular action of erythrocyte breakdown products. Stroke 15, 60-64 (1984)

20. Paul, K.S., Whalley, E.T., Forster, C., et al.: Prostacyclin and cerebral vessel relaxation. J. Neurosurg. 57, 334-340 (1982)

21. Pickles, H., Brown, M.M., Thomas, M., et al.: Effect of indomethacin on cerebral blood flow, carbon dioxide reactivity and the response to epoprostenol (prostacyclin) infusion in man. J. Neurol. Neurosurg. Psych. 47, 51-55 (1984)

22. Quintana, L., Konda, R., Ishibashi, Y., et al.: The effect of prostacyclin on cerebral vasospasm: an experimental study. Acta Neurochir. 62, 187-193 (1982)

23. Sasaki, T., Wakai, S., Asano, T., et al.: The effect of a lipid hydroperoxide of arachidonic acid on the canine basilar artery. J. Neurosurg. 54, 357-365 (1981)

24. Sasaki, T., Murota, S., Wakai, S. et al.: Evaluation of prostaglandin biosynthetic activity in canine basilar artery following subarachnoid injection of blood. J. Neurosurg. 55, 771-778 (1981)

25. Tanabe, Y., Sakata, K., Yamada, H., et al.: Cerebral vasospasm and ultrastructural changes in cerebral arterial wall. An experimental study. J. Neurosurg. 49, 229-238 (1978)

26. Uchida, Y., Murao, S.: Role of prostaglandin I_2 and thromboxane A_2 in recurring reduction of carotid and cerebral blood flow in dogs. Stroke 12, 786-792 (1981)

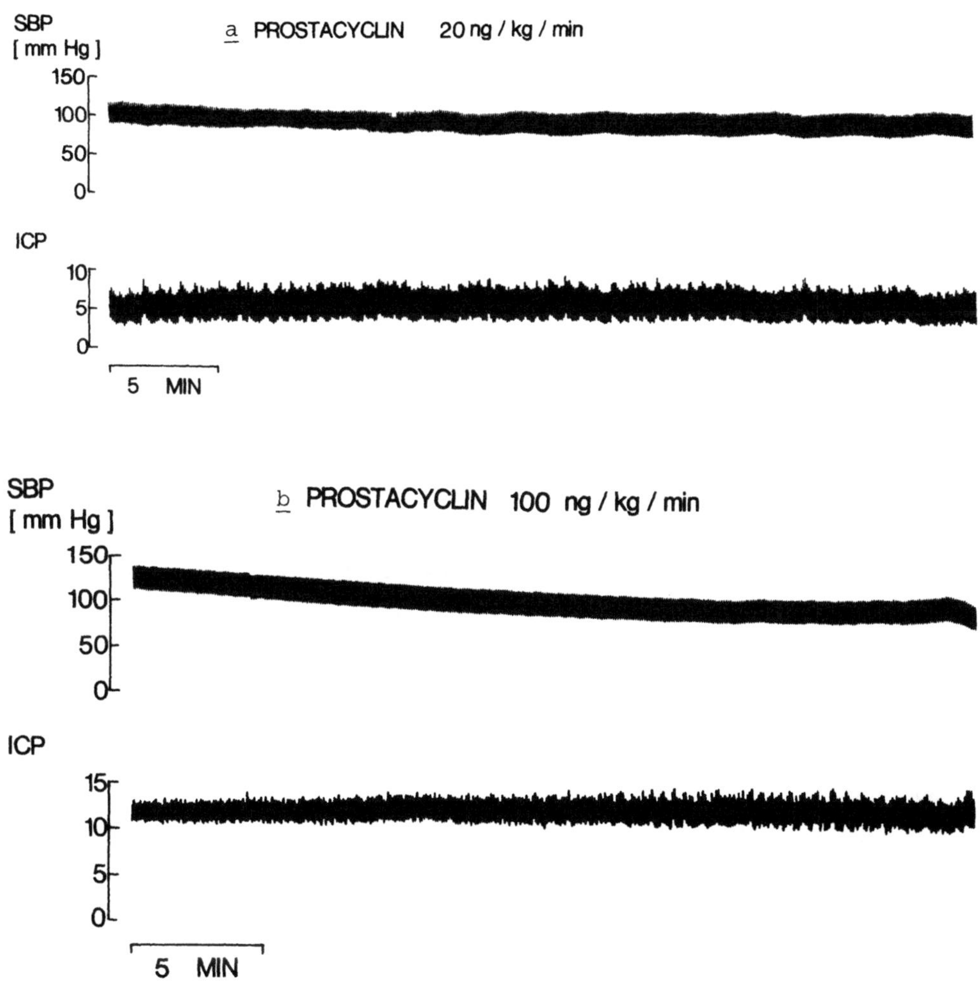

Fig. 1a,b. Original recordings of SBP and ICP during the first 30 min of administration of a 20 and b 100 ng/kg prostacyclin per minute

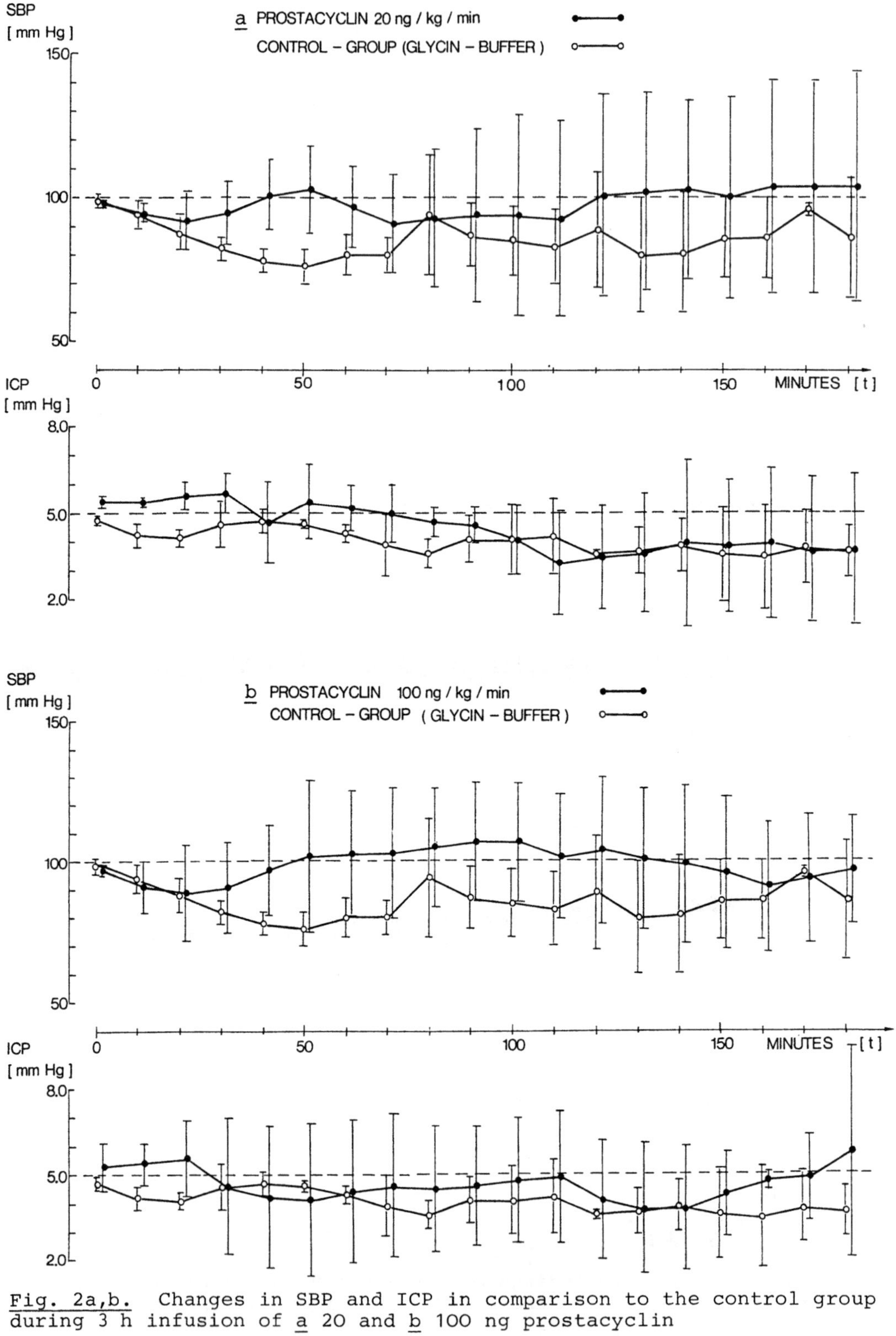

Fig. 2a,b. Changes in SBP and ICP in comparison to the control group during 3 h infusion of a 20 and b 100 ng prostacyclin

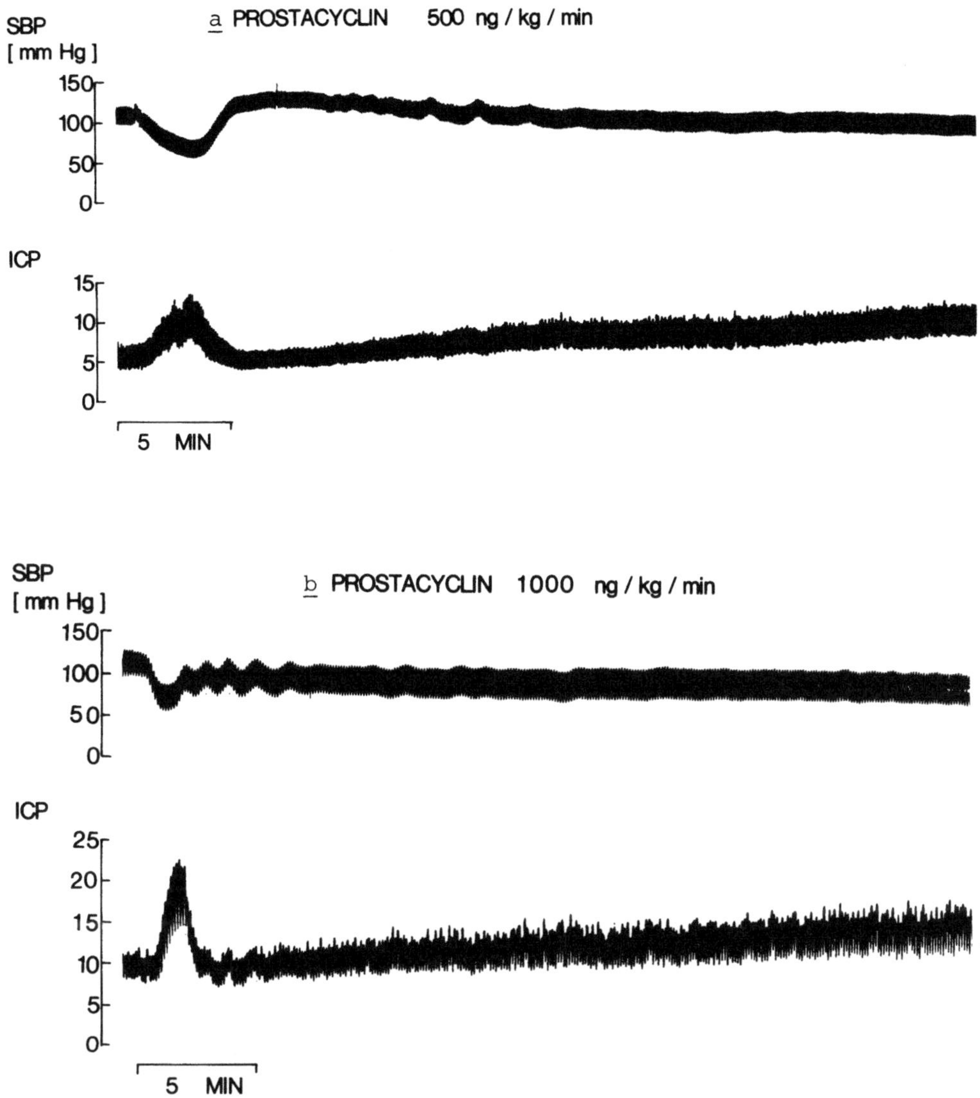

Fig. 3a,b. Original recordings of SBP and ICP during the first 30 min of administration of a 500 and b 1000 ng/kg prostacyclin per minute

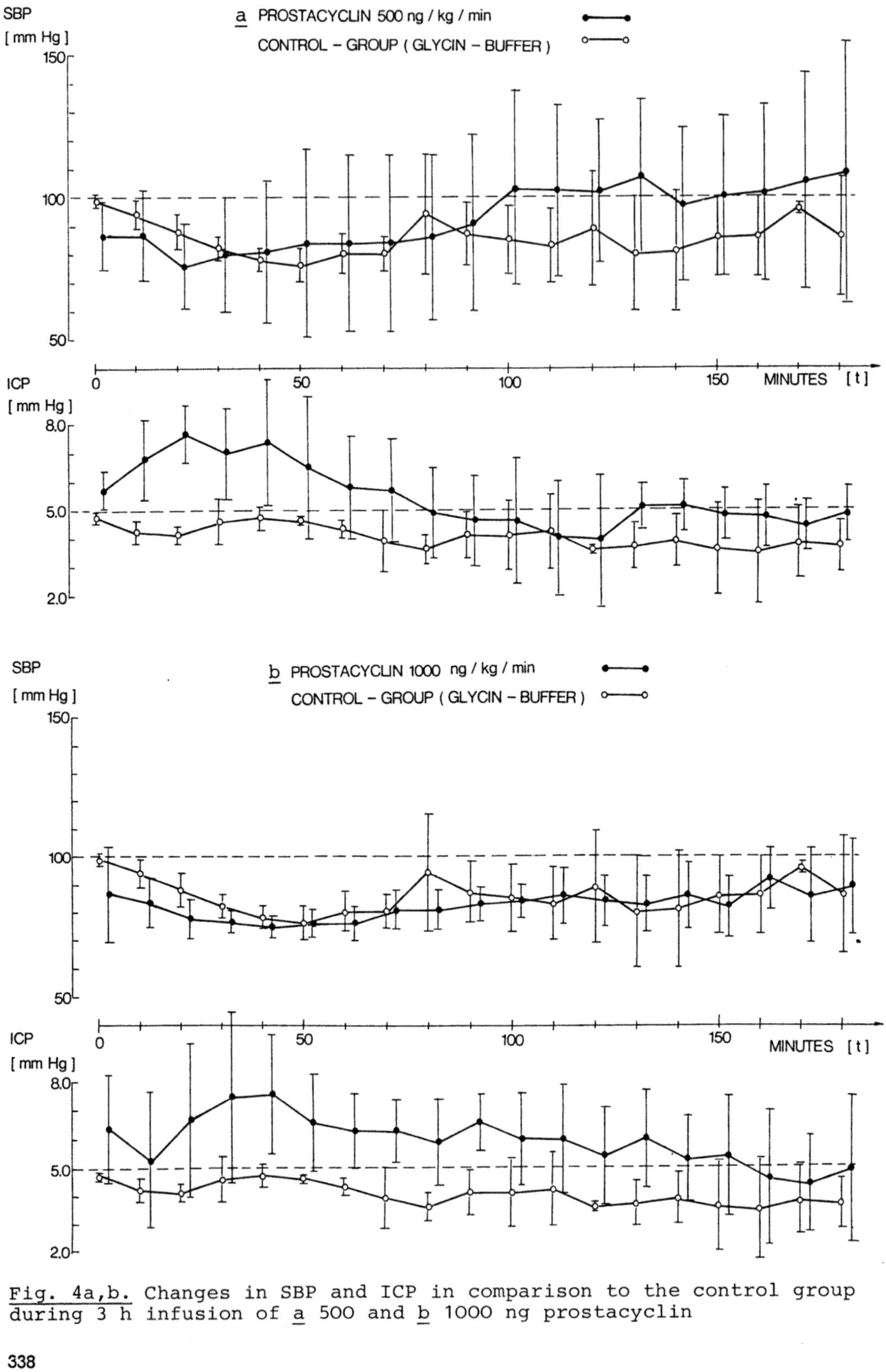

Fig. 4a,b. Changes in SBP and ICP in comparison to the control group during 3 h infusion of a 500 and b 1000 ng prostacyclin

Skin Testing – The First Step to Selective Chemonucleolysis

H. M. Mayer, M. Brock, and H. H. Görge
Neurochirurgische Klinik, Klinikum Steglitz, Freie Universität Berlin,
Hindenburgdamm 30, D-1000 Berlin 45

Introduction

Intradiscal injection of chymopapain has become a valuable therapeutic alternative in the treatment of lumbar disc disease (1, 4, 5, 9). Besides technical problems, which have almost completely been solved, one major concern, namely hypersensitivity to chymopapain, still remains. An easy diagnostic skin test to detect hypersensitivity to chymopapain prior to chemonucleolysis (CNL) has been reported recently (6, 7). We have been using a modified skin test routinely in our department since September 1983. This paper reports the results of the first 100 patients submitted to this test, and discusses its applicability and reliability.

Materials and Methods

Test Solutions

The following solutions were used to test cutaneous sensitivity: (1) histamine-dihydrochloride (concentration 1:1000), (2) Discase (D), (3) Chymodiactin (CD), (4) Solutrast 250 M (Iopamidol 510, 3 mg), and (5) buffer. The buffer solution was composed of sodium chloride (0.5%), sodium bicarbonate (0.275%), and phenole (0,4%) (6). Two milliliters of the buffer solution were added both to CD and to D as dry substances and stored at room temperature for 24 h to become enzymatically inactive. These solutions were then diluted with glycerol (50%) to a final concentration of 25%. The buffer solution served as a negative control to exclude false-positives due to hyperergic predisposition. Histamine-dihydrochloride, on the other hand, was used as positive control. All solutions were stored at 4°C and renewed weekly.

Tested Patients

A total of 100 patients, ranging in age from 20 to 62 years [40.8 ± 9.2 ($\bar{x} \pm s_x$)], were tested under identical conditions in the period between 21 September 1983 and 31 January 1984. Seventy-five (45 males, 30 females) were tested prior to CNL. Twenty-five (16 males, 9 females) were submitted to test prior to "open surgery" from six days to eight months following unsuccessful intradiscal therapy with chymopapain. Twenty-one of these patients had also been tested prior to CNL and had had a negative test result.

Advances in Neurosurgery, Vol. 13
Edited by H. Dietz, M. Brock, and M. Klinger

Test Procedure

All tests were performed in the operating room immediately before CNL in local anesthesia or before surgery with an anesthesiologist in "standby". One drop of each solution (Nos. 1-5) was placed on the palmar face of the patient's forearm (Fig. 1). The buffer (B) was applied most distally and the histamine (H) most proximally. After application of the drops, cutaneous scarification through the center of each drop was made with a 5/8-inch 25-gauge needle. Twenty minutes later, the drops were gently wiped off and each site was examined, searching for a wheal and/or erythema. The results were classified into three categories: (1) *Negative:* none of the solutions 2, 3, 4, and 5 produced a wheal or erythema (see also Fig. 1). (2) *Positive:* wheal and erythema caused by histamine (No. 1) *and* by CD (No. 2) *and/or* D (No. 3) *and/or* contrast medium (No. 4) but *not* by the buffer (No. 5). (3) *Dermatographic* reaction: all five test solutions (thus also the pure buffer) induced erythema or a wheal. During the test, an electrolyte solution was infused i.v. and vital parameters controlled continuously.

Results

Tests Prior to CNL

1. Negative Test Results (Fig. 1). A total of 45 male and 30 female patients were tested prior to CNL. Seventy-two of them (95.8%; 43 m, 29 f) had a negative response to both CD and D (Table 1, Fig. 1). Either D or CD were applied in the usual dosage to all these patients without any kind of adverse reaction.

2. Positive Test Results (Fig. 2). Two patients (2.7%) had a positive cutaneous response to both CD and D. There were another two positive responses, one to CD only and the other to D only. Both patients who had been positive to CD and D were treated with collagenase (Nucleolysin) at L4/5 and L5/S1, respectively ("selective chemonucleolysis"). The patients who had been positive either to D or CD were treated with the test-negative substance under prophylactic antiallergic medication.

3. Dermatographic Reaction. One of the test-negative patients showed a severe dermatographic reaction to all substances tested, including the buffer solution (Fig. 3).

Tests Following CNL

A total of 25 patients (16 m, 9 f) were tested following CNL with chymopapain (D or CD). All tests were performed prior to open surgical treatment because enzyme therapy had failed. Twenty-one of them had had negative skin tests prior to CNL; the rest (four patients) had not been tested before.

1. Negative Test Results (Table 2). Sixteen (64%) patients had a negative skin test result despite previous intradiscal application of chymopapain. In 12 (75%), time lapse between CNL and surgery was either less than two weeks ($n = 7$) or more than 12 weeks ($n = 5$).

2. Positive Test Results (Table 2). Nine patients (36%; 4 m, 5 f) had a positive test result following CNL either with D ($n = 5$) or with CD ($n = 4$).

Table 1. Skin tests *prior to* chemonucleolysis with chymopapain

	Negative response			Positive response		
	Male	Female	Total	Male	Female	Total
Discase	43	29	72	2(4.7%)	1(3.4%)	3(4.2%)
Chymodiactin	43	29	72	2(4.7%)	1(3.4%)	3(4.2%)
Discase + Chymodiactin	44	29	73	1(2.3%)	1(3.4%)	2(2.7%)

Table 2. Skin tests *following* chemonucleolysis with chymopapain

	Negative response			Positive response		
	Male	Female	Total	Male	Female	Total
Discase	12	4	16	4(25%)	5(55.6%)	9(36%)
Chymodiactin	12	4	16	4(25%)	5(55.6%)	9(36%)
Discase + Chymodiactin	12	4	16	4(25%)	5(55.6%)	9(36%)

Table 3. Time dependence of positive responses to the skin test performed *following* chemonucleolysis with chymopapain

Weeks after chemonucleolysis	1 - 2	3 - 4	5 - 12	13 - 24	24+	Total
Total number of tests	7	7	5	2	4	25
Positive test results to Discase and Chymodiactin	0	5 (71.4%)	3 (60%)	0	1	9 (36%)
		88.9% of all positive tests				

With only one exception, all positive skin reactions (i.e., 8 out of 9 = 88.9%) were observed between the second and twelfth week after enzyme application. As shown in Table 3, development of allergy to chymopapain appears to be time dependent. Only one out of 13 patients (7.7%) tested less than two or more than 13 weeks following CNL had a positive prick test, while this was the case in eight out of 12 (75%) patients tested between two and 12 weeks following CNL. Altogether, this means a tenfold increase in sensitivity during this period.

Discussion

The incidence of sensitivity reactions to chymopapain after intradiscal application has been reported to be between 0.35% (3) and 1.5% (5, 10). Altogether, complications of CNL may reach 3% (5, 10), allergic reactions, thus being responsible for half of them. To avert this potential hazard, two commercially available in vitro tests have been developed (8). It appears, however, that a prick test such as is commonly used to detect hypersensitivity to other drugs or materials would best combine the advantages of simplicity and safety.

The overall sensitivity rate of 4.2% (three out of 74 patients) prior to CNL is slightly higher than that of 2.5% reported by McCULLOCH et al. (7). On the other hand, sensitization occurred in 36% of the patients previously submitted to intradiscal treatment with chymopapain. Eight of the nine positive skin tests in this group were observed between the second and twelfth week after CNL. These results suggest a time dependence of sensitization to chymopapain. In our series, only one patient showed a positive skin test more than six months after CNL. This patient had not been tested prior to CNL. Even if we assume that, after such a long time, IgE levels would be too low to trigger a skin reaction to chymopapain, the patient could just as well have had exposure to one of the commercially available chymopapain-containing substances (1) in the meantime.

Conclusions

1. In our opinion, the risk of anaphylaxis to chymopapain decreases after a period of three months following CNL, provided that there is no renewed exposure which might have a booster effect on IgE production.

2. Chemonucleolysis should not be performed or repeated in patients with a positive skin reaction.

3. At present, three enzyme preparations are available for intradiscal application (Discase, Chymodiactin, and Nucleolysin). This raises the question of performing a selective chemonucleolysis according to the skin-test result.

Our data are still too limited to present an answer, but we believe that *selective chemonucleolysis* might broaden the field of application of this procedure by increasing the number of patients who benefit from it.

In closing, we have observed three late adverse reactions following chemonucleolysis with chymopapain. In two of these cases the skin test prior to chemonucleolysis had been positive to Chymodiactin and to Discase and Chymodiactin, respectively. Both patients had been treated with Discase at L4/5 under antiallergic premedication.

References

1. Brock, M., Mayer, H.M., Görge, H.H.: Die Chemonukleolyse mit Chymopapain. Deutsches Ärzteblatt (1984) (to be published)
2. Görge, H.H., Curio, G., Brock, M.: Chemonukleolyse als Alternative zur offenen chirurgischen Behandlung des lumbalen Bandscheibenvorfalls. Dtsch. Med. Wschr. 109/2, 68-72 (1984)

3. Hall, B.B., McCulloch, J.A.: Anaphylactic reactions following the intradiscal injection of chymopapain under local anesthesia. J. Bone and Joint Surg. 65-A/9, 1215-1219 (1983)

4. McCulloch, J.A.: Chemonucleolysis: Experience with 2000 cases. Clin. Orthop. 146, 128-135 (1980)

5. McCulloch, J.A., MacNab, M.B.: Sciatica and chymopapain. Williams & Wilkins, Baltimore London 1983

6. McCulloch, J.A.: Personal communication

7. McCulloch, J.A., Canham, W., Jolovich, J.: Skin testing for chymopapain allergy – a preliminary report. J. A. M. A. (submitted for publication)

8. Nordby, E.J.: Current concepts review: chymopapain in intradiscal therapy. J. Bone and Joint Surg. 65-A/9, 1350-1353 (1983)

9. Smith, L.: Enzyme dissolution of the nucleus pulposus in humans. J. Am. Med. Ass. 187, 137-140 (1964)

10. Watts, C.: Complications of chemonucleolysis for lumbar disc disease. Neurosurg. 1/1, 2-5 (1977)

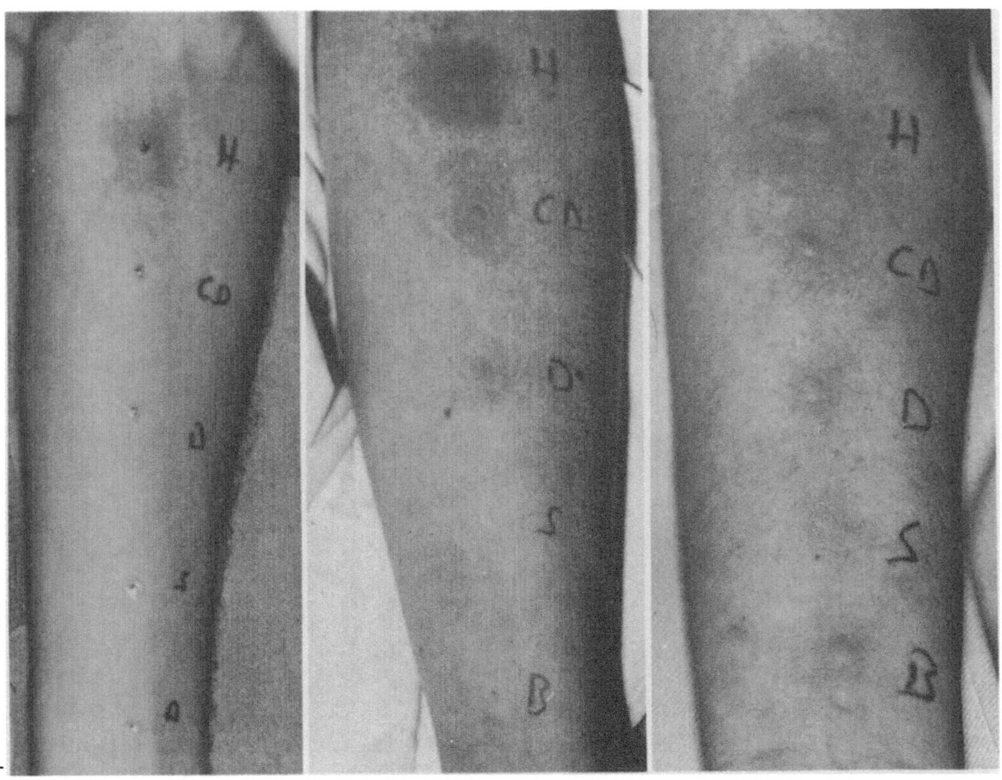

1,2 3

Fig. 1. Negative skin test to Discase, Chymodiactin, and Solutrast 250 M

Fig. 2. Positive skin test to Discase and Chymodiactin

Fig. 3. Dermatographic reaction at all test sites

Subject Index

GPSR Compliance

The European Union's (EU) General Product Safety Regulation (GPSR) is a set of rules that requires consumer products to be safe and our obligations to ensure this.

If you have any concerns about our products, you can contact us on ProductSafety@springernature.com

In case Publisher is established outside the EU, the EU authorized representative is:

Springer Nature Customer Service Center GmbH
Europaplatz 3
69115 Heidelberg, Germany

Batch number: 10607330

Printed by Printforce, the Netherlands